Management
for psychiatrists

T0332281

Management for psychiatrists

4th edition

Edited by Dinesh Bhugra, Stuart Bell
and Alistair Burns

RCPsych Publications

RCPsych Publications is an imprint of the Royal College of Psychiatrists,
21 Prescot Street, London E1 8BB
http://www.rcpsych.ac.uk

British Library Cataloguing-in-Publication Data.
A catalogue record for this book is available from the British Library.
ISBN 978-1-909726-65-9

Distributed in North America by Publishers Storage and Shipping Company.

The views presented in this book do not necessarily reflect those of the Royal College of Psychiatrists, and the publishers are not responsible for any error of omission or fact.

The Royal College of Psychiatrists is a charity registered in England and Wales (228636) and in Scotland (SC038369).

Printed by Bell & Bain Limited, Glasgow, UK.

Contents

Part III: Personal development

Contributors

Gwen Adshead, Consultant Forensic Psychiatrist at Ravenswood House and Visiting Gresham Professor of Psychiatry, Gresham College

Oyedeji Ayonrinde, Consultant Psychiatrist, South London and Maudsley NHS Foundation Trust

Martin Baggaley, Medical Director, South London and Maudsley NHS Foundation Trust

David Baldwin, Professor of Psychiatry and Head of Mental Health Group, Faculty of Medicine, University of Southampton

J. S. Bamrah, Medical Director, Manchester Mental Health and Social Care Trust

Stuart Bell CBE, Chief Executive, Oxford Health NHS Foundation Trust

Sabyasachi Bhaumik OBE, Honorary Professor of Psychiatry, University of Leicester

Dinesh Bhugra CBE, President, World Psychiatric Association

Nick Brindle, Consultant Psychiatrist, Leeds and York Partnership NHS Foundation Trust

Alistair Burns CBE, Professor of Old Age Psychiatry, University of Manchester and National Clinical Director for Dementia and Older People's Mental Health, NHS England

Jerome Carson, Professor of Psychology, University of Bolton

Eleanor Cole, Consultant Psychiatrist and Associate Medical Director, South London and Maudsley NHS Foundation Trust

Peter Conradi, Foreign Editor, *Sunday Times*

Alastair Cook, Associate Medical Director for Mental Health and Learning Disability Services and Director of Medical Education, NHS Lanarkshire

Sarah Cornick, Specialist Registrar, General Adult Psychiatry, South London and Maudsley NHS Foundation Trust

Tom Edwards, Consultant Psychiatrist, Walsall Assertive Outreach Team and Walsall North Community Recovery Service, Dudley and Walsall Mental Health Partnership NHS Trust, Walsall, West Midlands

Judith Harrison, ST4 in Psychiatry and Welsh Clinical Academic Training Fellow, Cardiff University

Michael Holland, Deputy Medical Director, South London and Maudsley NHS Foundation Trust

Frank Holloway, Emeritus Consultant Psychiatrist, South London and Maudsley NHS Foundation Trust

Adrian James, Registrar, Royal College of Psychiatrists and Consultant Forensic Psychiatrist, Devon Partnership NHS Trust

Kate Jefferies, Consultant Old Age Psychiatrist and Lead Consultant for Older Adults, Surrey and Borders Partnership NHS Foundation Trust

Verity Kemp, Director of Healthplanning Ltd, Associate of the Welsh Institute for Health and Social Care, University of South Wales

Mike Kingham, Consultant Forensic Psychiatrist, Kent and Medway NHS and Social Care Partnership Trust

Greg Lydall, Consultant Psychiatrist, Castel Hospital, Guernsey

Amit Malik, formerly Consultant Psychiatrist and Commercial Director at Surrey and Borders Partnership NHS Foundation Trust

Charles Marshall, Director, Healthskills

Roy McClelland, Professor Emeritus of Mental Health, Queen's University Belfast and Consultant Psychiatrist at Belfast City Hospital

Samuel Menon, General Practitioner, Brondesbury Medical Centre, London

Stephen Morris, Development Adviser, Public Health England

Adrian Neal, Consultant Clinical Psychologist, Head of Employee Well-being, Aneurin Bevan University Health Board, NHS Wales

Edward Noble, ST6 Registrar in General Adult Psychiatry, Support and Recovery Service, Southern Health and Social Care Trust, Northern Ireland

Ross Overshott, Consultant Psychiatrist, Greater Manchester West Mental Health NHS Foundation Trust

Luca Polledri, Consultant Psychiatrist, Liaison Psychiatry Service at Whipps Cross University Hospital, North East London NHS Foundation Trust

Rob Poole, Professor of Social Psychiatry, Centre for Mental Health and Society, Bangor University, Wales

Rosalind Ramsay, Consultant Psychiatrist and Associate Clinical Director, South London and Maudsley NHS Foundation Trust

Zoë Reed, Director of Organisation and Community, South London and Maudsley NHS Foundation Trust

Diana Rose, Professor of User-Led Research, Institute of Psychiatry, Psychology and Neuroscience, King's College London

Mark Salter, Consultant Adult General Psychiatrist, East London NHS Foundation Trust

Jill Sandford, FuturePositive

Mike Slade, Professor of Mental Health Recovery and Social Inclusion, Institute of Mental Health, School of Health Sciences, University of Nottingham

Bryan Stoten, Chairman UKPHR (Public Health Register), Halford, Warwickshire

Graham Thornicroft, Professor of Community Psychiatry, Institute of Psychiatry, Psychology and Neuroscience, King's College London, London

Alex Till, Psychiatric Core Trainee, Health Education North West (Mersey)

Manel Tippett, Policy Administrator, Royal College of Psychiatrists in Wales

Koravangattu Valsraj, Consultant Psychiatrist and Associate Clinical Director, South London and Maudsley NHS Trust

Antonio Ventriglio, Honorary Researcher, Department of Clinical and Experimental Medicine, University of Foggia, Italy

Jonathan Waite, Consultant in the Liaison Psychiatry of Old Age, Nottinghamshire Healthcare NHS Trust

Ellen Wilkinson, Medical Director, Cornwall Partnership NHS Foundation Trust

Richard Williams OBE, Emeritus Professor of Mental Health Strategy, Welsh Institute for Health and Social Care, University of South Wales

Figures, tables and boxes

Tables

Boxes

Preface

It is indeed a great pleasure to bring out the fourth edition of this book. When the first edition appeared, in 1992, management in general and medical management in particular were seen as dirty words, and clinicians who became medical managers were seen as having gone over to the dark side. Over the past quarter of a century, management by doctors has become respectable, and leadership and management skills have taken on a certain degree of prominence. There is no doubt that management and leadership skills have a degree of overlap, but by and large they are separate activities, as detailed in this book.

The entire volume has been completely revised, with many new chapters reflecting the current medical management and leadership skills. The changes in the National Health Service and resulting changes in working conditions have also meant that clinicians must be aware of competing interests and demands and yet forge a way forward in their professional lives. We very much hope that readers of all seniorities will continue to find this book useful. For early-career psychiatrists and trainees, the book will provide an introduction to the skills they need; and for more senior clinicians, it will provide an opportunity to keep up to date and continue professional development. We persist in believing that the relationship between personal skills and clinical management needs to become mainstream.

We are most grateful to our authors, who, in spite of (or perhaps because of) their busy schedules, have led from the front and delivered material which is not only a pleasure to read but also helpful and provocative in equal measure.

We thank Andrea Livingstone for her sterling support and project management of the book; her gentle and persistent style in communicating with the authors has proved to be extremely successful.

Thanks are also due to Dave Jago, Andrew Morris and the staff in the publications department of the Royal College of Psychiatrists for their help.

Dinesh Bhugra, Stuart Bell, Alistair Burns

Part I
Theoretical overview

CHAPTER 1

History and structure of the National Health Service

Ross Overshott, Alistair Burns and Dinesh Bhugra

It is perhaps important for everyone working in the National Health Service (NHS) to have some idea of the origins, development and current structure of what is one of the biggest and most complicated organisations in the world. A detailed analysis of the NHS and its history is outside the scope of this chapter; suggestions for further reading are given at the end. Its purpose is instead to outline briefly how the NHS has evolved and to put into perspective the current changes.

Healthcare before the NHS

Until the middle of the 19th century, the state had virtually no control over the medical profession. Doctors had developed their own organisational structure which satisfied the need for self-protection. Members of the Royal College of Physicians mainly worked in the London teaching hospitals and treated those who could afford their fees. Members of the Royal College of Surgeons (which was the Company of Barbers a century before) were more experienced in the practice of medicine and treated patients both in London (in competition with the physicians) and outside. The vast majority of people were treated at the hands of members of the Society of Apothecaries, who basically prescribed medication. For a considerable time churches provided forms of treatment to people with mental illnesses.

The state became more involved in the health of the population and regulation of the medical profession throughout the 19th century and in the early 20th century. The 1834 Poor Law was the first acknowledgement that government had some responsibility for the care of the population. Among its effects was the statutory provision of a parish medical officer to care for the poor. These established that the parish workhouses should have sick wards where the able-bodied inmates could be treated when they became ill (Levitt, 1976). Free services were offered by boards of guardians to those who could pass a means test.

The Public Health Act 1848 established statutory powers that enabled a local medical officer of health (an official of the local authority) to cater for the health of the local population. Following the Poor Law reforms, the medical officers' responsibilities were extended to some Poor Law hospitals which were considered to be providing healthcare rather than welfare. By the 1930s, these included control over environmental hazards, infectious diseases, the school medical service and district nursing/midwifery services.

Local acts (e.g. in London and Liverpool) had proved the benefit of providing care for people suffering from infectious diseases and for those with mental illness and handicap. The establishment of the General Medical Council under the Medical Registration Act 1858 granted the profession self-regulation by establishing a basic qualification for doctors and instituting a register of qualified medical practitioners.

In the first half of the 20th century there were some important changes in the mode of delivery of healthcare and in the organisation of the medical profession (Stacey, 1988). The medical profession had gained prestige and status but lacked tools; these came about with the development of microbiology, which led to the establishment of a scientific basis for medicine.

The National Health Insurance Act 1911 was passed to ensure that workers were afforded some protection in the event of sickness. It involved compulsory contributions from the employee, the employer and the state. (The National Sickness Insurance Bill was to have been an early provision, but this was changed to the National Health Insurance Bill, from which the NHS took its name – had this not happened we might be referring today to a National Sickness Service.) The 1911 Act concerned mainly general practitioners (GPs) and the working classes; the middle and upper classes could afford their own care and the Act, which covered the cost of GP care and medication, did not include the cost of hospital care, nor did it cover workers' families.

Around this period GPs were perhaps the least contented of medical men, and were also the most vociferous (Stacey, 1988). The 'sick clubs' offered treatment to their members and sometimes their dependants. GPs were unable to choose their patients, and to be controlled by a committee of working men was 'not a pleasant matter for an educated gentleman to serve under' (*British Medical Journal*, 1875: p. 484). Before 1911, only a small proportion (5 million) of working-class people could afford GP care through membership of friendly societies or other agencies. The 1911 Act immediately covered 15 million people, and by the mid-1940s covered about 24 million (half the population).

However, the scheme was inefficient. Local insurance committees (the forerunners of family practitioner committees) and approved societies (private insurance companies, friendly societies and trade unions, all of which tended to be confined to a particular occupation or location) formed the administrative agencies. The approved societies brought the system into disrepute. As they were not allowed to be profit making, money was purposefully wasted by increasing the numbers of staff. They paid sickness benefit and were able to pay for specialist care only if there was a surplus at the end of a defined period, which was rare, especially in those occupations where morbidity was high and which caused the greatest drain on the resources of an individual society. Those earning over the income limit were excluded. Needless to say, this limit had to be changed regularly, always against the wishes of the doctors, because of inflation.

Whereas before the 19th century treatment was offered at home, by the next century treatment was gradually being shifted to hospitals, in the public domain. A major consequence of the increasing influence of hospitals was an increasing differentiation between GPs and the hospital consultants under the 1911 Act (Honigsbaum, 1979). Increasing specialisation among consultants and the development of a hierarchy were two major factors that were to affect the running of the NHS subsequently. Non-clinical advances contributed to the development of specific skills and interests in specialties such as psychiatry (Stevens, 1966).

By the time the NHS was formed, in 1948, there were about 2800 hospitals in England and Wales (just over 1000 were voluntary hospitals and the rest were municipal hospitals). The voluntary hospitals ranged from the London teaching hospitals, staffed by consultant specialists, to non-teaching hospitals with little money, staffed by local doctors who combined general practice with hospital practice. About one-third of the voluntary hospitals were larger hospitals where the beds were controlled by consultant specialists, who were unpaid and relied on private practice to generate income. An appointment to such a hospital was regarded as a stimulus to the recruitment of patients. This part of the hospital system was affected by the rise of specialism in the 19th century, as only very large centres were able to support all specialties.

Voluntary hospitals were run using money gleaned from endowments, donations, public appeals and schemes whereby care from the hospital was guaranteed by means of a regular weekly payment. The municipal hospitals provided about 80% of the total number of beds. They consisted of a number of Poor Law hospitals (the former workhouse infirmaries, handed over to the local authorities when the Poor Law was reformed, and run by the local medical officers of health) and local infectious disease hospitals. Mental asylums (also under local control) accounted for half the total number of beds. Although some of the Poor Law infirmaries were of a standard equivalent to that of the voluntary hospitals, they were mainly concerned with the care of the elderly and chronically sick.

The hospital component of the health service was therefore unsatisfactory. Many of the hospitals were old and ill equipped; scant provision was made for the ordinary worker and there was relatively little healthcare available between private medicine and the Poor Law; there was inequality in the distribution of services and a financial crisis developed in the London teaching hospitals towards the end of the 1930s.

The Emergency Medical Service (EMS) was an important development in the hospital system. It was established in 1939 by the Ministry of Health to coordinate the response to the expected number of war casualties and to arrange supporting services. The EMS took over financial control of the hospitals (but not ownership), divided England and Wales into 12 regions, and categorised each hospital by its particular function. Many of the voluntary hospitals became second-line hospitals (outside the main centres of population) and specialists worked in them on a salaried basis. It is interesting to note that by the time the NHS was formed in 1948, many hospital specialists had been paid on a sessional basis for a decade. Thus, the payment system was never a political issue in the same way that it was for GPs, who had maintained their freedom of practice despite the introduction of the National Health Insurance Scheme in 1911. It was the threat to this independence which was at the root of the GPs' suspicion of the introduction of the NHS. The EMS proved that the central administration of the hospital system could work, and it was the forerunner of the NHS.

The formation of the NHS

The NHS provides an administrative structure by which healthcare can be properly organised and financed. The essence of the NHS is that it provides, free at the point of service, healthcare to anyone who wants it, regardless of ability to pay. The idea of the NHS originated as far back as the Health Insurance Act 1911. The originator of the Insurance Bill (the then Chancellor of the Exchequer, Lloyd George) had the idea that the Act would be extended to cover dependants, specialist care and, eventually, hospital care.

With the creation of the Ministry of Health in 1919, an attempt at extending the bill was made, embodied within the Dawson report (after Lord Dawson, the leading physician of the day). The report had recommended that preventive and curative medicine be combined, that hospital inefficiency be corrected by elected regional authorities (each of which would have a principal medical officer in administrative charge) and, in an effort to increase standards, that all general hospitals be brought into line with teaching hospitals. No mention was made of the funding of these health services, but the report specifically warned of the dangers of a salaried service, suggesting that this would 'discourage initiative, diminish the sense of responsibility and encourage mediocrity'. However, the necessary political commitment to respond positively to the Dawson proposals was absent, and it took the threat of war and the consequent creation of the EMS in 1939 to resurrect these principles.

Sir William Beveridge produced his report *Social Insurance and Allied Services* in 1942. As part of an attack on the 'five giants' impeding social progress (want, disease, ignorance, squalor and idleness), he suggested that the burden of the cost of a health service should be borne by everyone, in the belief that such a service would make the nation healthier, thereby saving on social security payments and increasing national efficiency. However, he missed the point that better health, if it leads to longer life, inevitably leads during that longer life to a greater use of services (Godber, 1975).

The wartime coalition government accepted the principle of a national health service and set about finding a formula which would be acceptable to the medical profession, politicians, the voluntary hospitals and local authorities. The Minister of Health, Ernest Brown, proposed that the service would be administered by local authorities (with voluntary hospitals retaining their independence) and that GPs would be paid a salary. The doctors effectively rejected these proposals and they were dropped when Sir Henry Willink succeeded Brown in late 1943.

In February 1944, the government published a white paper on the NHS. The plan was to make local authorities responsible for health, directly in control of municipal hospitals, and to make contractual arrangements with the voluntary hospitals. Hospital doctors would be salaried and GPs would have the choice of a salaried service or capitation fees. The British Medical Association (BMA) held a postal ballot and doctors (especially GPs) came out strongly against the proposals. They were opposed to the idea of local authority control and to a scheme which would be available to all, free at the time of use, restricting scope for private practice. There was widespread general public acceptance of the proposals, in particular the fact that services would be free at the time of use.

Before a bill could be drafted on these proposals, a Labour government came into power with Aneurin Bevan as the Minister of Health. Bevan took a much harder line, claiming that Willink had merely cobbled together conciliatory proposals to keep everyone happy. He objected to the political erosion of the supremacy of Parliament and made the point that he should consult, but not negotiate with, outside bodies such as the medical profession. He felt that the Minister of Health should have total control of the service. The bill was put forward in spring 1946 and was opposed by both the Conservative opposition and the BMA. The former argued that the nationalisation of the hospitals and loss of independence of GPs discouraged initiative, and deprived the profession and voluntary hospitals of their freedom.

However, experience with the EMS had shown that central control of hospitals could be a success. The reasons why the medical profession objected were more complex – restriction of individual freedom was one – but it is possible that they were fuelled by resentment over the Labour government's attack on the middle classes, from which the medical profession generally drew its members. The objections spanned the spectrum from doctors being guardians of vested interests to doctors waging a war on the government on behalf of their class.

Both Bevan and the BMA (an incredibly complex negotiating machine where its leaders had very little room to manoeuvre) stood firm. The deadlock was broken when Bevan introduced an amendment saying that he could not introduce a fully salaried service for GPs without further legislation. Leaders of the BMA (helped by the Royal Colleges) saw the chance to save face and accepted the new service. Thus, on 5 July 1948, the NHS was born.

The principle of universalism which characterised welfare and health legislation in the post-war period was perhaps manifested most dramatically in the Health Service (Stacey, 1988). To provide good healthcare to the whole population without a financial barrier was the original aim of the NHS.

The Health Service in Scotland

The Scottish Health Service was created in May 1947, on the same tripartite principles as the Service in England and Wales. The hospital and specialist services were administered by five regional hospital boards with 65 boards of management. The community and environmental health services were provided by 55 local health authorities, and family practitioner services were administered by 25 executive councils. The Secretary of State for Scotland was responsible for the whole of the NHS in Scotland (Levitt, 1976).

Under the National Health Service (Scotland) Act 1972 health boards were created for each area of Scotland to act as the single authority for administering the three branches of the former tripartite structure. Two new bodies – the Scottish Health Service Planning Council and the Common Services Agency – were created.

1948–1974

The NHS developed a tripartite structure, as much because of vested interests as from an overall view that this structure was the most efficient. What the founders of the NHS thought they were doing and what in fact emerged are two distinct questions, for there were undoubtedly a number of unintended consequences (Stacey, 1988). Out of the negotiations leading up to the brave new world of 1948, the consultants overall, but especially those in teaching hospitals, did better than the GPs. The nurses did less well and the ancillary workers were not considered at all. The role and function of multidisciplinary teams needs to be addressed in the light of this historical development.

The hospital system was nationalised and taken away from local authorities (mainly as a result of the profession's unwillingness to work under local authority control). The Minister of Health was responsible for hospitals through hospital management committees (336 in number) and non-elected regional hospital boards (numbering 16). Teaching hospitals retained their independent status (not wishing to 'come down' to the level of all voluntary hospitals) and were responsible through 36 boards of governors to the Minister, independent of the regional hospital boards.

General practice was unaffected by the changes, retaining independent status. The Health Insurance Act 1911 was extended to cover the whole population and general practice was controlled by 134 executive councils (the successors of the local insurance committees). The rest of the service was left to the 174 local authorities' medical officers of health, essentially because no other influential medical interest wanted them. These consisted of the maternity and child welfare services, health visitors, health education and prevention, the ambulance service and vaccination/immunisation.

The problem of what doctors should be paid emerged soon after the creation of the NHS. Sir Will Spens chaired three committees dealing with the pay of GPs, consultants and specialists, and dentists. The committee on consultants' pay recommended that the salary for a consultant aged about 40 should be £2500, compared with £1300 for a GP of equivalent age (both 1939 prices). Consultants' pay before the NHS had such a wide range (from a consultant in a non-teaching voluntary hospital to one in a London teaching hospital with income from private practice) that a salary scale incorporating both ends of the spectrum was impractical. The distinction award scheme was introduced as a solution to this problem, with the top grade doubling the basic consultant salary. Much discontent still existed following the Spens committees and it took a Royal Commission into doctors' and dentists' pay (the Pilkington Commission) to recommend the establishment of an independent review body to advise the Prime Minister directly.

Another problem concerned the number of junior doctors. By 1950 there were 3800 registrars and senior registrars, but only double that number of consultant posts. There also existed the grade of senior hospital medical officer (devised at the inception of the NHS to employ those practitioners in hospital practice who were not of consultant calibre), many of whom were in competition for consultant posts. The Ministry of Health attempted to force hospitals to terminate contracts of time-expired senior registrars (after three years in higher professional training), but following an outcry from the profession it was decided that their contracts could be renewed annually. The suggestion was made that consultant numbers be expanded, but this was rejected by the Ministry on the grounds of cost, and by existing consultants for fear of added competition for private patients. The result was a review of the numbers of doctors required in the UK, conducted by Henry Willink (formerly the Minister of Health in the coalition government). The recommendation was a 10% reduction in intake to the medical schools. However, the review did not take into account the numbers of doctors emigrating and the increased numbers required because of advances in medical technology, and this led to a shortage of junior doctors in the 1960s, with an attendant influx of foreign graduates to fill posts in unpopular specialties, of which psychiatry was one.

The need for change

Almost as soon as the NHS was established, there was recognition that reorganisation was necessary. It was noted as early as 1952 – by Dr Ffrangcon Roberts in *The Cost of Health* (see Watkin, 1978) – that Sir William Beveridge was wrong in assuming that the demand for healthcare was limited. The aphorism of the NHS, 'infinite demand, finite resources', was born. A committee was set up under the chairmanship of the Cambridge economist C. W. Guillebaud, with the remit of reviewing the cost of the NHS and to make recommendations for changes in administration which would make the service more efficient. The committee's conclusion was that the service was not wasteful and that a major change in organisation was unnecessary.

Inequalities in the distribution of resources both geographically and within medical specialties highlighted deficiencies in the system, the latter causing embarrassment to successive Ministers of Health because of scandals concerning ill treatment in mental and geriatric institutions. Klein (2010) argues that the NHS in 1948 was as much a product of messy compromises as of inspired visions, and the same remains true today.

In 1968, the government published a green paper on reorganisation, the basic proposals being integration of all services under 50 area boards (each to have 16 members) with responsibility for all hospital, general medical and health community services. Objections raised included the remoteness of the regional boards to local services, the problem of the continued independence of GPs, and the mismatch of the 50 area boards with proposed local government reorganisation that would result in 90 local government units. A second green paper in 1968 set out that there would be 14 regional health councils advising the Secretary of State on planning and 90 area health authorities (the word 'authority' having replaced 'board' without explanation) would coincide with 90 local government districts set up earlier in the year. The functions of the service were to be divided between health and local government, based on the skill of the provider rather than the needs of the user (e.g. all social workers were to be employed by local government, all nurses by the Health Service).

1974–1989

In 1971, the Conservative government published a further document, the thrust of which was embodied in the NHS (Reorganisation) Act 1973. The reorganisation came into being on 1 April 1974, which coincided with the reorganisation of local government. The reformed service was to have two characteristics: it was to be an integrated service and there was to be responsibility upwards, to managerial authority. The reorganisation led to the formation of regional health authorities, which had the responsibility to plan all services. The reforms led to a 30% increase in administrators and the influence of managers increased, leading to the creation of a managerial hierarchy.

The doctors insisted on retaining clinical autonomy, and this was noted: 'The distinguishing characteristic of the NHS is that, to do their work properly, consultants and general practitioners must have clinical autonomy, so that they can be fully responsible for the treatment they prescribe for the patients' (Department of Health and Social Security, 1972). This notion of a one-to-one doctor–patient relationship has been challenged by Stacey (1988). The clinical autonomy and security of tenure for the consultant were seen as advantageous (Beeson, 1980).

However, the final document differed from the second green paper in that regional health authorities were in line management with the area health authorities and the 90 family practitioner committees (replacing the executive councils) were coterminous with the local government areas. Community health councils became essentially watchdogs of the Health Service. There were also 'district' management teams under the 1974 organisation. Some regions had 'single district areas', but more commonly each area had several such teams. The aim of the reforms in 1982 was to abolish this duplication.

Readers are recommended to read the account by Draper *et al* (1976) on the influence of the 1974 reorganisation of the NHS. A detailed analysis of the political and practical ramifications of the relationship between central and local government and their representation on the authorities is given by Forsyth (1982).

The Conservative government also introduced general management of hospitals following the Griffiths report in 1983. Sir Roy Griffiths, a supermarket executive, had been commissioned to review the management of hospitals. He concluded that the traditional NHS management by senior consultants and administrators had led to 'institutionalised stagnation'. The report's recommendations, including that hospitals be managed by general managers, were accepted and in the middle of the 1980s they took over the role of managing hospitals. This change in emphasis brought about a large increase in general or senior managers in the NHS, from 1000 in 1986 to 26000 in 1995, with spending on administration rising dramatically over the same period (Webster, 2002). This also resulted in a number of managers being 'classified' into their primary professions, for example nursing, also indicating that a number of people from professions were brought into management.

There was also a new business/commercial culture in the NHS, which led to the policy in the 1980s of 'contracting out' or 'outsourcing'. The clinical work of the NHS was retained in the public sector but, to reduce costs, support services such as laundry, cleaning and catering were contracted out to private service providers. The number of non-clinical NHS employees had nearly halved by the end of 1980s. To ensure they could make a profit, the private companies paid the support staff less, while quality of service reduced – and in fact, the cleanliness of hospitals is still a major issue for the NHS.

From the changes to the NHS in the early 1980s four themes emerged which had a lasting influence (Klein, 2010). First, there was a sharp turn towards centralisation. This led to the second theme – that of managerialism and bureaucratic rationalisation. Third, the expansion of private medicine continued apace, along with privatisation of ancillary services within the NHS. Fourth, there was increasing consumerism within the health sector. The demand for increased NHS funding was accompanied by the development of healthcare as a public policy issue. A consumer-led service was being emphasised rather than a professional-led care system (Davies, 1987). Klein (2010) argues that the 'politicisation' of the NHS between 1974 and 1989 was also to do with shifting accountability from local to central authorities.

A crisis in the NHS developed in the second half of 1987. Since 1979, resources for the NHS had been increased by the Conservative government and the cost of the service had increased from £7.7 billion in 1979/1980 to £18.35 billion in 1988/1989. Despite this, the service was not doing well. Although resources were increasing, demand was outstripping this. The increasing elderly population, advances in medical technology and priority objectives (e.g. kidney transplants) meant that services had to be increased by 2% per annum just to keep up.

To reduce costs and stave off a crisis, some services provided by the NHS were effectively privatised in the late 1980s. Resources for dentistry in the NHS were reduced and as dentists were, like GPs, mostly 'independent contractors' they stopped taking on NHS patients and worked increasingly in the private sector, where they could earn more money. In 1989 routine eye examinations became free only for children and the elderly. It was argued by the government that people could now afford to pay for tests but the new policy led to a major reduction in examinations. Long-term care from the NHS was also eliminated, which stimulated the growth of private nursing and residential homes throughout the 1990s. These measures were implemented to reduce costs, in an attempt to avert the financial meltdown of the NHS. They also, however, compromised one of the founding principles of the NHS – to provide a comprehensive service.

Following the June 1987 election, when Margaret Thatcher was returned for a third term, a financial crisis began facing the health authorities. Beds began to close, charities began to shore up NHS operations, cancer patients were being denied operations and both the Institute of Health Service Management and the King's Fund announced their own independent reviews of NHS funding.

In early December 1987, the lack of heart operations on children in Birmingham was publicised and nurses from St Thomas' Hospital in

London picketed the Houses of Parliament in their uniforms. Probably the most significant event, and certainly a historical one, was when the Presidents of the Royal Colleges of Surgeons, Physicians and Obstetricians and Gynaecologists issued a joint statement suggesting that the NHS was almost at breaking point (Hoffenberg *et al*, 1987). The BMA supported the Presidents and added to the media clamour for increased resources. The government responded on 16 December by announcing an extra £100 million for the NHS, but despite this the crisis continued and more nurses began to strike.

The Prime Minister reassured the public that the NHS was in safe hands and was not about to be abolished. She, however, was still advocating tax cuts to encourage private health insurance. It was generally accepted that a government review of the NHS was inevitable.

1989–1997

The results of the government's review were initially announced in the white paper *Working for Patients*, published on 31 January 1989. A year later the NHS and Community Care Act followed. These two policy initiatives instigated what was at the time the most radical reform the NHS had undergone since its inception in 1948. The policies were criticised for containing a lack of strategic planning and many were unhappy that there had been no consultation inside the NHS.

The main reforms were:

- *Self-governing hospitals*. Stand-alone hospital trusts were established which were separate from the health authority and were accountable directly to central government. These NHS hospital trusts were to be managed by a board of directors with a chair appointed by the Secretary of State for Health. The hospital trusts were able to contract out services and buy and sell assets, borrow capital, employ staff on local terms and advertise their services. The government's idea was to move decision-making to as near to patients as possible.
- *Fund-holding GPs*. Fund-holding GPs were created, who were given their own budget which they used to buy hospital services directly from source. The scheme was voluntary for GPs but provided financial incentives to encourage them to sign up. Initially only practices with lists of at least 11 000 could apply to be fund-holders and their budgets covered just elective surgery, out-patient and diagnostic services, prescribing and staff costs.
- *The internal market*. To create an internal market, the NHS was split into 'purchasers' (health authorities and fund-holding GPs) and 'providers' (hospital and community trusts and non-fund-holding GPs). It was envisaged that providers, which were still all part of the NHS, would compete with each other to secure contracts with the purchasers by offering higher-quality, more responsive and more efficient services.

The internal market did not lead to the benefits the government thought it would produce. Hospitals could not truly compete with each other as the government could not, for political reasons, allow less competitive hospital trusts to go out of business, as would happen in the commercial world. GP fund-holding was also an unpopular policy. Being a fund-holding practice offered many financial advantages but it was available only to larger practices, which were already better resourced. A two-tier system was therefore created. Fund-holders' contracts with healthcare providers gave fund-holders' patients quicker access to hospital services than patients from non-fund-holding practices. There were distinct advantages for patients whose GP belonged to a fund-holding practice (the 'haves') over patients whose GP was part of a non-fund-holding practice (the 'have-nots'). The reforms of 1989 severely compromised the premise of equity that the NHS had been founded on.

The Conservative government under John Major won the 1992 general election and continued to develop the internal market in the NHS. Many still feared privatisation, as part of the 1989 reforms had allowed hospital trusts to raise income from other sources, such as private beds. The collectivist model of the NHS was being threatened, although the 1992 white paper, *The Health of the Nation*, appeared to readdress the government's responsibilities for the health of the country. The document moved towards health promotion and set out 25 specific policy targets, including reducing the suicide rate by 15%. There were also targets to reduce the proportion of the population who were obese, smokers and heavy drinkers. The white paper was criticised for setting targets that were easily achievable and for failing to address the effect poverty, inequality and unemployment have on health. Kearney (1992) concluded that the policy had no strategy at all and was merely 'window dressing'.

The Patient's Charter (Department of Health, 1991), implemented in the early 1990s, reinforced the consumerist model the government had been encouraging. The document set out explicitly patients' rights, some of which reflected the original philosophy of the NHS, for example with the statement that people have the right to receive healthcare on the basis of clinical need, regardless of ability to pay. Standards were promised for patients, such as waiting no more than 2 years once placed on a waiting list and to be seen within 30 minutes of a specific out-patient appointment time. A performance guide in relation to *The Patient's Charter* was published by the Department of Health in 1994 and hospital trusts were rated on whether they had achieved its standards, using a five-star system. This system gave the public information on how their local NHS services were performing, but gave little true power to choose between different NHS providers: only to opt out of the NHS or to choose private services, which they would have to pay for.

The reforms of the 1990s moved the power base of the NHS, for the first time in its history, away from hospitals and towards primary care. The advent of GP fund-holders altered the relationship between hospitals and GPs. The hospitals were now in effect answerable to the GPs and therefore, in essence, the patients. Community service providers were also encouraged to establish themselves as separate trusts from acute hospital services, which further promoted community services over hospitals. The multitude of reforms did not lead to an improvement in services, however. GP fund-holding was a moderate success as a relaxation of entry requirements had allowed approximately 50% of GPs to become fund-holding by 1996. Many, however, had joined under duress, as they felt they would be left behind if they did not become fund-holders. The cost of reorganisation (e.g. purchaser and provider) had been covered by two short-term increases of funding to the NHS in 1992/1993 and 1994/1995. The extra money was quickly absorbed and no benefits were seen to services. The government remained prudent but its belief that the NHS would become more efficient and save money if there were strict financial pressures was misguided.

Further reorganisation was implemented and by 1996 regional health authorities had been abolished and replaced by eight regional offices of the NHS Executive. There were 425 NHS trusts, which acted as 'providers' of services, and 8500 GP fund-holders, who were 'purchasers'. In addition to fund-holders, there were non-fund-holding GPs, who were still under the management of 100 health authorities. This division of the NHS into purchasers and providers made it difficult for the NHS to plan and distribute resources on the basis of the population's health needs. Many NHS trusts were failing financially and waiting lists remained static. The NHS had lurched from reform to reform, nearing a crisis so many times that on the eve of the 1997 general election the *Sun* newspaper implored its readers that they had '24 hours to save the NHS' (*Sun*, 1997).

1997–2010

The 1997 Labour Party general election victory brought new hope to the NHS, which in many people's eyes had been in a permanent state of crisis for over 20 years. Eighteen years in opposition had forced the Labour Party to instigate major policy reform. Traditional party beliefs of nationalisation, central planning and state paternalism, which the creation of the NHS was based on, were abandoned. The new government adopted what was to be known as 'the third way', mixing notions of equality and social justice with privatisation and free market competition (Blair, 1998). The 'third way' of running the NHS was based on partnership and driven by performance and led to the biggest period of reforms in its history.

The newly elected government had committed to sticking to the overall expenditure plans of the previous Conservative government for the first 2 years of its term. An extra £1.2 billion was, however, invested immediately into the NHS, which was just the beginning of increased resources. Following the Wanless report (Wanless, 2002), which recognised that the NHS was and had for many years been under-funded, UK taxes were increased to finance extra NHS expenditure, averaging an increase of 7.4% a year in real terms for the next 5 years. This raised total health spending in the UK from 6.8% of gross domestic product (GDP) in 1997 to 9.4% in 2007/2008, which made the UK one of the higher spenders on health in Europe (Stevens, 2004).

Extra investment in the NHS coincided with a programme of major reforms, which focused on reorganising services and raising standards of health and care. In 1997 the UK's first Minister for Public Health was appointed. Subsequently, the policy document *Our Healthier Nation* (1998) was published to replace *Health of the Nation*. The new policy set a national target of saving 300000 lives over the next decade, focusing on cancers, coronary heart disease and stroke and mental illness. *Our Healthier Nation* shifted focus away from the policies of the 1990s, based on the principle that individuals were responsible for improving their health, and recognised that there needed to be a framework to empower individuals as well as strategies to decrease inequality and poverty.

The first significant set of reforms by the new Labour government were set out in a white paper *The New NHS: Modern, Dependable* (Department of Health, 1997), which was published at the end of 1997. The paper proposed the dismantling of the internal market but many components of it were maintained. The purchase–provider split remained but the emphasis was on cooperative relationships rather than competition. GP fund-holding was abolished and instead all general practices were obliged to join primary care groups (PCGs). PCGs covered populations that varied in size from 30000 to 250000 and functioned as both providers of primary care and purchasers of secondary care. They were still led by GPs, although their boards also contained representation from community groups and the local health authority. PCGs were set up so they were able to retain any surplus from their budgets, which could be spent on services or facilities of benefit to patients. Although competition was disapproved of by the Labour government, purchasers (i.e. PCGs) were still able to switch to other providers if they were dissatisfied with the services they received.

The 1997 white paper also began to address quality and standards in the NHS and was expanded upon by *A First Class Service: Quality in the New NHS* a year later (Department of Health, 1998*b*). Clinical governance, which was seen as a radical idea, was introduced to the NHS and placed a statutory responsibility for the quality of care upon trust and health authority chief executives. Hospital trusts and PCGs developed systems and committees to meet the clinical governance requirements of quality assurance, audit and risk management. There has been criticism that the implementation of clinical governance in the NHS was impeded by lack of time and resources – too much change, too quickly – and a lack of clear guidance (Roland *et al*, 2001).

The government also set up two new national bodies: the National Institute for Clinical Excellence (NICE; which in 2013 became the National

Institute for Health and Care Excellence, after some interim changes of name and specific responsibilities, while retaining the acronym unaltered) and the Council for Health Improvement, which evolved into the Commission for Health Improvement (CHI) in 2000. In 2002, the CHI was replaced by the Commission for Health Audit and Inspection (CHAI), which combined its work with that previously done by the Audit Commission. The CHAI also had responsibility for regulation in private healthcare (e.g. private nursing homes and hospitals). The work of the CHAI was in turn taken over by the Healthcare Commission in 2004 and later conducted by the Care Quality Commission (CQC). In simple terms NICE was expected to set standards while CHAI enforced them. NICE's aim to address the lack of national standards and resultant wide variations in quality of healthcare was at first very popular. There had been growing public concern over 'postcode prescribing', where the availability of effective treatment depended on where in the country the patient lived. NICE's assessment of the effectiveness of drugs and other medical technologies led to it recommending their use in virtually all cases. A large part of NICE's remit was to attempt to limit the growth of the NHS drug bill, but even when its experts asserted that the anti-viral drug zanamivir had little therapeutic benefit, they back-tracked on their original judgement and recommended its use. Moreover, CHI/CHAI inspections proved truly effective only when discovering gross incompetence and negligence, as they had few solutions to offer still under-resourced trusts which were not meeting the performance standards (Day & Klein, 2002).

Other innovations to modernise the NHS and change the ways it had previously worked included NHS Direct and the National Programme for Information Technology (NPFIT). NHS Direct was a nurse-led 24-hour health advice phone service. Five years after its inception in 1998 it was handling over half a million calls a day and expanded into an equally busy online service in 2001. The NPFIT was an ambitious project which originally aimed for NHS trusts to have electronic records in place by 2005 (NHS Executive, 1998). However, it was riddled with logistical and technical difficulties, and failed to meet its aim (Hendy *et al*, 2005). Critics of the Labour government of this period often cite the project as an example of NHS mismanagement and wasting precious public investment.

The NHS Plan

The New NHS: Modern, Dependable (1997) was only the beginning of the reforms the Labour government intended for the NHS. Its full programme to modernise the NHS was announced in July 2000, in *The NHS Plan* (Department of Health, 2000a). This described the government's vision for the NHS for the next 10 years and led to unprecedented change. The plan was enterprising, impressive in scope and in places daring. It concentrated on the areas of capacity, standards, delivery and partnership, but at its core was the aim of creating a patient-led Health Service. It proposed an NHS that responded to the needs and preferences of patients, rather than their choice being prohibited by 'the system' or health professionals. Significant improvements were expected to proceed from the new investment:

- *More health professionals.* Over a 5-year period it was expected to provide 7500 more hospital consultants (a rise of 30%), 1000 more specialist registrars and 2000 extra GPs and 450 more trainees. There would also be 1000 more medical school places each year, on top of 1000 places that had been announced before the NHS Plan.
- *More hospitals and beds.* Provision was made in the Plan for 100 new hospitals over a 10-year period and 7000 more hospital and intermediate-care beds.
- *National standards for waiting times.* By 2005 the maximum waiting time was expected to be 3 months for out-patients and 6 months for in-patients. No one should be waiting more than 4 hours in accident and emergency departments by 2004. It was also promised that all patients would be able to see a GP within 48 hours by 2004. Waiting lists for hospital appointments and admissions would be abolished by the end of 2005 and replaced with a booking system designed to give patients a choice of a convenient time.
- *Performance monitoring.* The performance of hospital trusts and primary care groups would be rated by CHI, using a traffic light system: 'green light' organisations, the 'best performers', would receive funds from the National Performance Fund and be given more autonomy; a 'red light' rating would lead to intervention from government agencies and if necessary the installation of new management. (The traffic light system was later replaced by the equally loathed star rating system, whereby trusts were evaluated against performance standards such as finances and waiting lists and awarded up to three stars.)
- *Expansion of nursing roles.* To make up the shortfall of doctors, the NHS Plan also proposed training for around 20000 nurses so that they would be able to prescribe a limited range of medicines.

To implement the NHS Plan, the government set up the National Modernisation Agency and local modernisation boards for each regional office of the NHS. The *Implementation Programme for the NHS Plan* was published at the end of 2000 and included provisional milestones and key targets for the early years of the Plan (Department of Health, 2000*b*). More targets followed and many working in the NHS felt overwhelmed by the pace of change.

Another reorganisation of the NHS

The NHS Plan promised greater power and authority for patients and the public. *Shifting the Balance of Power* (Department of Health, 2001) attempted to give that greater authority to patients as well as to decentralise decision-making. The NHS Executive was dismantled and all English and Welsh health authorities were abolished. They were replaced with 28 new strategic health authorities (SHAs), which had a strategic role in improving local health services and also monitoring the performance of local health trusts.

Primary care groups evolved into new primary care trusts (PCTs), which inherited the health authorities' powers, responsibilities and resources. PCTs became the new powerhouses of the NHS. They were responsible for health improvement, and developing and delivering primary care, but also for commissioning hospital services. PCTs held approximately 75% of the NHS resources. While there were nearly 100 health authorities, there were over 400 PCTs, each covering an average population of 175 000.

One of the most controversial reforms during this period was the formation of foundation trusts. Initially, only top-performing trusts could apply for foundation status, but it was envisaged that all hospital trusts and PCTs would eventually be eligible. Becoming a foundation trust offered more financial freedom, as they were allowed to retain operating surpluses and to access a wider range of options for capital funding to invest in new services. They could also recruit and employ their own staff. Although they still had to deliver on national targets and standards, they were not under the direction of the Department of Health and the regional strategic health authorities. There had been much resistance to the introduction of foundation trusts, however, as many felt they indicated the break-up of the NHS, with individual hospitals having almost complete independence and determining their own priorities.

The NHS and the private sector

For the NHS to reach the targets of the NHS Plan it needed to increase its capacity, but extra resources to build new hospitals were unavailable. Previous governments had used the Private Finance Initiative (PFI), whereby private capital was used to build hospitals and hospital trusts would then lease the buildings from the private companies, under contracts lasting 25 years or more. The NHS gained new buildings without raising taxes, as the public's payment was deferred, although over the long term the arrangement was more expensive than if the buildings had been built using public money. The 2002 white paper *Delivering the NHS Plan* announced that 55 major hospital building schemes would be carried out, mostly through the PFI system (Department of Health, 2002). The PFI schemes were later renamed 'public–private partnerships' (PPPs).

Some NHS services, such as psychotherapy, were contracted out to private companies. This was done in the hope of increasing capacity and meeting targets. Most contracts involved elective surgical procedures or diagnostic tests. The primary concern of private healthcare providers is profit and so they were too prone to choosing activities that would yield a profit and leaving less financially attractive services to the NHS. There were also concerns about the quality of work provided by the private companies and so contracts included expected performance levels. During this period there were sustained concerns that the NHS was slowly being privatised through PPPs, although at the time the government was committed to a maximum of 15% of the NHS's output being provided by the private sector. For an in-depth discussion of the relationship between the NHS and the private sector, readers are recommended *NHS plc* (Pollock, 2005).

The results of increased investment

There was massive investment in the NHS in the period 1997–2006: NHS spending increased from £46 billion a year to £94 billion a year. This investment led to some modest improvements, including nearly 200 000 extra front-line staff. However, over half the extra money was spent on pay and pensions for staff, most significantly in increased National Insurance contributions. GPs and hospital consultants received new contracts, which, while increasing the scrutiny and accountability of their work, considerably increased their pay. UK doctors became some of the highest paid in the world outside the USA. However, as perhaps was to be expected, with increased salary came increased public expectations. There was also a contradiction that with the new GP contract patients had access to new clinics and general practices had extended their opening hours but the contract also allowed GPs to opt out from out-of-hours work. The government was perhaps surprised by the high proportion of GPs who took that option and there was concern about the quality and cost of the night visiting services that were commissioned to replace the patients' regular GPs.

There were some successes from the increased investment. The number of patients on waiting lists, a favourite marker of success for politicians, fell to an all-time low, although the average out-patient waiting time was reduced only to 6.6 weeks, compared with 7.7 weeks in 1997. The government set a new target in 2008 that patients would wait no more than 18 weeks from referral to treatment. This was an ambitious aim, as only 10 years before there had been over 280 000 patients waiting for more than 6 months for admission to hospital and it was not uncommon to wait more than 2 years (Nicholson, 2009). From 2009, patients were also given the right to choose where they would be treated, from a menu of providers which included private healthcare companies.

There had been improvements on many measures of NHS activity following the implementation of the NHS Plan and subsequent policies. However, there was a general feeling that too much had been spent on delivering too little. NHS productivity had not increased enough and the Service ended up costing more and delivering less value for money. Even before the worldwide economic downturn following the collapse of the banking industry in 2008 there were concerns about the future financing of the NHS. In 2006 the NHS in England had a net deficit of £512 million, which at the time was equivalent to 0.8% of its turnover.

This led to services being cut in some areas. The introduction of the 'payment by results' funding scheme, where hospitals were paid only for the work they did, rather than given a budget at the start of the year, also increased competition between providers. Each procedure, whether it be a surgical operation or an out-patient follow-up appointment, had an attached national tariff/price and the hospital received this payment only if it completed the activity. This change in funding, along with patients being able to choose their provider, led to increased financial pressures for some hospitals as they struggled to attract enough work and compete with other hospitals. The hospitals that faced the worst financial adversity already had financial deficits and were tied into long, expensive PPP contracts for the construction of new buildings.

In 2009, the then NHS chief executive, David Nicholson, established the QIPP (quality, innovation, productivity and prevention) programme to deliver efficiency savings to the NHS of £15–20 billion between 2011 and 2014 (Nicholson, 2009). This put further emphasis on NHS organisations redesigning their services and making savings while maintaining patient safety and standards of care.

Patient safety and clinical standards

The Labour government was aware that it would not be able to continue increasing funding for the NHS to the same degree. To set out a strategy for the NHS for the next 10 years, a review was conducted by the then health minister in the House of Lords, Lord Darzi, who was also Professor of Surgery at Imperial College London. The Darzi report had the advantage of presenting a clinician's vision as well as being informed by an extensive consultation with 60 000 staff, patients and stakeholder groups. Lord Darzi's final report, *High Quality Care For All* (Darzi, 2008), reflected, but also developed, many existing policies, including patient choice, the role of NICE and competition. However, importantly, it changed the emphasis of policy and highlighted the need to increase quality of care and ensure patient safety. It also promoted the involvement of clinicians to lead and manage improvements in the services in which they worked.

The Darzi report also set out the values contained in the first NHS Constitution (Department of Health, 2009) in the form of patients' rights and pledges that the NHS would strive to deliver. It also set out the responsibilities which the public, patients and staff owe to one another to ensure that the NHS operated fairly and effectively. It enshrined the principle that access to NHS care was based on clinical need and not the individual's ability to pay and the principle that patients have the right to be treated with dignity, respect and compassion.

The positive impact of the NHS Constitution was reduced by one of the biggest scandals to ever hit the NHS, which occurred in the same year. The Healthcare Commission investigated the high mortality rate in Stafford Hospital and uncovered 'appalling' standards of care (Francis, 2010). It was a reminder that despite increased resources, new policies and values, there was still unacceptable variability in the standard of care provided by the NHS. This added to the next government's argument that major reform in the NHS was required.

Developments since 2010

No party had an outright majority after the 2010 general election which led to the Conservative–Liberal Democrat coalition government being formed. Neither party set out any significant reform for the NHS in its election manifesto. The Conservatives promised that, despite the need for a programme of austerity measures to address the country's financial crisis, they would 'ring-fence' the funding for the NHS. Before the election they also guaranteed that, if they were in power, there would be 'no top-down reorganisation of the NHS'. Politicians and the public alike were almost universally shocked that in its first year in government the coalition presented the first draft of the Health and Social Care Bill, which set out the most wide-ranging reforms of the NHS since it was formed in 1948. The bill received a strong reaction, including claims that it would lead to the privatisation of the NHS.

The comprehensive organisational changes contained in the bill included:

- A new NHS Commissioning Board (NHSCB) was to be directly responsible for the day-to-day running of the NHS, rather than the Department of Health.
- The PCTs were to be abolished and replaced by several hundred clinical commissioning groups (CCGs), made of consortia of GPs. They would receive 60% of the NHS budget and, with other clinicians and support from managers, commission services on behalf of the local population to meet its specific needs.
- The strategic health authorities were also to be abolished, with the CCGs being accountable to the NHSCB.
- All NHS providers of hospital and community services were to become foundation trusts. Foundation trusts were to be allowed to generate up to 49% of their income from private patients.
- Monitor, the organisation that oversees the running of foundation trusts, was to become the economic regulator for the healthcare sector. It was specifically set the task of promoting competition as well as licensing providers and setting prices through a national tariff, with price competition allowed.
- A new body, Public Health England, was to lead on public health at a national level, while local authorities were to take the lead at a local level.
- A new national patient body, Health Watch, was to be set up, with local Health Watch groups.

There was a strong negative reaction to the bill and many saw it as the dismantling of the NHS, and ultimately its privatisation. It was feared that the entitlement to free health services would be curtailed (Pollock *et al*, 2012). There was also a fundamental change in the role of the Secretary of State proposed in the bill, whereby they would no longer have a duty to provide a comprehensive health service but instead have a duty to 'promote' a comprehensive service. The bill also transferred from the Secretary of State to CCGs the power to determine what is 'appropriate as part of the health service' for certain individuals. Those against the bill felt that it would ultimately lead to some patients being excluded from parts of the NHS and that it would lead to an increase in the services that could be charged for.

The provisions of the original bill were extensively debated in Parliament and some 2000 amendments were made before it was passed. The duty and accountability of the Secretary of State to provide, and not 'promote', comprehensive healthcare was maintained. The original duty on Monitor to 'promote competition' was dropped and amendments were made to rule out competition on price, while other safeguards were added to reduce the emphasis on competition. However, despite these amendments there was still strong opposition to the Health and Social Care Act, as it was still felt that the emphasis on competition would lead to greater privatisation and fragmentation of the NHS.

The government's appraisal of the need for such a radical reorganisation was not supported by the public's view of the NHS. When the coalition came into power in 2010, the NHS had its highest public approval rating, at 70% of respondents, since the start of records in 1983, and had the support of 97% of the population (Taylor, 2013). However, satisfaction fell by 12 percentage points in 2011 when the bill was published, which was the biggest fall in 1 year ever recorded, although the satisfaction rate was still the third highest recorded.

Other concerns about the Health and Social Care Act included that the radical restructuring of the NHS would be a major distraction for clinicians and managers at a time when it faced the biggest financial challenge in its history. The government claimed that the proposed reforms would save at least £1.5 billion. However, others suggested that abandoning the Act would actually have saved £1 billion (Walshe, 2012). The NHS had been struggling to address the 'Nicholson challenge' of saving £20 billion over 4 years. NHS organisations' efforts to make efficiency savings had largely been disappointing and what was still required was a real and painful reconfiguration of services.

The Health and Social Care Act was unpopular in many quarters but the coalition government had consistently highlighted that it shared many values with the policies of the previous Labour government. Clinicians, mainly GPs, were still central to the commissioning of services, while the Darzi report had encouraged the empowerment of clinicians to be involved in the design, change and structuring of services. The Act also increased competition between healthcare providers, which, it was presumed, would increase quality and efficiency. Critics of the Act believed that such a major reorganisation of the NHS was not needed. However, the coalition's case for change to improve quality of care was supported by the Francis report on the Mid Staffordshire NHS Foundation Trust (Francis, 2010) (see above). He reported examples of appalling nursing care and an extra 500 deaths that occurred between 2005/2006 and 2007/2008. Francis made 290 recommendations to improve the NHS, with the focus being on putting patients' needs first and avoiding a fixation on financial issues and targets.

The scrutiny of the Health and Social Care Act highlighted the inequalities across the NHS as a consequence of devolution. The universal, national service that the NHS was set up as had already been diminished prior to the Health and Social Care Act and there were now essentially four different NHS organisations across the four jurisdictions of the United Kingdom. This has led to a variability in the provision of services. An example of this is the NHS in Scotland, where the Scottish National Party government introduced a policy of free prescriptions, which is not the case elsewhere.

Conclusion

It is hoped that this brief précis of the history of the NHS will act as an introduction to the subject for doctors interested in the management and the complex organisational structure in which we work. Two things can be learned from taking this historical overview: first, that history repeats itself and it is remarkable how recent plans for the NHS are similar to earlier ideas; second, as an administrative machine the NHS is continually evolving, and that should be borne in mind by all of us who intend to plight their troth to it for the vast majority of our professional careers.

It will be several years before we know whether the most recent policies for the NHS will 'save' it, as the government hopes, or be the beginning of the end of the NHS, as others fear. History perhaps tells us that they are most likely to do neither.

Changes in NHS management structure since 1974 are summarised in Table 1.1.

References and further reading

Allsop J (1986) *Health Policy in the National Health Service.* Longman.

Beeson PB (1980) Some good features of the British National Health Service. In *Readings in Medical Sociology* (ed D Mechanic): 328–34. Free Press.

Blair T (1998) *The Third Way: New Politics for the New Century.* Fabian Society.

British Medical Association (1989) *Special Report on the Government's White Paper 'Working for Patients'.* BMA.

British Medical Journal (1875) Provident institutions and hospitals. II: Outpatient reforms. *British Medical Journal*, 483–84.

Table 1.1 Some important changes in NHS management structures since 1974

Year	Initiative
1975	*Better Services for the Mentally Ill*, a white paper based on a report of the Audit Commission
1982	The Korner report, from the Department of Health and Social Security's Steering Group on Health Services Information, concerning the collection and use of information on hospital clinical activity
1982	Abolition of NHS area health boards
1983	Management budgeting experiment started
1984	Griffiths report on Health Service management
1986	Introduction of the Resource Management Initiative
1987	*Achieving a Balance* published by the Department of Health and Social Security, making recommendations for staffing levels for doctors
1988	NHS review announced
1989	*Working for Patients* and *Caring for People*, white papers leading to the 1990 Act
1990	The NHS and Community Care Act (reforms effective 1 April 1991) and introduction of the purchaser–provider split
1991	Postgraduate and continuing medical education introduced
1991	First wave of trust hospitals
1992	Second wave of trust hospitals
1993	Managing the new NHS – new proposals
1994	Fourth wave of trust hospitals
1997	*The New NHS: Modern, Dependable* published: GP fund-holders abolished; moves away from competition; PCGs established
1998	*A First Class Service* introduced clinical governance
2000	The NHS Plan increased resources and introduced performance monitoring (traffic light system)
2001	*Shifting the Balance of Power* launched: primary care trusts set up; NHS Executive replaced by strategic health authorities
2002	Wanless report – highlighted under-funding of the NHS
2003	Health and Social Care Act presented the concept of foundation hospitals
2008	Lord Darzi's *Next Stage Review* published, based on a consultation involving 60 000 staff, patients and members of the public
2009	*The NHS Constitution* published, outlining patients' rights
2010	The *Liberating the NHS* white paper set out putting patients at the heart of everything the NHS does
2012	The Health and Social Care Act set up care commissioning groups and disbanded the strategic health authorities and primary care trusts

GP, general practitioner; PGC, primary care group.

Darzi A (2008) *High Quality Care For All: NHS Next Stage Review. Final Report.* HMSO.

Davies C (1987) Things to come: the NHS in the next decade. *Sociology of Health and Illness*, **9**: 302–17.

Day P, Klein R (2002) Who nose best? *Health Service Journal*, April: 26–9.

Department of Health (1989) *Working for Patients.* HMSO.

Department of Health (1990) *The Community Care Act.* HMSO.

Department of Health (1991) *The Patient's Charter.* HMSO.

Department of Health (1992) *The Health of the Nation.* HMSO.

Department of Health (1994) *Hospital and Ambulance Services: Comparative Performance Grade 1993–1994.* HMSO.

Department of Health (1997) *The New NHS: Modern, Dependable.* TSO.

Department of Health (1998a) *Our Healthier Nation.* TSO.

Department of Health (1998b) *A First Class Service: Quality in the New NHS.* TSO.

Department of Health (2000a) *The NHS Plan: A Plan for Investment, A Plan for Reform.* TSO.

Department of Health (2000b) *Implementation Programme for the NHS Plan.* TSO.

Department of Health (2001) *Shifting the Balance of Power Within the NHS.* TSO.

Department of Health (2002) *Delivering the NHS Plan: Next Steps on Investment, Next Steps on Reform.* TSO.

Department of Health (2009) *The NHS Constitution: The NHS Belongs To Us All.* TSO.

Department of Health and Social Security (1972) *Management Arrangements for the Re-organised Health Service.* HMSO.

Draper P, Grenholm G, Best G (1976) The organization of health care: a critical view of the 1974 reorganization of the National Health Service. In *An Introduction to Medical Sociology* (ed D Tuckett). Tavistock.

Forsyth G (1982) Evolution of the National Health Service. In *Management for Clinicians* (eds D Allen, D Grimes): 18–35. Pitman.

Francis R (2010) *Inquiry Report into Mid-Staffordshire NHS Foundation Trust.* TSO.

Godber G (1975) *The Health Service: Past, Present and Future.* Athlone Press.

Godber G (1988) Forty years of the NHS. *Origins and early development. BMJ*, **297**: 37–43. (Subsequent articles in the same issue, pp 44–58, are also of interest.)

Hampton JR (1989) White paper – white elephant? *Hospital Update*, April: 245–6.

Hendy J, Reeves BC, Fulop N, *et al* (2005) Challenges to implementing the National Programme for Information Technology (NPFIT): a qualitative study. *BMJ*, **331**: 331–6.

Hoffenberg R, Todd IP, Pinker G (1987) Crisis in the National Health Service. *BMJ*, **295**: 1505.

Honigsbaum F (1979) *The Division in British Medicine: A History of the Separation of General Practice from Health Care 1911–1968.* Routledge & Kegan Paul.

Honigsbaum F (1989) *Health, Happiness and Security: The Creation of the National Health Service.* Routledge.

Kearney K (1992) Strategy for improvement or window dressing? *Guardian*, 9 July.

Klein R (2010) *The New Politics of the National Health Service: From Creation to Reinvention* (6th revised edition). Radcliffe Publishing.

Levitt R (1976) *The Reorganised National Health Service.* Croom Helm.

NHS Executive (1998) *Information for Health: An Information Strategy for the Modern NHS 1998–2005.* NHS Executive.

Nicholson D (2009) *The Year 2008/2009: NHS Chief Executive's Annual Report.* Department of Health.

Pollock A (2005) *NHS plc.* Verso.

Pollock A, Price D, Roderick P (2012) Health and Social Care Bill 2011: a legal basis for charging and providing fewer health services to people in England. *BMJ*, **344**: e1729.

Roland M, Campell S, Wilkins D (2001) Clinical governance: a convincing strategy for quality improvement? *Journal of Management in Medicine*, **15**: 188–201.

Stacey M (1988) *The Sociology of Health and Healing.* Unwin Hyman.

Stevens R (1966) *Medical Practice in Modern England: The Impact of Specialization and State Medicine*. York University Press.

Stevens S (2004) Reform strategies for the English NHS. *Health Affairs*, **23**: 37–44.

Sun (1997) You have 24 hours to save the NHS. 4 May.

Taylor R (2013) *God Bless the NHS*. Faber & Faber.

Timmins N (1988) *Cash Crisis and Cure: The Independent Guide to the NHS Debate*. Newspaper Publishing.

Walshe K (2012) The consequences of abandoning the Health and Social Care Bill. *BMJ*, **344**: e748.

Wanless D (2002) *Securing Our Future Health: Taking a Long-Term View. Final Report*. Her Majesty's Treasury.

Watkin B (1978) *The National Health Service: The First Phase 1948–1974 and After*. George Allen & Unwin.

Webster C (2002) *The NHS: A Political History*. Oxford University Press.

CHAPTER 2

The politics, funding and resources of the NHS in England

Luca Polledri, Samuel Menon and Stephen Morris

There is probably never a sensible time to write about NHS resources. Indeed, the current stepwise rolling reform introduced by the Health and Social Care Act 2012 makes its full implications elusive. Part of the problem is that reforming the financing of the NHS is a long-term project, whereas politics is not. Equally difficult for politicians is the requirement that they understand in full the effect their policies have; they might better be piloted on a smaller scale, with some honesty about what works and, more importantly, what does not. As a result, over its nearly seven decades of existence, the NHS has seen many incomplete attempts to reform its finances, but none has overcome the perception of many who deliver services that, at best, resource allocation is unfair and illogical.

The level of spending on the NHS consistently increased ahead of inflation until the recent economic crisis (Fig. 2.1). The spending in real terms (adjusted for inflation) increased from £60 billion in 1996/1997 to nearly £140 billion in 2009/2010 – an extraordinary 12 years by any

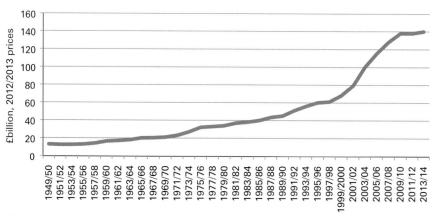

Fig. 2.1 NHS spending in real terms (2012/2013 prices) from 1949/1950 to 2013/2014. Adapted from Nuffield Trust (2012)

standards, especially when the first 2 years saw a very low rate of growth by historical standards. Yet the National Audit Office showed a significant fall in productivity in the NHS during the Blair era (partly because of pay rises), suggesting that there is still a significant productivity gain that could be achieved. Even after the economic crisis, the NHS has largely been protected from the 'austerity' imposed on the rest of the public sector. The £20 billion saved by the NHS during the period 2011/2012 to 2014/2015 was achieved in major part by reducing pay increases rather than by restricting services or cutting waste.

Two questions spring to mind.

- For HM Treasury (and the electorate), what did we get, and what do we get now, for our money?
- For healthcare professionals and all those working directly with patients, where did all the money go?

Right now, mental health services are complaining loudly about 'cuts' and yet more cash is being spent on mental health services than it was 10 years ago. It seems that despite the amount invested, it is never enough to meet the needs of service users.

Because of the dominance of a performance management regime that focuses on an increasingly small number of national targets, we can provide better answers than in the past to the first question. Targets are themselves a reflection of the key government priority to know what it is getting for the cash being injected. They have caused quite a stir. Most accept that they work (look at the numbers), but it is a problem if what is important to you and your service is not included, and if the effort made to measure or achieve them draws resources away from clinical work. Mental health may well have cause for complaint in the absence of such clear performance indicators as waiting time for elective surgery.

Since 1997, performance indicators associated with targets have been impressive, as demonstrated by the international interest in them, not least from overseas politicians. Waiting times for elective surgery and in accident and emergency departments – the cause of the public's greatest expressed concern – have been reduced significantly.

Mental health has been slower to introduce such performance indicators and targets: it is only recently that patient-reported outcome measures (PROMs) and patient-reported experience measures (PREMs) have been developed on a large scale and started to be trialled in most trusts. This delay leaves us with little information on which to assess the impact of the Blair years of Labour government on our specialty. Measures such as suicide rate or negative media coverage (as a measure of degree of stigma and discrimination) have been used at times; however, these are too spurious to allow for reliable interpretation. For example, the Blair era saw a steady yearly decrease in suicide rates as well as an improvement in the media treatment of high-profile mental health cases, such as homicides committed by people with mental health problems. Mental health services have a clear role in tackling suicide, stigmatisation and discrimination: has the targeted resource allocation to services such as early intervention, liaison and home treatment teams worked, therefore? It seems unlikely that anyone would wish to make such a simple connection. This illustrates the great difficulty for the NHS, and its decision-makers and leaders, in making sense of the politics, finance and funding needed to improve performance, and in understanding why there is such pressure for the systematic application of outcome measures.

Before considering in greater detail the financial policy environment that has emerged since 1997, and in particular after the Health and Social Care Act 2012, let us first discern the priorities for spending in the NHS. It is not always clear whether services are free at the point of delivery, and mental health services are strongly affected by other costs and charges. For service users there are benefits and social care costs that are means tested, but there is also the need to budget everyday living costs, often on a very small income. Should the NHS spend more on prevention, or more on treatment? Should the agenda be driven by those who make the most noise (who generally seem to call for attention to be paid to issues such as waiting times, acute episodes of mental illness, heroic surgery and pioneering drug therapies for terminal cancer) or by properly researched and tested interventions that deliver real population health improvements? There is a reasonably sound evidence base for both war and improving the performance of the local football team in preventing suicide. Perhaps that is why these decisions are best left to the politicians.

The NHS since 1997

The election that brought a Labour government into power in 1997 provides a useful starting point for assessing the development of recent health policy as it relates to finance and resources. Labour returned to power just in time to celebrate the 50th birthday of what some might see as both its problem child and its greatest achievement: the NHS. The issues facing the NHS and the government might not have changed dramatically in this time, but the expectations of the electorate, NHS staff and the Labour Party itself were now extremely high. And the obstacles to fulfilling these hopes were now daunting.

The years that followed with Labour in power, up to 2010, can be summarised with the help of three milestones: the Wanless report, the NHS Plan and the Health and Social Care (Community Health and Standards) Act 2003.

The Wanless report

The Wanless report, commissioned by the Treasury and published in 2002, provided the government with a quasi-independent assessment that a health service, centrally funded through taxation and with services free at the point of delivery, is indeed the best system for the UK. It specifically rejected an insurance-based system and any of the alternatives used in other parts of the developed world. Notably, it painted a picture that fitted well with the government's view of individual rights balanced by responsibilities. In the Wanless 'fully engaged' scenario, individuals would be enabled to take responsibility for lifestyle choices that have an impact on their health, and would be encouraged and given the opportunity to actively manage their own healthcare. This had the double advantage of supporting the government's goal of improving the nation's health while at the same time reducing the incidence of avoidable illness, so that the NHS could concentrate its resources on tackling disease and improving the health of the population.

The NHS Plan

The NHS Plan, set out by the Department of Health in the document *The NHS Plan: A Plan for Investment, a Plan for Reform* (2000), overlapped with the preparation of the Wanless report. It translated into political recognition that the NHS needed a substantial increase in funding, and that this increase had to be matched by an absolute requirement for tangible and measurable results. It set ambitious targets across the Health Service; these reflected the public service agreement negotiated by the Department of Health with the Cabinet Office.

The Plan started a major reorganisation of the NHS. The regional offices and health authorities were abolished and replaced by 28 strategic health authorities (SHAs) and 302 primary care trusts (PCTs). The SHAs were given three roles: performance management, increasing capacity and supporting strategic development. The PCTs received the majority of the funding and were charged with 'commissioning' services that were sensitive to local needs and that delivered the centrally determined targets of the NHS Plan.

Perhaps most profoundly, the government directly tackled the NHS's funding gap and increased National Insurance – a straightforward price increase for the NHS's services. This now meant that money was linked directly to targets. In 2007/2008 the total spend on healthcare reached 8.8% of gross domestic product, in line with the European average and the Prime Minister's commitment to matching the European average spend per head.

Significant achievements were made at the time: a decrease in waiting times both in accident and emergency departments and for elective surgery; and an increase in the numbers of general practices, hospital consultants, qualified nurses and extras in the NHS. Moreover, there was a significant modernisation of NHS buildings and hospitals and a renegotiation of contracts with all NHS staff; the new contracts allowed for much greater flexibility of the workforce but added significantly to salary costs.

Health and Social Care (Community Health and Standards) Act

The final stage marked a move to a 'self-sustaining' system that rewarded performance, was independently regulated and promoted choice and contestability. Its initiation can be seen with the Health and Social Care Act 2003 and the publication of the NHS Improvement Plan in June 2004.

The Act introduced NHS foundation trusts, public interest companies no longer accountable to the Department of Health but independent, with some (initially very limited) ability to raise capital commercially. They were regulated by a newly created independent body, Monitor, which acts as the licensing body with sole discretion in the suspension of their authorisation. The government's intention was that the introduction of these trusts would mean a better management of performance, when rigorous top-down performance management targets alone appeared to cause excessive bureaucracy and dent the smooth running of the health delivery system. Foundation trusts have a 'council of governors' that acts as a link between the board of directors and the community. The majority of the governors must be elected by secret ballot and the constituencies include staff, patients and other members of the public. This is meant to ensure that hospitals, now accountable to the membership of the local NHS foundation trust, are more locally accountable.

Whatever the reasons and however limited their margin to manoeuvre, the birth of these foundation trusts represented a huge cultural shift and was not spared harsh criticism: it was the first significant step towards setting the NHS free from central government. To their opponents, these trusts represented a back-door privatisation that could destabilise the NHS and introduce a two-tier service.

Overview

Overall, during Labour's reign, the NHS made significant progress not just in terms of waiting times but also in terms of reduced morbidity for cancer, coronary heart disease and suicides. Waiting times in accident and emergency departments and for elective surgery quickly disappeared from the front pages of tabloids and broadsheets alike. Yet, when the financial crisis and a reduction in resources started to hit, signs of a reversal of these improvements appeared quickly: not only was there a deterioration of performance indicators such as waiting times, but also, and most worryingly, some NHS trusts were forced into administration. The NHS failed to change and learn how to negotiate the containment of costs within projected resources.

So why did these reforms fall short? Perhaps they were not brave enough, or lacked direction. Or was it simply that the financial crisis hit before they could be realised? It is hard to say. What is clear, however, is that the NHS did not look hard enough at its resource base. And once funding growth returned to more neutral levels, the NHS was not ready. Even though efforts were made – such as looking at length of stay, effectiveness of community interventions, case management of long-term conditions, and better and closer working between primary and secondary care – these were too shy and not considered a priority. Indeed, mental health services have attempted to work on them, but a lack of time – these things do not happen overnight – and a lack of a systematic approach got in the way.

The coalition government and the Health and Social Care Act 2012

The Health and Social Care Act 2012 (HSCA) followed the appointment of the coalition government in 2010. It was preceded by the publication of a white paper in 2010 and the Health and Social Care Bill in 2011, and was claimed by the *Daily Telegraph* (26 February 2012) to be 'the most extensive reorganisation of the NHS ever undertaken'. The HSCA aims to foster competition in the provision of healthcare and notably introduces the scope for 'any qualified provider' to be commissioned for a specific service by the commissioning authorities. This principle is highly controversial when applied to health and, perhaps not surprisingly, has been met with strong opposition by associations such as the British Medical Association (BMA), the Royal College of Physicians and – although less vehemently – the Royal College of Psychiatrists.

The Act represented the coalition government's attempt to introduce structural changes to the NHS and to shift its culture towards a competition-based system, by loosening the monopoly of the NHS in the delivery of healthcare. In the government's view, the NHS should continue to move away from central control, and this reform strongly encouraged its autonomy.

If we consider the structuring reforms introduced, the most notable is the creation of clinical commissioning groups (CCGs) at the base of the commissioning structure. These are GP-led organisations with additional representation by a hospital doctor, a nurse and several community representatives. They are in charge of buying and providing healthcare for their local populations in what is a fundamental change in the balance of power within the NHS: the control of the budget has shifted from the administrator-led PCTs to bodies with a strong clinical base, inside which GPs have a prominent role. As a direct consequence, PCTs and SHAs have been abolished. Notably, CCGs have been empowered to make decisions and to shape services by their allocation of the majority of NHS funds: every year CCGs receive between £60 and £80 billion, or roughly 60–80% of the total NHS budget. They use this to buy services for their local community while bodies called commissioning support units help them with practical tasks ranging from transactional services, such as payroll and information technology services, to equipping CCGs with the complex population-level data required to inform commissioning decisions.

The reform gives CCGs the power to choose: from different providers within the NHS to, crucially, 'any qualified provider' (AQP) that they deem able to offer effective services. Therefore, external providers such as charities and private agencies can compete with the NHS in the delivery of healthcare. Providers willing to achieve the 'qualified' status need to be licensed by Monitor (or to meet equivalent assurance requirements in some particular situations), by undertaking an approval process that includes registering with the Care Quality Commission (CQC), meeting the terms and conditions of the NHS standard contract, and accepting NHS prices.

The NHS Trust Development Authority oversees the performance management and governance of NHS trusts that are yet to attain foundation status. As per the Act, this is a temporary body, as all trusts must achieve this status. With a view to enabling them to compete in the market, foundation trusts are granted increased autonomy over their budget: the proportion of income that NHS foundation trusts can now source from private patients has risen to 50% of their total income. This should improve their market competitiveness.

This new scenario of competitors and commissioners is a fundamental overhaul of the system and is bound to lead to deep modifications in the healthcare system in England and Wales. It is hardly a surprise that the reform generated a fierce debate. Alongside calls for the bill, and then the HSCA itself, to be scrapped, the debate focused on what providers would be allowed to compete on, that is, what the rules of the game are. What principles will determine commissioners' choice of provider? What will stop them from commissioning the cheapest provider against the best quality? In the consultation period that followed the publication of the bill, the initial proposal to allow for price competition was abandoned; the HSCA now stipulates that competition is solely *quality based*. Providers are paid a fixed amount for each service: this is either set by Monitor in the national tariff or, where this does not apply, set by the local commissioners. All providers in the area are paid the same tariff.

The wave of reforms did not stop at the base of the NHS: structural reforms were introduced at the top of the health commissioning structure too. A new national body, NHS England, was created from the NHS Commissioning Board, while Monitor received a broader range of powers and functions. Together they have an overarching role in facilitating and completing the role of CCGs.

NHS England is a politically independent agency. It absorbs the commissioning responsibilities historically located within the Department of Health and oversees the work of CCGs. NHS England is responsible for supporting, developing and holding CCGs to account. Among its functions, NHS England allocates funds to CCGs and ensures that they work in a cohesive way. It also directly commissions a number of services where an organisation at regional or national level is thought to be more efficient, as is the case for highly specialised services. The Act enables the Secretary of State for Health to set priorities for the NHS through a mandate to the board of NHS England (to which that body is legally obliged to adhere).

NHS England hosts the clinical networks that advise on specific conditions or patient groups where improvements can be made through an integrated, whole-system approach. The networks advise local commissioners, help reduce variation in services and encourage innovation.

Monitor has become the healthcare-specific economic regulator. It has been given the mandate to guard against 'anti-competitive' practices. Monitor is now responsible for licensing every healthcare provider, regulating prices for NHS services, and addressing restrictions on competition that act against patients' interest. It can suspend and revoke licences, or fine providers for licence breaches. It sets prices for services, and these are published in the national tariff. Ultimately, it has the mandate to enforce the use of transparency on providers; this is meant to prevent the use of 'cherry-picking' strategies such as turning away complex (and less profitable) patients on non-clinical grounds.

The Act addresses the governance of public health by placing the duty to protect the people of England on the Secretary of State, with central responsibility for health protection and response to emergencies. The national leadership for public health is transferred to a new executive agency of the Department of Health, named Public Health England (PHE). PHE is directly accountable to the Secretary of State for Health.

It is evident that competition may test the healthcare system's ability to deliver integrated care to service users, with the risk of compartmentalisation and fragmented care. In response to these concerns, the government progressively introduced agencies tasked to protect and facilitate communication and integration of care. Among them are the 'health and wellbeing boards'. These are established and hosted by local authorities and work to bring together the NHS, public health, adult social care and children's services. The members of the boards include an elected representative, representatives of Healthwatch and local CCGs, the local directors of adult and child social services and of public health, alongside a representative of NHS England. The local Healthwatch organisations are new public bodies that act as a point of contact for service users, community groups and voluntary organisations when dealing with health and social care. The health and wellbeing boards have the duty to encourage integrated commissioning. During their meetings, they plan how best to meet the needs of the local population and tackle local inequalities.

So far, we have seen how the reform has introduced several new bodies and shifted power and functions within the NHS. But what is the gist of the reform – the underpinning philosophy of the government's choice of direction? It is helpful to analyse the reform in the light of the four classical domains of healthcare management: market incentives, empowering users to shape services from the base, top-down performance management, and increasing capability and capacity. So how does the HSCA take these levers into account?

Marketing incentives

The HSCA's most controversial effect on the healthcare system is the strong boost of marketing incentives as a drive to shape the NHS. This includes:

- increased competition
- greater autonomy and buying power for commissioners
- implementation of the payment by results (PbR) system
- independent regulation.

Introduced by the previous government and already piloted for acute providers, the PbR system has now been extended to a broad range of services, including mental health. It is the mechanism by which hospitals are rewarded for the work they actually do. For this to be open and transparent, payment is made on the basis of a fixed tariff, so that more efficient hospitals are rewarded. Furthermore, the PbR tariffs allow for data collection, which commissioners will use to inform their choice in the allocation of services.

With regard to regulation, the CCGs, Monitor and NHS England are all independent bodies. This is meant to provide assurance that NHS and non-NHS services compete in an open market to offer high-quality and cost-efficient care.

Empowering users to shape services

Following the blueprint of previous reforms, the HSCA gives special emphasis to patient choice. It is meant not only to improve the patient experience but also to act as a lever for competition. In theory, patients choose the best services; this encourages poorer-quality services to improve in order to compete for patients and funding, thereby driving up standards across the NHS. Competition and choice are therefore inextricably linked. Under the motto 'no choice about me without me', the HSCA states that CCGs, NHS England, and Monitor must all act with a view to enable patients to make choices about their healthcare and the health services provided to them. How patients will be given the relevant information to enable them to make an informed choice between different providers remains to be tested, and will probably play a crucial role in determining the success of the reform.

Patient choice is expanded by both opening the healthcare system to AQPs and allowing a broader range of patients to choose between providers. Mental health patients who require an elective mental health referral (i.e. excluding patients detained under the Mental Health Act) are to be offered choice with regard to their first out-patient appointment. They may choose:

- any clinically appropriate provider that has a contract with a commissioner
- any clinically appropriate consultant-led team that is employed by that provider.

Patients are also allowed to choose their GP regardless of where they live, which naturally has repercussions for mental health services.

Top-down performance management

Perhaps less central in the HSCA, top-down performance management is assured by the CQC and through accountability.

The CQC (which pre-dates the HSCA) is the quality regulator for the health and social care system. It sets the standards of care and inspects services to ensure compliance with the requirements. All NHS and non-NHS providers must be registered with the CQC. If providers do not meet the standards of care, the CQC has the power to issue fines, issue a warning, stop services from caring for new patients, stop services from caring for any patients and to close services.

In relation to accountability, the Secretary of State for Health retains the duty to promote a comprehensive health service and can intervene if there are 'significant' institutional failures of the national bodies. NHS England and the CCGs are required to promote the NHS Constitution (Department of Health, 2009), which describes the rights and responsibilities of patients, staff and trust boards. CCGs must include two lay members, in order to champion public involvement, and adhere to the Nolan principles, which guide the ethical standards of public life: these are selflessness, integrity, objectivity, accountability, openness, honesty and leadership (see Chapter 35).

Increasing capability and capacity

When applied to the healthcare system the terms 'capability' and 'capacity' refer to leadership, workforce development and organisational development. To lead on these, the reform has created a new authority, Health Education England (HEE), whose role is to provide national leadership and coordination for education, training and workforce development. Working alongside HEE are 12 clinical senates, tasked with providing multi-professional clinical leadership in the new NHS structure.

Health Education England

This body promotes high-quality education and training that is responsive to the changing needs of patients and local communities. Professional regulators are still responsible for setting and upholding standards. HEE has six professional boards. Its medical board is responsible for ensuring that training posts are filled by high-quality candidates, that curriculum-based training is delivered, that academic medicine's needs are recognised, and that there is enough capacity in the NHS to deliver high-quality training.

It helps healthcare providers and clinicians to take greater responsibility for planning and commissioning education through the development of local education and training boards (LETBs). These are statutory committees of HEE responsible for workforce planning, education and training at a local level. They bring together all healthcare and public health providers of NHS-funded services, education providers, professional bodies and local government and universities or research centres. They will host postgraduate deaneries and their functions.

Clinical senates

The clinical senates are 12 multi-professional steering groups allocated to 12 broad geographical areas. They provide independent and strategic clinical advice and leadership to CCGs, health and wellbeing boards and NHS England. The nerve centre is the Clinical Senate Council, which is responsible for coordinating and formulating advice. In addition, the Clinical Senate Assembly is a broad multi-professional forum that provides the Council with ready access to experts in all tranches of healthcare, including patient representatives.

Critics of the reform

Critics of the reform have not been shy or isolated. A large number of trade unions and Royal Colleges embraced the fight against it, as it was perhaps logical to expect from an extensive reorganisation vowing a change of culture in the healthcare system. Alongside a perceived threat to the values that constitute and support the NHS, the main battlefield has been a lack of evidence supporting competition as a way to improve efficiency – with some evidence supporting the opposite – and the costs and disruptions that such a wholesale reorganisation creates. The BMA called for the HSCA to be scrapped and was supported by a survey in which only 5% of its associates felt that the HSCA had improved the quality of service for patients. In the same survey, 57% felt that it had made it harder to work collaboratively. The trade union warned that the core message of the reform, namely to allow marketisation and competition in healthcare, was eroding the core principles of the NHS and would lead to fragmentation in the delivery of care (BMA, 2016).

With regard to the healthcare system, the reality is that there is little evidence available either way. The principle of competition as a means to boost quality and efficiency is widely accepted in other sectors of the economy, but this does not have to be true for healthcare, where the 'product' is much harder to measure. The evidence currently available for healthcare suggests that the best cost–benefit ratio is achieved when services have a high level of integration. Competition, by its nature, is a drive towards fragmentation, and policies that promote competition are a 'waste of precious resources' (BMA, 2014) that would otherwise be better invested in the promotion of 'seamless not fragmented care' and in putting 'Integration before competition', to quote the BMA (2016). It is almost invariably true that if we look at other more liberal healthcare systems in the Western world, such as the United States, higher costs and increased inequality are associated with involvement of the private sector. Nevertheless, the question of how comparable these systems are, and how reliable the evidence against controlled and well-regimented competition is, remains. In theory, a national healthcare system such as the NHS should perform highly on prevention, and yet the UK is lagging behind most countries when preventable diseases such as obesity and diabetes are considered. After all, the NHS itself was pretty much an untested experiment when it was first rolled out in 1948.

With regard to mental health, the Royal College of Psychiatrists (2012) stopped short of calling for the Bill to be withdrawn. Despite describing the bill as 'fundamentally flawed', it agreed to engage in its review process. The College did not oppose the principle of competition once it had been established that it would be a function of quality, and the College agreed to work with the government in championing the need to safeguard integration of care.

Two reports published during the development of the HSCA marked the College's views. The first, *Bridging the Gap* (Foley, 2013), outlined how a disjointed commissioning system may lead to loss of cost-efficient integrated services if adequate safeguards are not in place.

The second, *Whole-Person Care: From Rhetoric to Reality* (Royal College of Psychiatrists, 2013), called instead for a reduction of health inequalities and requested the recognition of parity of esteem between mental health and physical health. The document issued key recommendations on how to achieve parity of esteem. These included: the need for broad mental health representation at provider and council boards; improved access to mental health treatment; inclusion of parity in the NHS Constitution and Mandate; increased commissioning of psychiatry liaison services; and parity of funding and research. The principle of parity of esteem has been widely accepted since and its implementation has been incorporated as a duty of the Secretary of State for Health. In its *Five Year Forward View*, the chief executive of the NHS mentions the achievement of parity of esteem between mental and physical health by 2020 as one of the objectives of the NHS Plan (NHS England, 2014). Actions do not always follow words but this commitment was a huge achievement for the College.

Finally, several Royal Colleges expressed concerns over how the new system will provide high-quality education and training when the workforce is split over competing providers. Moreover, the NHS's monopoly allows clinicians a flexibility to undertake work for the benefit of the wider system. In a scenario of multiple providers, this may be harder to achieve.

What's next? The *Five Year Forward View*

Are these reforms here to stay? Simon Stevens, appointed chief executive of the NHS in April 2014, did not waste time in confirming that there would be no going back. The NHS will continue to shift from the holistic provider of healthcare it used to be to a position of a leader among several players. In the prospective report *Five Year Forward View* he vowed not to undertake any further 'wholesale structural reorganization'. Instead, he confirmed that the NHS is going to continue to shift from the position of the sole provider of healthcare towards the one of leader among several.

This was far from ruling out further change. The document estimates that if the NHS fails to modernise there will be a £30 billion gap between patients' needs and resources available by 2020. In order to avoid this, it suggests a three-pronged approach.

First, the NHS will reduce demand by strengthening both primary and secondary prevention. It will seek stronger links with local communities to incentivise healthier behaviour and support local democratic leadership over public health. By working more closely with the third sector and social care, the NHS will also treat more people safely in the community. Promoting formal and financial recognition of the role of carers is an example.

Second, the NHS will increase efficiency, aiming for a performance improvement of 2–3% per year. Once again, local communities, CCGs and patient choice will be at the heart of it. CCGs will see their mandate extended while they increase their control over the NHS budget. They will drive the experimentation of new care models in the belief that diverse realities in the country will be better served by a diverse set of care models as opposed to a 'one size fits all' view. The traditional divisions between primary and secondary care, mental and physical health, and health and social care will become more flexible. GP consortia may be able to hire consultants, and take control over parts of hospitals, or even entire hospitals. Patients will have easier access to their records and possibly have allocated budgets with a say in how this is spent. An example of this will be integrated personal commissioning (IPC), an integrated 'year of care' budget for people with long-term need. IPC will blend together health and social care funding and could be managed by the patients themselves.

Third, the document recognises that, even in the more optimistic scenario, the NHS will need an increase in funding if it is to maintain its renowned standards. It is estimated that if the NHS is to perform at its best, there will still be a gap of £8 billion in 2020 without increased funding. It is hard to know at present what the level of funding will be – in part due to its dependence on changes in politics and the economy. In terms of future funding these are the three most likely scenarios. (1) Flat real-terms NHS spending (i.e. adjusted for inflation) would represent a continuation of the previous budget protection. (2) Flat real-terms NHS spending per person would take account of population growth. (3) Flat NHS spending as a share of gross domestic product would differ from the long-term trend in which health spending in industrialised countries tends to rise as a share of national income.

Overall, while endorsing the current structure, the *View* vows to implement measures to render the NHS more open and transparent, improve the set of targets providers are audited on and redesign parts of its payment system in order to reward quality.

Managing resources in the current environment

In conclusion, it is important to emphasise that the requirements to manage effectively as a doctor – whether as a consultant, clinical director, medical director or chief executive – remain little changed. Furthermore, as set out at the start of this chapter, almost no government policy survives long enough to see an absolute conclusion to the introduction of its planned benefits. This is likely as true for the present system reforms as it is for the economy. In politics, it is events – in particular those unforeseen – that count. All we can be certain of is that we do not know what these are likely to be. Whoever predicted in 1995 that the NHS would receive the biggest cash injection in its history, with a tripling in funding over the next 13 years, would surely have been referred, choice or not, to a local mental health service. The rest is speculation and belongs more to the lounge bar than the boardroom.

Finally, by way of a straightforward and practical guide, set out below are the key elements of successful financial management for clinicians in the NHS:

- *Don't overspend.* It can look very tempting; after all, why should you care, and surely users' needs are the ultimate law? Two cautions: first, if you overspend, then you will always be concerned about recovering the position and the pressure will throw current and longer-term plans into disarray; second, in the end it is staff, and mainly nurses, who pay for overspends, through reduced head count, because that is where the money is tied up.
- *Argue for parity of esteem.* Parity of esteem is the new fashion in politics, so go for it! It is now widely accepted as a principle by healthcare authorities. However, beware: spot the right opportunity, select your words well and be mindful of your time. Given the complexity of healthcare funding and the relative shortness of life, developing epidemiologically brilliant demonstrations of funding shortfalls on the basis of comparative and absolute population information can be a huge investment, but not always the right one.
- *Do highlight efficiency.* All investors want to know that what they are buying is good value for money. So show it. Always consider the

possible cuts in costs your project may lead to and why resources are better spent on it. Then, do not be shy in presenting these findings, even when they are minimal: showing to commissioners that you made a thorough economic evaluation prior to launch of your project will give you credibility.

- *Do act opportunistically.* This is not the same as acting unethically but instead it is about not looking gift horses in the mouth. Funding often arrives on the back of some half-baked initiative or under-spending. Have ready-made projects and ideas that show that money spent with you really is value for money.
- *Do work with partners.* Social services, other mental health services and the local acute trust are all sources of extra resources if you find ways of allying your goals with theirs – resources are about much more than just money. Endorsement by a clinician, buildings, expertise, kind words – these are all tradable commodities, so use them.
- *Do reward productive behaviour.* Groups of human beings are good at thinking up better ways of doing things. The resource you already control is often the easiest, and least noticed, source for funding new initiatives and getting improvement.
- *Do hire a first-rate manager/management team.* Someone numerate, determined, good at negotiating and focused on the needs of your service is critical to achieving a healthy and wealthy service. But do not forget that it is clinical decisions that determine the vast bulk of how resources get used. Clinicians may not like it, but they are the ones who determine success or failure for their services. You are a critical part of management.

And if there is time after getting that sorted out, worry about the politics of resource allocation.

References

BMA (2014) NHS cannot afford to support competition. Press release at https://www. bma.org.uk/news/2014/june/nhs-cannot-afford-to-support-competition-says-bma (accessed May 2016).

BMA (2016) Health and Social Care Act … it's not working! Web page at https://www. bma.org.uk/collective-voice/policy-and-research/nhs-structure-and-delivery/hsca (accessed May 2016).

Department of Health (2009) *The NHS Constitution: The NHS Belongs To Us All.* TSO.

Foley, T. (2013) *Bridging the Gap: The Financial Case for a Reasonable Rebalancing of Health and Care Resources.* Royal College of Psychiatrists. Available at http://www.rcpsych.ac.uk/ pdf/bridgingthegap_fullreport.pdf (accessed May 2016).

NHS England (2014) *Five Year Forward View.* Available at https://www.england.nhs.uk/ wp-content/uploads/2014/10/5yfv-web.pdf (accessed May 2016).

Nuffield Trust (2012) *NHS and Social Care Funding: The Outlook to 2021/22.* Available at http://www.nuffieldtrust.org.uk/sites/files/nuffield/publication/120704_nhs-social-care-funding-outlook-2021-22-update2.pdf (accessed May 2016).

Royal College of Psychiatrists (2012) College clarifies its position on the Health and Social Care Bill. Press release at http://www.rcpsych.ac.uk/press/pressreleases2012/ hscbillposition.aspx (accesssed May 2016).

Royal College of Psychiatrists (2013) *Whole-Person Care: From Rhetoric to Reality. Achieving Parity Between Mental and Physical Health.* Available at http://www.rcpsych.ac.uk/pdf/ op88summary.pdf (accessed May 2016).

CHAPTER 3

Medical management

Martin Baggaley

Psychiatrists are key members of staff in mental health trusts and the relationship between them and the trust management is crucial to the day-to-day running and development of the organisation. Ideally, psychiatrists should work together with the management team in a collaborative way, in pursuit of a common goal. Unfortunately, in some cases this happy circumstance does not occur and there can be mistrust and antagonism between the two groups.

In most mental health organisations, psychiatrists have a management position, as a medical director, a clinical director or a lead consultant. Such psychiatrists usually continue to have some clinical responsibility. Indeed, one of the challenges of these positions is to retain credibility with both clinical and management colleagues. Without continuing clinical work, it is difficult to have either credibility or up-to-date knowledge of issues 'on the ground'. However, this dual responsibility can often cause tension and conflict. Effective medical managers can play an important role in developing a collaborative way of working and encourage psychiatrists to have a degree of corporate responsibility while maintaining professional standards.

The role of a medical manager is usually very challenging and can be stressful but at the same time can be exciting and enjoyable. It is important that a medical manager must not become too closely identified with one or other constituency. In other words, he or she must not become too much of a manager nor too much one of the consultant body. The difficulty of the job will depend on the context of the service at the time. It is easier to do the job at times of stability and development of services; it is less easy when money is short and services are contracting. The current environment is particularly challenging.

Medical director

Role of a medical director

The portfolio of the medical director can vary from trust to trust. In a foundation trust the medical director is one of the mandated executive directors who sit on the main trust board. Medical directors usually have the responsibility of ensuring that appropriate systems and mechanisms are in place to safeguard the quality of the clinical service. They have a key role of providing to the board assurance of service quality. In some trusts the director of nursing has this responsibility or it is held jointly. Often the medical director is the only person on the board who still practises clinically. The various responsibilities can be divided into corporate responsibilities, specific trust responsibilities and external liaison for the trust.

Corporate responsibilities

Medical directors are responsible for:

- quality of the service
- service policy development
- response to a major clinical problem
- clinical risk management
- medical workforce planning.

Specific trust responsibilities

These include:

- having a leadership role for psychiatrists
- clinical governance
- appraisal and revalidation of psychiatrists
- performance management of psychiatrists
- managing psychiatrists
- managing clinical services.

External liaison

Medical directors are responsible for external liaison with:

- the media
- commissioners
- clinical networks
- the local authority
- service users' and carers' groups
- the deanery and Royal Colleges.

Being a medical director

As can be seen, the remit of the medical director role is wide and demanding. It requires a broad range of skills and competencies. In many trusts some of the responsibilities are delegated to other managers, either medical or non-medical. For example, one or more associate medical directors may be appointed who have responsibilities for specific areas such as clinical governance or revalidation. There may well be one or more clinical directors who can be delegated tasks. They, together with associate medical directors, can form a supportive group of medical managers within the trust as well as providing some cross-cover for sickness and leave absence.

The medical director usually sits on the trust board as a director and becomes a key member of the trust board and executive. The relationships with the chief executive and chair of the trust in particular are crucial to being a successful medical director. It is virtually impossible to be a medical director without the support and backing of the chief executive and chair. In foundation trusts the medical director will have regular contact with the council of governors.

Corporate responsibilities

Quality of the service

The medical director has a key role in delivering a high-quality service through:

- the recruitment and retention of the best doctors
- ensuring they retain high morale
- ensuring they are well trained and have appropriate skills through excellent and well-funded continuing professional development (CPD)
- ensuring that they are appraised and engage with the revalidation process
- ensuring that they remain registered with the General Medical Council (GMC) and keep their 'approved clinician' and section 12(2) status up to date
- ensuring they work well with colleagues of different disciplines in multidisciplinary teams
- ensuring that they operate the latest evidence-based practice
- ensuring that they work with the highest ethical standards
- ensuring that they understand, help develop and work towards the objectives and policies of the trust.

In a large trust it can be difficult to know how one individual can implement such a list of worthy objectives. However, the behaviour of consultant colleagues is often strongly influenced by the culture of the organisation, which in turn is influenced by the behaviour of those at the top. The medical director, together with other members of the trust executive, therefore has a key role in modelling appropriate behaviour. If the medical director has great vision and strategic direction, the consultant workforce is likely to have similar attributes.

Clinical risk management

Risk is an integral part of psychiatric practice and the medical director has a role in ensuring that all clinicians, including psychiatrists, are appropriately trained in clinical risk management and that their practice incorporates effective risk management principles. Success in this area can reduce the number of serious clinical incidents which medical directors are asked to investigate. Part of the process of risk management is ensuring the organisation has robust systems to examine what has gone wrong after a serious untoward incident and why, and to try to prevent it happening again.

Workforce planning

The medical director has a responsibility for ensuring that the trust has the appropriate numbers of medical workforce with the necessary skills. Historically, the NHS has struggled do workforce planning well and psychiatry has struggled to attract sufficient numbers of good doctors. There will be periods when there is a shortage of good candidates for consultant posts. The medical directors (and clinical directors) have a key role in recruiting and retaining high-quality doctors. This can be achieved by ensuring that the morale of the consultant workforce is high, by making the individual jobs manageable and by giving consultants a feeling of being valued by the organisation and giving them a voice. In addition, attention should be paid to the experience of doctors coming through the organisation in training posts, as this is often the best way of ensuring that there are high-quality candidates for more senior posts. One of the skills is to realise that not all doctors should be managed in the same way, although they should be treated equally. In other words, understand that each consultant is different and what motivates one may put off another.

Specific trust responsibilities

Appraisal

All psychiatrists require an annual appraisal and it is the responsibility of the medical director (and individual consultants) to ensure that this occurs. If the medical director is the responsible officer, he or she cannot undertake appraisals. Appraisers have to be appropriately trained and the quality of the appraisal process has to be audited.

An appraisal serves a number of purposes, including preparing for revalidation. There is a separate process for job planning (see below). In an ideal world, an appraisal should be an enjoyable experience, and one of the key guiding principles of appraisal is that there should be no surprises. That is, if there are major performance issues which need to be discussed, these should be known about before the actual appraisal meeting. Many consultants genuinely believe that their job is the busiest, least-supported and most stressful job in the trust. All consultants cannot be correct about this. It is important, therefore, for as much objective information as possible to be available in order to inform discussion. The appraisal and revalidation process is usually supported by a software system to allow the documentation and portfolio to be kept electronically.

Consultant job planning

The job planning process in relation to the consultant workforce is a way of meeting the needs of the service more effectively, because the day-to-day working practice of the consultants can be changed to meet the needs of the clinical team. This process should be managed by negotiation and, ideally, mutual agreement. It was anticipated that the introduction of the new consultant contract would increase consultant productivity in return for increased pay. However, to date, there is little evidence that the new contract has delivered the increased productivity from consultant psychiatrists which had been hoped for by the Department of Health.

The majority of consultants in England have moved onto the new contract. This is based on a 10-session week, of which 7.5 sessions typically involve patient contact and 2.5 supporting activities. Each session is 4 hours. Consultants with extra responsibilities such as clinical tutor may have some of their sessions for supporting activities dedicated to this purpose. Consultants may negotiate extra sessions if they can demonstrate they are working the required number of hours, but these are not pensionable and need to be reviewed each year. There is inevitably pressure to bring most consultants down to 10 sessions with the introduction of the new contract and consultants are not supposed to be appointed with more than 10 sessions. The contract places specific expectations on consultants and in theory at least allows the trust more control over how consultants spend their time.

It must be borne in mind that there is a shortage of consultant psychiatrists. It is therefore important to ensure that similar policies exist across neighbouring trusts to discourage consultants moving trust on purely financial grounds.

Performance management of psychiatrists

One of the most challenging roles of a medical manager is to deal with situations where a psychiatrist is not performing appropriately. There may be one particular incident such as a serious complaint from a service user or colleague. Alternatively, there may be a long history of minor complaints or comments. Many difficulties relate to problems of personality and being unable to work easily in a multidisciplinary team. Some performance issues may relate to illness or to criminal behaviour. It is important to work closely with the trust's human resources/medical staffing director and to follow the appropriate trust policy (which should of course be in line with national policy).

The first step is to investigate the facts fully and this is best done by an independent team. The next step is to reach a decision. It is important to follow the process through to its conclusion, which may be a disciplinary hearing and dismissal, although the latter outcome is rare. It is important to keep detailed notes at every step.

Managing clinical services

This is typically delegated to clinical directors (see below), although it usually involves managing psychiatrists within clinical services rather than managing complete operational services.

External liaison

This should be one of the more enjoyable roles, although appearing as a spokesperson following a homicide by a service user under the care of one's trust would not be.

It is important to build up relationships with other medical directors and board members in neighbouring trusts (both mental health and acute). At times of crisis, it is much easier if one has a good personal relationship with someone senior who is in a position to lend advice and support. In some parts of the country, for example London, there are regular formal meetings of mental health medical directors.

Key relationships with external groups and organisations include those with the Royal College, the Department of Health, the regional office of NHS England, the clinical commissioning groups, Academic Health Science Centre networks and the postgraduate training organisations.

The medical director also has a responsibility to develop good relationships with local stakeholders such as carers, service users' groups and the local authority.

Clinical director

Organisations vary in terms of their structure and therefore the exact role of the clinical director will differ. Some services are arranged along directorate lines (i.e. adult services, old age services, etc.), others along geographical areas (e.g. a borough, clinical commissioning group) and others along service lines or clinical academic groups (CAGs).

Role of a clinical director

Management of a directorate, service line or CAG

Clinical directors have operational responsibility for the doctors in the directorate. They may become involved in the organising of rotas and in ensuring complaints are dealt with. They may be required to resolve issues such as who is responsible for which patient in cases of dispute. They usually have responsibility for the medical budget. In practice, the majority of the budget is taken up by salaries and there is therefore often little control over this. It is helpful if the clinical director has a good relationship with the financial director or accountant and understands how to read a budget report. Locums can be very expensive, especially from agencies. It is useful for the clinical director to have good networks with colleagues who run the local training schemes, as such individuals may know of doctors interested in doing a locum and they can be employed directly, which can be considerably cheaper than using an agency. It is important for trusts to have a clear sickness policy and to hold return-to-work interviews for doctors who have had time off, as this is supportive of staff and can reduce absenteeism.

Responsibility for individuals

Clinical directors manage the doctors within their area of responsibility, and this includes ensuring that they are appraised. They have a role to play in the recruitment and retention of consultants. They should know their colleagues well and be able to identify their strengths and weaknesses and be aware when they are particularly stressed or under pressure. It is important for clinical directors to treat all colleagues equally and be open and transparent. Although they may be tempted to respond to colleagues who complain the most, it is better to reward good behaviour.

Clinical governance.

The clinical director may have responsibility for issues of clinical governance as it relates to medical staff. This role is carried out in conjunction with the trust's clinical governance structures. There is a formal part of the role in ensuring that appropriate meetings are held and minuted. The less formal part of the role is more difficult: it includes inspiring and encouraging clinical teams and psychiatrists within clinical teams to understand fully and take up the challenge of what clinical governance means at a local level.

Corporate responsibility

The clinical director is responsible for helping develop the directorate and taking forward the trust vision. This involves engaging colleagues in the agenda and direction in which the trust is moving. This involves trying to explain the 'bigger picture' to colleagues and giving an explanation and justification for the change. Consultant psychiatrists can be surprisingly unaware of organisations and issues at board, local health community or national level. They may take pride in their clinical work but be dismissive of other things. It is the job of the clinical director to inform colleagues of important developments and suggest which policy statements can be skim-read and which are important enough to give some time to read and digest.

Succession planning

There are often few psychiatrists who are prepared to take on the role of a medical manager, or have the skills to do so. On some occasions it is possible to externally recruit medical managers, although it can be difficult to attract suitable candidates and there may be problems of acceptance of an external consultant by the existing consultant group. Therefore it is important to identify, encourage and develop any potentially suitable internal candidates and engage in succession planning.

Leadership

A successful medical manager must show strong leadership skills. Leadership is a much misused term, and it is often most noticeable when absent in a clinical or medical director. The King's Fund, the NHS Leadership Centre and other organisations such as Keele University run courses to help clinicians develop leadership skills. The process of mentoring by or coaching from a fellow medical director or suitably qualified person may help a manager develop the necessary leadership skills. Kouzes & Posner (2002) suggest that 'Leadership is the art of mobilising others to want to struggle for shared aspirations'. Others have suggested that managing consultant psychiatrists is more akin to attempting to herd a group of cats.

Creating a career pathway

One of the difficulties of becoming a medical manager is planning a satisfactory career. It has been a tradition for a doctor to become a clinical or medical director for a number of years and then stand down. Some organisations have an informal system of taking turns. This can lead to very unsuitable medical managers being appointed, to the detriment of their own working life and the smooth running of the trust. It is not always easy to return to being an ordinary consultant after being a leader and manager. It can also be awkward for the colleague who assumes the role to have to manage the ex-director. In addition, there is usually extra remuneration associated with the role, which may not be easy to simply forgo.

Training in medical management

Psychiatrists in training, usually specialist registrars, often request experience in management, which should be encouraged considering the importance of succession planning. This can include attendance at various management meetings, attendance at courses run for example by the King's Fund and specific projects. Some psychiatrists undertake a master's degree in business administration (MBA) in preparation for a career in medical management.

Relevant organisations

- Faculty of Medical Leadership and Management (https://www. fmlm.ac.uk). The FMLM was set up after the demise of the British Association of Medical Managers.
- NHS Leadership Academy (http://www.leadershipacademy.nhs.uk). This is for all staff but provides courses and other resources for medical managers.
- King's Fund (http://www.kingsfund.org.uk). This is an independent charitable foundation working for better health, especially in London. It runs a number of leadership programmes for medical and clinical directors.

Reference

Kouzes J, Posner B (2002) *The Leadership Challenge*. Jossey-Bass.

CHAPTER 4

Doctors and managers

Stuart Bell

The historical background

The Association of Medical Officers of Asylums and Hospitals for the Insane met for the first time in 1841 at the instigation of Dr Samuel Hitch, resident physician of the Gloucestershire General Lunatic Asylum. It was a gathering of the medical men in charge of asylums across the UK. The Association met with increasing regularity, until in 1865 it changed its name to the Medico-Psychological Association. That was an important step in the organisation's development from arranging gatherings at which members aimed 'to cooperate in collecting statistical information relating to insanity and above all ... assist each other in improving the treatment of the insane' and towards becoming a professional body for doctors with an interest in the study of insanity (Bewley, 2008). In 1926, following the grant of a Royal Charter, it became the Royal Medico-Psychological Association, and in 1971 it became the Royal College of Psychiatrists. Over the course of 130 years it evolved from being a body brought into being by those who were in effect the managers of the mental health services of the country to being a professional Royal College for specialist doctors.

That pattern of evolution is part of a more general trend described by the social historian Harold Perkin in his 1989 book *The Rise of Professional Society*. He describes the change which took place in England between the 1880s and the 1980s and which established professions as a dominant form of social structure, especially in the workplace. In 1880, he notes, 'there were still only twenty-seven qualifying associations ... (counting the four Inns of Court for barristers and the two Royal Colleges and the Society of Apothecaries for medical doctors), but thereafter there was enormous expansion'. By 1970 another 140 had been added, plus an even larger body of non-qualifying but professionally oriented associations. Society, in short, had become professionalised, reflecting both the growing specialisation of skills following the Industrial Revolution and the growing role of government and its agencies in everyday life. As the roles and numbers of professions grew, so by turn more and more people became correspondingly 'lay' with respect to an increasing number of areas of expertise.

That rapid development of specialisation is understandable if one takes into account the exponential growth in the scale and complexity of health services over that period, although, thanks to the development of the public asylums, mental health services in the UK were a rather unusual case. They were almost exclusively run by publicly funded bodies; much of the rest of healthcare depended heavily, until the advent of the welfare state, on charitable contributions or on self-payment. Institutionally and organisationally, the asylums were separated from the rest of health service provision, and their professional structures were relatively straightforward, with one single medical specialty clearly dominant, the other main group being a branch of nursing that was, for much of the 19th and early 20th centuries, remote from the leadership and prestige given by Florence Nightingale and her followers. The medical superintendents of the large Victorian asylums, often living in spacious and comfortable villas built in the hospital grounds, were obviously 'in charge', directing much of what happened within, and answering for that to the local authorities from which they received their funds.

The leadership structures of the big voluntary hospitals which dominated acute care in the Victorian cities were more elaborate, with overall authority being exercised by governing committees of 'the great and the good' (not least because that helped to raise funds); senior medical staff, who would often have significant personal private practices, were visitors to the hospital ('consultants' – the origin of the term) rather than having any significant role in its direction. As these hospitals grew in scale and complexity, experts in their day-to-day administration – 'house governors' or 'hospital secretaries' (secretaries, that is, to the boards of governors) – emerged and took a growing role in decisions over the getting and spending of funds.

Other professions emerged and although none challenged medicine for dominance, nursing acquired prestige and numbers, and as the technology of healthcare developed, its delivery became increasingly dependent on therapists and technicians of all varieties. Medicine itself became more a collection of subspecialties, each with its own interests and objectives, and it became increasingly difficult for anyone to be able to comprehend the whole, so the success of the institution depended on professions and their subgroups being able to work together in collaboration, respecting each other's area of expertise. There were undoubtedly some strong and charismatic individuals, who by virtue of their personalities exercised a great and sometimes a controlling influence, but there was rarely someone who by virtue of their job was in executive charge of the whole organisation.

Gradually, as the asylums also grew in size, in some cases to well over 2000 patients, and as they became professionally more and more complex, it became less realistic for a single individual to exercise the traditional model of leadership, and they, too, moved towards groups of senior

53

individuals from a range of different backgrounds exercising joint control. That trend was of course accelerated as the transition began towards a more community-based model of mental healthcare, away from the asylums.

Looking back, it appears as though the high point of this professional dominance may have been the establishment of the welfare state in the aftermath of the Second World War, when the very institutions of the state's social welfare programme itself were shaped around pre-existing or rapidly developing professional groups. The education system developed around teachers and lecturers, family and individual welfare around social workers, and so forth. In the NHS before the mid-1980s, separate, professionally determined hierarchies existed for hospital doctors, public health doctors, general practitioners, nurses, administrators and accountants and, at less senior levels, for the other clinical professions. No one was in overall charge and each of the different groups had substantial autonomy to run its own realm. Where decisions required agreement between the different groups, deadlock was always possible. Doctors probably were the most powerful and influential of these groups, even though they rarely operated as a homogeneous whole, but they did not have overall executive control, and the means by which they could be held to account for exercising such authority as they possessed informally was vague, except in the most general terms, so long as the enterprise was able to get by within the overall resources made available to it. Perhaps there was no longer an impetus towards maintaining overall executive control, since the very structures of the industry, as they became established at the time, through the mechanisms of the welfare state, allowed people to exercise authority sufficiently, purely through their professional status.

Regulation and the setting of standards was left, by and large, for each of the relevant professional groups to determine for itself, and so professional bodies like the Royal Colleges exerted considerable influence over NHS policy – it was expected that they should – and when the Department of Health needed advice on policy it would turn first to them. The notion of management, as we understand it today, could not easily be separated or identified as being distinct from the structures of these professional hierarchies; indeed, there were no such people as 'managers' in the NHS (or for that matter in many other public services) prior to the mid-1980s.

That began to change, partly because it became progressively more difficult to operate a system less and less able to keep the status quo gently ticking over. That system faced more and more contentious decisions about service change, resource allocation and reconciling the different roles of the myriad of professions within healthcare – an industry which is almost uniquely rich in the range of professional identities it encompasses. The change was also a consequence of the growing size and complexity of the institutions of healthcare, and an emerging restlessness among politicians and patients about the sense of a lack of accountability in the professionally dominated model. The professions began to be portrayed by some as doing what suited them, closed shops, which closed ranks and protected their own, rather than being held to account and serving the public good.

A key point in that change in the NHS was the publication of a report by Roy (later Sir Roy) Griffiths in 1983 (see Chapter 1), who was asked by the government of the day to review the organisation of the NHS, and who famously noted that if Florence Nightingale returned to visit the NHS of the day she would struggle to identify who was in charge. That was true. Not only did the various local health authorities which brought together the leaders of the different professional hierarchies have no individual in overall executive charge, but the organisation of the NHS as a whole had no head office and no overall executive authority: matters were devolved from the Department of Health and Social Security to 14 regional health authorities. The only body in the NHS which truly operated at a national level ran its pension scheme!

Griffiths introduced the concept of 'general management': at a local, regional and national level one individual should be clearly in overall executive charge, able to take a decision if consensus had failed. He also proposed that someone should be in overall charge of the NHS itself, distinct from the Department of Health. The implementation of Griffiths' proposals prompted the first attempt to introduce, at scale, management skills from the private sector to the NHS, on the principle that good managers would be able to manage effectively in any industry, and that, as there had been no general management in the NHS historically, an injection of new skills would be necessary if the concept was to take hold. In the event, that produced limited and rather mixed results, and by far the majority of the new general management roles were filled by individuals from across the range of professions already in the NHS. The majority came from the pre-existing administrative hierarchy, although in mental health services it was common at that time for senior nurses to become the new general managers, and comparatively few doctors made the transition.

It is worth noting that Griffiths himself commented:

> 'the nearer that the management process gets to the patient, the more important it is for the doctors to be looked upon as the natural managers. This should be more explicitly recognised: in the doctors' training – undergraduate, postgraduate, in-service, and in preparation for particular clinical management posts' (Griffiths, 1983).

He was not, however, of the view that general managers could or should come only from a specific professional background: 'in identifying a Unit General Manager we believe that the District Chairman should go for the best person for the job, regardless of discipline'.

Writing in the late 1980s, after these changes had started in the NHS and in other parts of the welfare state, Perkin (1989) sought to explain the apparent challenge to the autonomy and dominance of professional groups which was then beginning to emerge. Doctors, teachers, lawyers and others were all being enjoined to become more accountable and began to lose some of their traditional privileges. Rather than seeing this as a turn against the historical trend towards the gradual dominance of professionalisation across society as a whole, he interpreted it as part of a struggle for hegemony between the older established groupings and newer, emerging professions, such as economics, marketing and accountancy. The paradox is that as society has become more and more dominated by professions, following the lead established by the law and medicine, so the power and authority of each individual profession has been relatively weakened and the rivalry between them has grown. When governments have required advice on health policy, since the 1980s they have turned successively to civil servants, NHS managers and management consultants before settling most recently on think-tanks and policy specialists (often drawing on economics for their inspiration, rather than specific expertise in healthcare or biomedical science), whose principal purpose in life is to develop policy rather than to put it into practice. Their profession is about coming up with innovative ideas and bringing them to the attention of decision-makers, rather than expertise in any particular field of public service delivery.

The long period when different professions, including doctors, nurses and administrators, had broadly coexisted in the NHS without obvious struggle for overall dominance had ended. Whatever professional background they happened to come from, the general managers had been put in charge, though quite how far their accountability and their authority were to extend is something which emerged only gradually over the next two decades. But the subject of 'doctors and managers', and indeed the concept of 'doctors as managers', had emerged.

The nature of management

It is arguable whether management itself constitutes a profession, in the sense that accountancy, economics and perhaps even management consultancy do, never mind medicine, nursing and the law. There have undoubtedly been attempts to cast it as such, and there are subcomponents of managerial activity which have certainly become professionalised, such as the use and application of information technology or various forms of analysis and modelling – economic and otherwise. Nevertheless, management in its most general sense has proved remarkably resistant to traditional professional categorisation. It remains, in the UK and much of the rest of the world, an unrestricted occupation – anyone can become a manager. The body of knowledge which can be formally imparted at the heart of any self-respecting profession is, in the case of management, hard to pin down. Its 'mystery', as Shakespeare's rustic players might have put it, sometimes sounds rather more like common sense, than any formal body of knowledge. Attempts in recent times to establish management as a quasi-profession – the Management Charter Initiative in the 1990s, for example – have never really gained traction.

Management, in short, fails to meet the essential criteria to be a profession, although it does draw on, and is heavily influenced by, bodies of knowledge and theory developed by some of the newer professions – psychology for instance, with which it is often closely connected. This view, I should say, remains contentious, partly because there are some managers who would very much like their occupation to be, or to be seen to be, a profession, and partly because there are those who might wish, for business reasons, to turn it into a 'mystery' which is inaccessible to those who are not initiates – that, after all, is the basis of much management consultancy. This argument about whether management is a body of knowledge which can be taught or acquired and tested through formal processes has become particularly acute in the world of management education, especially in the context of the master's degree in business administration (MBA) – surely the first litmus test of any modern profession is the qualifying degree?

Henry Mintzberg, a distinguished US professor of management, who was instrumental in the development of the MBA as a qualification, now argues that its dominance has distorted our understanding of the nature of management:

> 'It is time to recognise conventional MBA programs for what they are ... specialized training in the functions of business, not general educating in the practice of managing. Using the classroom to help develop people already practising management is a fine idea, but pretending to create managers out of people who've never managed is a sham' (Mintzberg, 2004: p. 5).

Mintzberg goes on to argue that management is a blend of three distinct elements: the craft – experience; the art – insight; and the science – analysis. The MBA really trains people only for the last of these, and gives a misleading quasi-professional veneer, which at best partially equips them for managerial jobs, while at worst giving them an inflated sense of their preparedness and competence to undertake them. Instead, he argues that management is neither a science nor a profession, and therefore it cannot be taught to people without experience – 'there is no one best way to manage; it depends on the situation'.

Above all, then, management is dependent on, and must respond to, context. It is perhaps also worth making the point (as it is often missed) that as well as drawing on some of the newer professions for its techniques and models, where longer-established professions are an important part of that context – as in the NHS and, indeed, in any of the services established by the welfare state in the 1940s – those involved in management will, sometimes indiscernibly, assimilate much of the thinking behind those professional traditions. In health, of course, that will not be confined to the profession of medicine – nor should it be – but it is often underestimated how much it matters to the ability to manage health services to have a deep knowledge of the way the 'industry' works, in detail, at the clinical level. That, surely, was Roy Griffiths' point back in 1983.

Management in the NHS

So, over the last 150 years healthcare, particularly mental healthcare, has moved away from being an industry in which there was little distinction between being a senior doctor and being responsible for overall direction of an institution. That period saw the rise of new professions and the subdivision of existing ones; institutions became so complex that it was difficult to point to any one individual being in charge, because senior professionals, collectively, shared responsibility. Finally, from the mid-1980s, the concept of general management was brought into the NHS, as into much of the rest of the public sector, creating a leadership and accountability role, in overall executive charge of a given healthcare organisation, not dependent on holding any particular professional qualification.

In practice, by far the majority of general managers in the NHS have come from within, not from the private sector, and the change has opened the door to clinicians from a very wide range of professional backgrounds to take on managerial roles; indeed, a frequent criticism of this phenomenon is that progression to senior positions now depends upon clinicians forsaking their professions and moving into a managerial role rather than being able to progress through clinical hierarchies. There remain a substantial number who in the past would have been part of the administrative tradition, but who would now perhaps be referred to as 'career managers', who undertake managerial roles at every level of healthcare, but without having any clinical professional background, although they should have a deep knowledge of healthcare as an industry.

The other very significant change, which emerged in the 1990s, was the separation, at least in the NHS in England, of the provision and the commissioning of services. This created two distinct managerial tasks, which, as they have evolved, have acquired their own bodies of knowledge and skill sets. For the first 15 years or so of this 'internal market' most of the individuals in managerial roles in the newer commissioning organisations would have had some experience of responsibility for the provision of health services at some point in their careers, but of late that has been much less the case. There is now a significant cadre of managers whose only experience is in commissioning organisations or those which exist to support or monitor them, and who have never actually been involved in the delivery of healthcare, which is where most, if not quite all, professional preoccupations remain. That does make an important difference because it creates a tension between theories of how health services ought to be able to work, and the practice of delivering them on the ground, which in times of constrained resources can become hard to reconcile, and which is located at the interface between commissioners and providers. At its worst it can appear as if people who do not actually have any experience of doing something are telling those who are experts at doing it how best to go about it, on the basis of an ill-digested and dubiously sourced cocktail of theory and anecdote, in the teeth of reality. That does not motivate people to change their ways, or even to work harder, and it usually fails rather dismally!

Thoughtful commissioners, by contrast, are very skilled at drawing on the experience, knowledge and motivation of those involved in delivering services to do a better job, but it does depend on possessing the humility, as Donald Rumsfeld might have put it, of 'knowing what you don't know'. And that underscores the fundamental point that good health service management must be informed by a deep understanding of the industry in which it operates, including the values and ideas of the professions which inhabit that world, and must be realistic about the dominance or wisdom which management may assume at a particular point in time.

Does this, though, mean that management itself is inherently devoid of underlying values and principles? Perhaps so, but that is a very different thing from individual managers being devoid of either. On the contrary, it is difficult to manage any group of people, never mind a large organisation, for a sustained period of time without being able to generate some sense of shared purpose, which must, in the end, be more than a short-term tactical or transactional community of interest, but which must give a strong sense of shared collective values and ambition. The difference is that 'management' as such does not necessarily come with a pre-set collection of values to be applied to whoever and whatever is managed, irrespective of the circumstances.

Those values will come from the individuals involved, the context of the industry and the nature of the task at hand. There is now also a well-established body of management theory which managers can use, examining how and why people and systems work together more or less successfully. It draws on a wide range of other disciplines and ways of thinking but, in the end, individual managers will need to formulate their own views about how their managerial world works – what the external environment looks like, what motivates the people they work with, what sets the culture, and what of that is to be built on and what must be challenged. In doing so, they will be obliged to address issues of principle and to set out their values; if they are purely synthetic and designed solely for the particular circumstances, that is very likely to be detected – people are very good at spotting inauthenticity – and it will not work for long. That is why there are some people who are good at being managers, and some who are bad at it.

How, then, is this phenomenon – 'management' – not properly a profession? It is eclectic in its choice of theory, hugely sensitive to context and difficult to pin down precisely – viewed from the standpoint of a much more clear-cut profession like medicine, which apparently enshrines a carefully cultivated scientific evidence base, which assimilates an ever-expanding body of knowledge and which is guided and regulated by professional codes of conduct. A common response is to judge management as though it were a conventionally understood profession and to find it lacking: either they don't know what they're doing, in which case they're useless, or they do know what they're doing, in which case they're not telling us about it. This misses the essential point that we are examining a fundamentally different phenomenon. Managers often make the same mistake in reverse – exasperated by the apparent rigidity of professional groups in the face of what appears to them a decisively changed context, they can see the characteristics of a profession as a set of rather selective and perhaps even self-serving constructs designed to preserve the status quo and to resist necessary change.

Where this mistrust occurs, it creates problems – of divergence of priorities, poor-quality decision-making, failure to tackle issues which must be faced, putting off that which must be done sooner rather than later, with delay leading only to problems of even greater intractability. Such failure of mutual understanding is also susceptible to exploitation by others – by other professions, which can be tempted to use mutual incomprehension between doctors and managers to advance their own positions – and perhaps most of all by the external world, be that in the form of politicians, the media or the general public. Notice how often the tactic is used of fastening on to the rather abstract notion of the number of managers in the NHS in order to distract attention from an uncomfortable debate about some other aspect of healthcare. What is the correct number? How does it compare with other healthcare systems or comparable industries? These questions are rarely part of the discussion. A favourite alternative device is to portray the apparent intransigence of doctors as a professional group – conservative, self-interested and shroud-waving – again as a distraction from a significant issue or as a way of weakening influence.

It is worth noting that these characteristics are most closely associated with publicly funded and nationally organised healthcare systems. In part, perhaps, the extent of political and media involvement in a publicly funded system creates a requirement for a general management role which is distinct from the professions, simply in order to deal with the burdensome requirements it creates. In some parts of the world there is a much older and more established tradition of the direct involvement of doctors in managerial activity – the development of specific branches of the profession for those who undertake such roles on a more or less full-time basis, for example. The extent to which healthcare is provided or funded directly by the state makes a significant difference – the model of the independent practitioner being paid for specific interventions by insurers leads to a very different tradition of management, not least because the task of management is not the same. Interestingly, however, the impulse towards a much more managed approach to care in the USA is being driven as much by concerns over the quality and reliability of care as by the need to manage resource use, which is familiar to us in state-funded systems (Lawrence, 2002). As expenditure on healthcare comes under greater pressure, and as the boundary between state and privately funded systems becomes more permeable, internationally this convergence is likely to continue.

Doctors and managers

The advent of the concept of general management in the NHS, while it led to quite a lot of clinical professionals from non-medical backgrounds being drawn into general managerial roles, has seen relatively few doctors taking up such generic positions. It has, however, seen the emergence of a predominantly medically led clinical leadership structure, with the widespread establishment of the roles of clinical director and medical director across most service provider organisations. It is required by law for any NHS foundation trust to have someone fulfilling the role of medical director as an executive member of its board, and most clinical subdivisions of a trust will have at least a part-time clinical director with some leadership responsibilities. Clinical director roles are increasingly not confined to individuals who hold medicine as a profession, and their accountability arrangements may vary, in terms of both the level of seniority to which they report directly and the extent to which they are part of operational management or professional hierarchies.

Typically, a clinical director will sit alongside a senior manager or service director (and sometimes, in research-active organisations, an academic director) with whom they will share the responsibility for leadership for a service. Sometimes the managerial role will report to the clinical director as a member of their team; sometimes (though less often nowadays) it will be the other way round. The more generally managerial a clinical director role becomes – the more accountable they are for the totality of the operation of a service – the more likely they are to be part of a managerial hierarchy, reporting perhaps to a chief operating officer on a trust board, rather than directly to the medical director, although there will usually remain some 'dotted line' of professional accountability, especially if they combine with their role the professional leadership and accountability of doctors in their service. Similarly, where clinical directors are, by professional background, psychologists, nurses or other clinical professionals, there will need to be some role which undertakes the professional leadership and supervision of doctors in the clinical service concerned, in just the same way as there need to be equivalent arrangements for other professional groups where the clinical director is a doctor.

The development of this focus on the clinical/managerial leadership of clinical operations increasingly as the joint enterprise of doctors and managers together, alongside other professions, has two main drivers. The first is the growth of clinical governance. For many years the separation of the management of the institution from the management of clinical practice was a strong feature of the relationship between doctors and managers. At that time, the manager's responsibility extended to ensuring that an institution balanced its books overall; other than in exceptional cases, it did not play a key role in the operation of clinical practice. Where this emerged as a tension, it was perhaps as a question about the limits of 'clinical freedom', a concept which was much debated in the mid-1990s, or the effect of resource constraints on rationing. What was also significantly absent from debates at the time was any explicit concern about patients' experience of care or their interests. There has been a decisive change since then, with the advent of clinical governance, which very clearly places on an institution – an NHS board – the responsibility for the clinical quality of the services it provides; that is now just as much a part of its statutory duty as the need to manage its finances.

Alongside this there has been a growing challenge within professions, as part of their development as professions, to the notion that, once qualified, members are equipped to respond as they see fit to any circumstances they may encounter across their career. Instead, few would now challenge the notion of there being an increasingly well-defined body of appropriate practice, based on a systematic and regularly reviewed appraisal of the evidence available, as the test of what one would expect to see in the majority of cases, the exceptions being those where an alternative approach is explicitly justified. That has replaced the idea of individual professionals carrying around a personal body of knowledge which they then apply as they think best in a succession of individual circumstances, over which they hold considerable discretion, the adequacy of which was a matter principally for their professional peers to judge, but usually only in exceptional circumstances. Professionals now need to be managed, or at the very least supervised, in relation to their practice as professionals, no matter how senior, and throughout their careers.

This has been accompanied by changes in public attitudes towards all professionals, including doctors, reinforced by a number of public scandals: Bristol, Alder Hey, Shipman and Stafford Hospital being only the most notorious. Sometimes this is characterised as being a 'lack of trust' but as, Onora O'Neill (2002) notes, it is perhaps more correctly described as being part of a 'culture of suspicion'. Sir Donald Irvine, a past President of the General Medical Council (GMC), described, with an insider's insight, the medical profession's at times ambivalent response to this, and its internal struggle to overcome vested interests and retain the initiative in its own professional self-regulation. He looked forward to a 'new professionalism' which:

> 'starts by recognising the importance of the autonomous patient … it embraces now evidence-based medicine rather than clinical pragmatism, the recognition of the importance of attitudes and behaviour, partnerships with patients, and accountability rather than personal autonomy. At the same time, the new professionalism is about teamwork rather than individualism, collective as well as personal responsibility, transparency rather than secrecy, and empathetic communication and above all of respect for others. An unreserved commitment to quality improvement through clinical governance is fundamental' (Irvine, 2003: p. 206).

There is a growing willingness in society at large to challenge, or at the very least to expect justification for, aspects of professional practice.

The second driver of the joint enterprise of doctors and managers is the growth of guidelines and systematic reviews and, perhaps above all, the phenomenal growth in the sheer body of knowledge available – way beyond the capacity of any single individual to assimilate in its entirety. This can only be set to continue with the impact of new science, big data, and the potential of genomics and new digital technology to transform even our basic understanding and categorisation of illness, never mind its care and treatment. This phenomenon has had an interesting effect on the relationship between doctors and managers in the realm of clinical practice. On the one hand, there is much more mutual interest in good clinical practice for its own sake – how effective is it, how good is it, how unusual is it? It is no longer possible or even sensible to take an interest merely in how expensive it is. The discourse must now focus on the effectiveness of a particular treatment and on the opportunities for innovation in care. On the other hand, these questions are now legitimately – even, given statutory responsibilities, necessarily – in the managerial domain too. While that is some way from managerial determination of what constitutes good professional practice, even that is now much more of a collective than an individual decision. Such questions have also been opened up more widely in recent years, not least by patients themselves; and, as Irvine points out, if professions fail to give a lead, then someone else surely will.

There is also a growing international recognition that even when there are no constraints on individual doctors' activities – where they are paid for each specific thing they do – this:

> 'encourages doctors to do too much and rewards those who perform procedures and surgery instead of focusing on diagnosis, prevention and education. Dr William Richardson, Chair of the Institute of Medicine studies on quality and safety, describes that system as 'toxic to quality' (Lawrence, 2002: p. 25).

This shared and mutual interest – in safety and accountability through clinical governance, and in effectiveness and innovation through evidence-based medicine, managed care and the systematic engagement of scientific and technological discovery in the delivery of care – combined with a recognition of the long overdue need to focus on care as experienced from a patient's (and, just as important, from their carer's) perspective, has created a joint endeavour where doctors and managers must come together. At its heart is the achievement and constant evolution of consistently good, effective and positively experienced care.

Perhaps of all the medical specialties, psychiatry comes closest to many of the preoccupations of management: it has to deal with high levels of uncertainty; it draws from a wide range of theoretical traditions – biological, psychological and social; context is as important as technical diagnosis in understanding how to institute effective treatment. Are managers and doctors in mental health services closer together than at first sight might appear to be the case? This suggests great potential for even better mutual understanding and respect, but the two occupations are not the same, and sometimes there is a greater risk of misunderstanding between those who are closest together than between those where the differences are clear and distinct. Nevertheless, every opportunity exists for collaboration and the converse is true – where relationships are chronically poor between doctors and managers, the service and the patient and the business will suffer. There may be many reasons for poor relations where they occur, and a range of solutions, including, at the extreme, getting new managers, or new doctors, or both. It is no longer a state of affairs which can be tolerated for long. A basic task, however, for anyone who is interested in making things better, irrespective of whether they are good or bad to start off with, is to find ways of understanding what people are trying to do, the constraints upon them, and how they are viewed by their wider professional community and the forces and responsibilities which influence them.

How, then, can a psychiatrist find out more about what makes managers tick? Conventional medical training offers limited opportunities for this, and where they exist they tend to be at a relatively late stage – mostly just before people apply for consultant positions. There are of course a range of management programmes, some as part of training schemes but some also run by institutions like the King's Fund. These are worthwhile, but they can only ever provide a brief insight. There are, however, good opportunities in every trust to find out more by attending board meetings (they are held in public), by shadowing managers as they go about their work (and by having managers shadow clinicians as they go about theirs) and by undertaking projects which relate to management problems (as part of a special-interest module, for example). One of the most valuable experiences in my own development as a health service manager was working closely with a doctor – a medical administrator from Australia – and learning to see the functioning of a hospital from their perspective.

It is vital that trainees and other readers of this chapter explore some of those opportunities because, now more than ever before, success in healthcare can come only as a result of joint enterprise between doctors and managers, built on a sound, shared understanding of the world in which both work, and a good knowledge of what each brings to the task.

References

Bewley T (2008) *Madness to Mental Illness: A History of the Royal College of Psychiatrists*. Royal College of Psychiatrists.

Griffiths R (1983) *NHS Management Inquiry*. Department of Health and Social Security.

Irvine D (2003) *The Doctors' Tale: Professionalism and Public Trust*. Radcliffe Medical Press.

Lawrence D (2002) *From Chaos to Care: The Promise of Team-Based Medicine*. Perseus Publishing.

Mintzberg D (2004) *Managers not MBAs*. Prentice Hall.

O'Neill O (2002) *A Question of Trust. The BBC Reith Lectures 2002*. Cambridge University Press.

Perkin H (1989) *The Rise of Professional Society*. Routledge.

CHAPTER 5

Resources in the NHS

Stuart Bell

There are various potential sources of funds for the provision of healthcare. Patients can pay directly themselves for the provision of their own care or that of their families. Healthcare can be funded by insurance, which can be purchased voluntarily or be required by government-sponsored schemes. Public funding can provide for part or for the totality of the population and for partial or total payment for the range of treatments available. All of these systems impose some form of constraint upon the range and extent of care available. Self-payment is of course dependent upon the ability of the patient to pay, but illness itself can prevent many people from being able to fund their own care; this is particularly true of mental illness, both because it frequently affects the ability of patients to support themselves and because poverty can be a precipitating factor. Insurance schemes are sometimes available only to the working population and their dependants; even where they are government-sponsored and designed to provide coverage for the poor and the non-working population, they can create restrictions on access to care, depending on what is covered by the policy. That can have the perverse consequence that it is necessary for people to become quite ill in order to become eligible for funding for treatment, and immediately after that treatment is concluded the insurance coverage ceases to fund their care. Consequently, such funding systems make more difficult the maintenance of well-being, the prevention of relapse and early intervention in mental illness.

Where do resources for mental health services come from?

Publicly funded healthcare systems confront most directly the problem of the allocation of finite resources between competing health needs across the population as a whole. That can lead to rationing, either by the restriction of access to certain forms of treatment, for example high-cost drugs, or by the imposition of waiting times for treatment for non-urgent conditions. It can lead to different priorities being accorded to different types of illness, sometimes influenced by stigma and discrimination – sometimes referred to as 'disparity of esteem'.

Over recent decades, whatever the source of funding for healthcare, in high-income countries expenditure has tended to rise as a proportion of gross domestic product (GDP), reflecting advances in medical science, longer life expectancy and rising public expectations about what healthcare should be able to achieve. In general, publicly funded healthcare systems have been more successful at containing costs, and achieving better value for the investment made, than systems which rely on self-payment or insurance. A recent Commonwealth Fund report comparing healthcare systems across a number of high-income economies rates the NHS most highly in this respect and in a number of others (Davis *et al*, 2014). For instance, the US healthcare system is seen to perform significantly less well in terms of value for money and outcomes. It is increasingly widely recognised, especially in the light of the recent economic downturn, that it is unrealistic to expect continuing and potentially unlimited growth in expenditure on healthcare in high-income countries along the lines we have grown used to in recent decades, and therefore major challenges face all of the current funding models in terms of both absolute cost and long-term sustainability.

In low- and middle-income countries, and particularly in the newly emerging economies of South America, China, India and Southeast Asia, Russia and other states of the former Soviet Union, there are rapidly growing expectations of and demands for healthcare. In many of those countries, however, the infrastructure and capacity of the existing healthcare system, particularly with respect to the availability of skilled practitioners, are such that it is very difficult to replicate conventional high-income healthcare systems directly, even if it were wise to attempt to do so in the long term.

There is though the opportunity to leapfrog traditional models of healthcare, and to take advantage of emerging technologies which offer radically different ways of delivering effective treatments to meet the needs of large and rapidly growing populations at pace and scale, and at the same time to create systems which offer much better value for money than traditional models. There is a convergence of interest between these two major strategic issues. For high-income countries there is much to learn from developing healthcare systems in the rest of the world, which can then be applied to reformulating traditional approaches so that they can be sustainable economically in the longer term. For the low- and middle-income countries there is the opportunity to apply some of the novel approaches that established healthcare systems adopt to address their long-term funding pressures without having to go through a long and painful transition which makes the process of change all the harder.

This story is likely to be a dominant theme in healthcare internationally over the next few decades, especially when taken in conjunction with the exponential growth in scale and achievement of the life sciences and the opportunities brought by digital technology. For psychiatrists, as for most other healthcare practitioners, it implies a great deal of change to established expectations and working patterns, but equally it promises to be a very exciting time to live through. The tension between growing need (and the potential to offer greater benefit) and tightening constraints on further growth in funding is sometimes said to be resolvable through the provision of 'value-based healthcare'. It is described, notably by Professor Michael E. Porter of Harvard Business School, as being the ability 'to increase value for patients, which is the quality of patient outcomes relative to the dollars expended'. He goes on:

> 'Minimizing costs is simply the wrong goal, and will lead to counterproductive results. Eliminating waste and unnecessary services is beneficial, but cost savings must arise from true efficiencies, not from cost shifting, restricting care (rationing), or reducing quality.' (Porter & Teisberg, 2006: p. 98)

Value-based healthcare is a concept which is fundamental to anyone in a leadership role in healthcare, and especially perhaps to those in clinical leadership positions.

Resources in the NHS

As far as the position in the UK is concerned, the overwhelming majority of resources for healthcare are raised from general taxation and National Insurance contributions. That fact has a direct bearing on their size, their allocation, their use and how they are accounted for. Monies for the NHS are ultimately allocated by Parliament. The availability of public funds is of course shaped by the overall performance of the economy, and recent years have seen the effects of a period of economic austerity following the financial crash of 2007/2008. Healthcare has, however, tended to have a privileged status among public spending priorities, both before and after the financial crisis. Following the publication of the Wanless report in 2002, and the related decision to raise public spending on healthcare in England to a percentage of the nation's GDP comparable with the (then) European Union average, the resource limit for health, but for health alone, was set for a period covering two cycles of the Comprehensive Spending Review (the 3-year government-wide forward look across the totality of public expenditure) – that is, until 2008. That unprecedented period of clarity about future resources, combined with a commitment to raise expenditure as a share of the national cake, had the obvious advantages of enabling better planning and of protecting healthcare from the risk that other government spending priorities might take precedence. The disadvantages were that there was little sympathy from other public services for the plight of healthcare, which has consistently done better in terms of its share of public funding, and that within the healthcare system itself we became used to a pattern of continued growth, which perhaps bred a sense of false comfort and even complacency.

Over the past few years, the government's response to the financial crisis and its impact on public debt has been to impose a period of austerity across all forms of public expenditure. Nevertheless, spending on the NHS, alongside spending on schools and overseas aid, has had privileged status. Nominally, there has been a very small margin of growth, although that is disputed in practice, but that position has unquestionably been better than the scale of reduction seen on expenditure in welfare benefits, social care and even defence. Again, there is very little sympathy for the NHS from the rest of the public sector, which sees it as being cushioned and protected. There is, however, a great difference between the high levels of growth in funding seen prior to 2008 and the effects in practice of so-called 'flat cash' in more recent years. The need to fund from within that fixed cash envelope the effects of inflation (even though pay has been tightly constrained for much of the period), and to accommodate the impact of demographic changes – both a growing and an increasingly long-lived population – has required the achievement of a minimum of 4% efficiency savings year after year. Given that for most of the NHS's history the achievement of 2% efficiency would have been regarded as an outstanding result, this sustained level of cost improvement is unprecedented, and would be most unusual in other healthcare systems internationally. At the time of writing it remains to be seen how much longer that can be sustained before systemic financial problems emerge across the NHS. There is also a complex interaction between funding for health and social care which is becoming ever more problematic as local authority budgets, which fund child and adult social care, are reduced at a faster pace than those in health.

This situation has been exacerbated by recent changes to the structure of the NHS stemming from the Health and Social Care Act 2012, following the white paper *Equity and Excellence – Liberating the NHS*. That has had the effect of complicating and in some cases fragmenting the arrangements for distributing resources across the NHS.

How are resources distributed?

It used to be the case prior to the implementation of that Act in 2013 that the bulk of funding for health services was distributed by the Department of Health to local primary care trusts (PCTs). The sum allocated to each was based on a formula which started with the total population registered with general practitioners (GPs) serving the area of the PCT and adjusted for various factors to take account of morbidity – principally the age and sex structure, but refined in the light of research on other factors that can have an impact on health need, for example measures of social deprivation. That system had its problems – there was always a debate about the accuracy of the measurement of the population based on Office for National Statistics (ONS) data, which depended on estimates for changes during the period between the once-a-decade national censuses. Sometimes even the accuracy of the base data was challenged, particularly where there were high levels of population movement, for example in the major cities. Different methods of estimation can give substantially different results, particularly when applied to relatively small areas (such as those served by many of the old PCTs). In London, for example, the Greater London Authority's estimates of population growth in certain localities (which take into account new house building) differ by as much as 20% from ONS estimates over the same period. Both remain only estimates, but which more accurately reflects the likely requirement for the funding of health services, and which will be more nearly correct?

The other key issue was the relative weight given in the adjustment formula to social deprivation factors versus age structure. The calculation could be complex, but in very simple terms a greater weighting for social deprivation tended to favour urban populations and the north with greater resource allocation, whereas a greater weighting towards an ageing population favoured rural counties and the south of England.

Nevertheless, the great advantage of the system was that the bulk of the resources intended to be used for commissioning healthcare for a local population was under the control of one body, and those local bodies tended to align closely with the local authorities responsible for commissioning social care. There were, as there still are, some discrepancies between the resident population served in a particular area by the local authority and the registered population of the GPs in the same area, as general practice populations can straddle local government boundaries, especially in urban districts. But there was flexibility in the application of the healthcare budget. The commissioning body could, for example, relatively easily switch resources from expenditure on in-patient child and adolescent mental health services to investment in outreach services, which might provide a better alternative to hospitalisation for young people.

The new structure implemented in 2013 changed all that. Clinical commissioning groups (CCGs) – locally based organisations led by GPs – are the successors to the PCTs, and are accountable to the local, regional and national commissioning structures of NHS England, the new body responsible for the overall commissioning of healthcare in England; that commissioning in turn is in line with a mandate agreed annually with the Secretary of State for Health. CCGs are allocated resources by NHS England, using a formula essentially similar to the previous one to take account of the population served, although in recent years the weighting has tended to shift more in favour of age relative to social deprivation. In two very important respects, however, the resources allocated to CCGs have been reduced. First, a significant tranche of services are now commissioned nationally or regionally by NHS England itself, and so the funding for them is now no longer under the control of local commissioners. In some cases that has inhibited their ability to fund a whole pathway of care, so for example the funding of in-patient child and adolescent mental health beds is now controlled by NHS England nationally, whereas services which operate as alternatives to such admissions are funded by local CCGs. Consequently, the benefits of investing more capacity in local outreach services which offer alternatives to admission would not accrue to the CCG responsible for commissioning that part of the care pathway, but rather to NHS England, which would see lower demand for the in-patient admissions which it is responsible for funding. That perverse incentive, combined with the use of a rather arbitrary methodology to disaggregate resources for in-patient child and adolescent mental health services from local services (i.e. one based on a snapshot of usage over a short period of time, rather than an average over several years), has meant, in practice, that the capacity of outreach services has reduced and the demand for child and adolescent mental health in-patient beds has increased, although they cost more overall and provide a more institutionally based service for young people. It is a clear example of what Michael Porter's 'value-based healthcare' is intended to avoid, but it is unfortunately only one example of the perverse consequences of the fragmentation of healthcare funding.

The other important respect in which the resources previously controlled by PCTs have been reduced in the new system arises because CCGs are GP-led organisations. It is considered that there would be a conflict of interest if they were to be responsible for commissioning primary care services, for which PCTs, which were controlled by a more conventional board of directors, used to have responsibility. To prevent that conflict of interest primary care services are now funded by the local area teams of NHS England – that part of the organisational structure to which CCGs are immediately accountable. Again, this can compromise the ability to fund pathways of care, especially at the interface between primary and secondary care, and the same risk of perverse incentives can arise.

In both cases the problems which arose over the first couple of years of the new system have to some extent been recognised and a review of national specialist commissioning is being undertaken with the expectation that a significant part of the current portfolio of services which are NHS England's responsibility will be transferred back to CCGs. That is to be welcomed, but unfortunately the impact of the disjunction of the commissioning arrangements on services was significant and happened surprisingly quickly, and much will now need to be repaired. It is a salutary lesson which shows that how you choose to distribute resources really can have a direct impact on the care and experience of individual patients. The situation with regard to primary care commissioning is more complex because the conflict-of-interest issue is less easily resolved and so the solution being adopted is 'co-commissioning' of primary care between NHS England and local CCGs. There is an element of paradox in this because those with the most expert insight into how primary care can best be resourced and commissioned are of course GPs themselves.

The other major difference in the post-2013 resource allocation arrangements is that a significant element of the healthcare budget (around 4–5%) closely associated with public health functions has been transferred to the control of local authorities under the remit of directors of public health. This includes resources for drug and alcohol services, health promotion, school nurses and sexual health, and in due course will encompass health visiting. While it is under the control of local authorities it generally remains distinct from the arrangements for the distribution of social care funding for both adults and children, although there is obviously potential for improving their alignment.

While resources for the commissioning of clinical care distributed through these now quite complex routes form the bulk of NHS expenditure, they do not constitute all of it. The other significant categories are resources allocated to support staff training and to support research and development. Both have been subject to change in recent years, although the National Institute for Health Research (NIHR) system for the distribution of research and development funds pre-dates the most recent reforms.

Education funding, which is substantial, is now under the control of a national body called Health Education England (HEE). It has established a number of local boards (which strictly speaking are subcommittees of HEE) consisting of representatives of local healthcare employers and academic institutions responsible for training healthcare professionals. They also include the local deans responsible for postgraduate medical education. The bulk of their resources are used to fund courses through contracts with universities for the training of a wide range of healthcare professions, but excluding medical students, whose training is funded nationally by the Higher Education Funding Council for England (HEFCE) as part of its responsibilities for undergraduate education. The HEE local boards also fund the salaries of postgraduate trainee doctors and, through employers – largely trusts – a range of postgraduate and in-service training for the whole range of healthcare staff. This arrangement has been the closest the NHS has come to allowing employers to exercise substantial control and influence over the resources used for training their staff, an arrangement which would be normal in nearly all other industries. Historically, control over these matters has largely been exercised at a national level or through regional/strategic health authorities, all of which have been abolished under the new arrangements. The temptation to revert to national control is strong, however, and it would appear that HEE is starting a process of centralisation which will reduce and might undermine the influence of local employers and their academic partners.

Until 2006, NHS research and development funding was, on the whole, not allocated directly to research activity but was intended to recompense services for the additional cost borne by the NHS where significant amounts of research and development took place – mainly in major academic centres. The problems with the system were that the basis of allocation was largely historical, that it did not reflect the quality or value to the NHS of the research being undertaken, and that it had perhaps led to a culture of complacency and dependence in some cases. In a radical set of changes the old allocation arrangements were gradually withdrawn and an entirely new set of structures put in place, intended to bolster centres of excellence in both basic and applied research, to fund directly research activity of value and interest to the NHS, and to stimulate involvement in research and development and clinical trial activity across the NHS. On the whole, the new system has been successful in achieving those objectives, although some smaller (and one or two very large) clinical academic centres which had depended on the historical funding arrangements without necessarily being able to demonstrate commensurate output have seen significant loss of funding. Perhaps most significantly, this system has supported the development of a strong business case at national level for the benefits of investment in biomedical research and life sciences, which has protected their funding through the recent period of austerity.

How are resources allocated to service providers?

Prior to 1990 there was no difference between the funding, purchasing or commissioning of services and their provision in the NHS. Local health authorities had resources distributed to them using a similar formula to that in operation today, and they were directly responsible for the operation of local health services. The establishment of the 'internal market' in 1991 was influenced, in part, by the work of Enthoven in the USA (e.g. Enthoven, 1985), but followed a pattern which over the last 25 years has become increasingly widespread across public services in England. This model separates bodies with the responsibility for commissioning services from those with the responsibility for providing them, and it led initially to the establishment of NHS trusts as distinct and 'independent' providers of services, operating within a quasi-market in which they competed to provide services to GPs. Initially, the competition was intended to be between established NHS trusts, but as the internal market has developed over the years there has been increasing encouragement of plurality of provision, with a growing role for the independent and voluntary sector. The most recent reforms have brought the provision of health services in England within the scope of European competition law, and encouraged much more routine competitive tendering of contracts for services.

This is a fundamental change, and no incumbent NHS provider of healthcare can take it for granted that it will continue to be the provider of any particular service in future. Indeed, even if its commissioner is satisfied with the service the provider is offering, that commissioner may feel obliged, periodically, to test the market. In practice, the provision of mental and community health services seems to be more exposed to the tendency towards competitive tendering than are general acute hospital services, and when this happens services are often broken into small 'lots', which can have the effect of fragmenting pathways of care, with consequences which are similar to those following from fragmented commissioning.

The mechanism for the allocation of resources to specific service provision is therefore increasingly through competitive contracting, but how does that determine the relationship between the cost of services, their quality and the value they bring? During the period following the 1990s reforms, the 'market' was always substantially restricted, in terms of both the overall levels of resources available and the number of new entrants of providers. The new NHS trusts essentially competed with one another for broadly the same amount of money and work, and while there were some relative winners and losers among these nominally independent organisations, they all remained accountable to the Secretary of State for Health, who was, thus, still responsible for what happened across the totality of the public healthcare system, including the fate of individual provider NHS trusts if they got into financial difficulties. Changes to the flow of funds were largely at the margins of historical patterns. Costs and quality varied; indeed, criticism grew about the variation in services available from locality to locality – the so-called 'postcode lottery'. That was seen to stem from the changes made by individual GP fund-holders, who undertook micro-commissioning at a practice level for a limited range of services, but in fact that was probably much less significant than long-standing variations in practice, availability of services and patterns of treatment which went back well before the 1990s.

When the Labour Party took power in 1997, GP fund-holding was abolished, but the distinction between purchasing and providing was retained. Much stronger measures were put in place at a national level to tackle the problems of variability, in particular the establishment of national standards for services (National Service Frameworks), as well as interventions and treatments (under the auspices of what is now the National Institute for Health and Care Excellence – NICE) and through the establishment of a national body for the inspection of publicly funded health services, originally the Commission for Health Improvement, now the Care Quality Commission (CQC). A similar attempt was made to standardise costs, with the intention of moving to a system where providers competed solely on quality (supposedly over and above agreed national standards) as prices were the same. That marked a significant change – under GP fund-holding much of the negotiation between the practice and the provider was about the price of the service, and providers might well seek to offer additional capacity at the margin, knowing that their costs would be marginal too. That had also been true of the contracts between the larger health authorities and individual providers – there was variation in prices and agreements to buy additional care at marginal cost were widespread. The system introduced to achieve standardisation of costs across the NHS was known as payment by results (PbR).

Payment by results

Payment by results was introduced gradually, starting with acute elective surgery, where it was specifically intended to increase the quantum of surgical procedures in order to reduce waiting times. Historically the NHS had relied on waiting lists to manage demand – it was a *de facto* method of rationing – but the scope for that had been removed in the case of elective surgery by the advent of national standards progressively reducing maximum waiting times. There was a strong, politically driven impetus to increase the volume of activity to achieve waiting time targets. Acute interventions were classified into 'healthcare resource groups' (HRGs), and over a transitional period prices were standardised, based initially on national averages, but increasingly shifting towards so-called 'best practice' tariffs. This sounds, and indeed is, very technical, but its significance extends well beyond its increasingly complex detail. First of all, it marks a decisive shift away from the traditional compromise in the distribution of resources between the historical pattern for a given population or service and the corresponding rationally derived 'correct' allocation. The tariff is based on a nationally determined formula, with some adjustments made to reflect the different costs of premises and salaries around the country. The acute PbR tariff is what a provider gets paid for a particular service: if it can provide it for less, then it can keep the difference; if it costs it more, then the provider must (very quickly) find savings to cover the difference, or stop providing a service it cannot afford to run, or go out of business.

The relationship between the volume of activity and resources is paramount, in a way that had never been the case hitherto. More work means more income for a provider; less work, less income. That was the theory as PbR started, but the more it has developed away from its origins in acute elective surgery, the more those principles have been compromised. For instance, as PbR was extended to non-elective hospital care, the growth in emergency admissions, in part stimulated by the 4-hour waiting target in accident and emergency departments, placed an unsustainable pressure on commissioners. According to the theory, once work is undertaken it has to be paid for. There is no negotiation other than perhaps about exactly which category a particular intervention falls into, and therefore which tariff is applied, and whether the activity was properly coded and notified. Before too long, the Department of Health, which was responsible for setting the tariff, had to set limits for the anticipated growth in emergency admissions, beyond which full cost payment under the tariff would be reduced to a 30% marginal rate.

Increasingly, tariffs have been adjusted to reconcile the powerful incentive for providers to do more and more work, which commissioners have in practice relatively little scope to control, with the need for the system as a whole to operate within a fixed overall allocation.

Payment by results in mental health services

Payment by results has been the principal funding mechanism for acute services for around 10 years now, and for much of that period it has been national policy to extend the regime to all forms of care, including mental health services. Doing so has proved to be a knotty problem. There are a number of very important considerations which have for some years been central to mental health policy which have to be reconciled with a PbR regime. The first relates to the incentives created. As applied in general acute services, PbR creates an incentive to increase the consumption of hospital-based interventions, tempered only to the extent that commissioners are able to manage demand, either by not referring or by providing alternatives to referral. As a long-standing matter of policy, mental health services have been developed to encourage secondary services to support people outside hospital, with the aim of minimising the need for admission. That principle is all the more important in view of the existence, unique to mental health services, of the possibility of compulsion in treatment, specifically linked to hospital admission.

In any case, most resources in mental healthcare are spent on patients who are in treatment for relatively long periods of time and whose care is often funded by both health and social care authorities. It has been a central tenet of recent policy to accelerate the degree of integration between health and social care. Eligibility for social care, provided by locally elected authorities and funded, in part, through the local council tax (albeit substantially augmented by a wide range of central government grants), is dependent on being a local resident, or on a locally established responsibility for care. If people are being cared for in their own homes, community-based case management is likely to have limited scope for movement from one provider to another, but is more likely to require long-term coordination between a number of complementary agencies. The model is less one of competition but rather more of collaboration.

There are, though, some aspects of mental health services which are amenable to the acute hospital model of PbR. Out-patient-based episodic treatment – for example cognitive–behavioural therapy for anxiety disorders or depression and perhaps some psychotherapy – can readily be accommodated within the established model. A standard tariff can be applied to a particular course of treatment in relation to a particular disorder and, given the widespread acknowledgement of the under-treatment of common mental illness, there are powerful reasons for creating incentives to increase the consumption of interventions which are known to be effective. There are also few features of such services that bind potential patients to a particular geography or provider – they can go wherever the waiting time is shortest, the location and timing most convenient for them, and perhaps where the outcomes, where published, are best. The services that come under the programme of improving access to psychological therapies (IAPT) which has been rolled out nationally over the past few years are well suited to such a model.

For the most part, however, the reconciliation of established mental health policy with standard national tariff-based payment systems has proved challenging. That is perhaps why many other countries which have introduced tariff-based systems in acute care for distributing resources to providers have abandoned the attempt in the case of mental health services. Nevertheless, some progress has been made. At the heart of the regime which has emerged is the principle that rather than paying for a specific intervention for a particular diagnosis, a provider should be funded to meet the needs of a patient with an identified level of need over the course of a specified period. The risk associated with the amount of intervention required to meet that need therefore sits with the provider rather than the commissioner, because it is amenable to clinical decision-making, which the provider is able to control. That avoids the problem of creating incentives to admit patients to hospital unnecessarily, and deals to some extent with the difficulty of compulsion, although it is important to ensure that no perverse incentive is created which discourages admission when it is in fact necessary. It supports the principle of trying to keep people well, intervening early in the course of an illness and preventing relapse, and so to that extent financial incentives are aligned with policy objectives.

The next question is how to relate resources to identified levels of need, and indeed, how to categorise need itself. One of the problems often encountered in the various international attempts to develop tariffs for mental health services is the unreliability of HRGs (and their forerunners) as predictors of resource use in mental healthcare. There are a variety of reasons for that, but at the core it is because diagnosis is a much less reliable predictor of resource use in mental healthcare than it is in acute medicine. Even where it is clinically straightforward, two patients with ostensibly the same diagnosis may be much more or less likely to require admission to hospital, to need much more or less intensive levels of care, and indeed coercion, in their treatment, and to remain in hospital for longer or shorter periods, depending on whether they have supportive relatives or carers, whether they have had contact with the criminal justice system, whether they have their own accommodation and whether they have legal entitlement to residence, benefits or housing in the UK.

The solution which has been adopted is to group patients into needs-based 'clusters', which use an adaptation of the Health of the Nation Outcome Scale (HoNOS) to distinguish different levels of likely resource use. HoNOS, as its name implies, was originally designed as an outcome measure, not as a needs assessment tool, and there was initially some criticism of its use for a different purpose, but in practice the 21 clusters derived from it seem to have face validity as a way of categorising need, and it is easier not to have multiple systems. It also offers a much simpler system than the literally hundreds of HRGs involved in acute PbR, and one which is therefore less susceptible to unanticipated consequences when incremental changes are made.

It also creates a relationship between the process of clinical needs assessment as a part of care planning and the allocation of patients to particular resource groups; if the level of need changes and that is identified in a clinical review, then that can readily be translated into allocation of the patient to a different cluster, associated with a higher or lower level of resource use. It is helpful to establish a relationship between factors involved in resource allocation and routine clinical processes. It also means that the discussion about the appropriate cluster and the likely level of need offers some opportunity for the involvement of patients themselves, their carers and their referrers. Once a patient has been allocated to a cluster, it is the responsibility of the provider to manage the financial risk associated with delivering appropriate care within the agreed cost of that cluster. It is the commissioner's responsibility to bear the financial risk associated with the numbers of patients in any particular cluster referred for treatment, and in that respect the PbR system mitigates the liability for the overall costs of providing a service to a population which existed for trusts under the block contract system.

What has proved much more problematic is using the cluster system to establish a set of national tariffs, that is to say consistent national prices for each cluster, so that all providers pay the same for treating a patient within a given cluster. There are a number of reasons for that. There are both legitimate and unjustifiable reasons for variation in the cost of the treatment pathway between different providers and indeed between different geographies within the same provider. Legitimate reasons include a richer content to the pathway of care: one service may incorporate welfare benefits advice for example, whereas a neighbouring service may be able to refer patients to a well-established Citizens Advice service which happens to exist locally. In the first case both commissioners and providers might have agreed that it is worth investing in the welfare benefits advice because it results in shorter lengths of stay in hospital and promotes greater independence and support for patients – it demonstrates the principles of 'value-based healthcare' in other words.

Unjustifiable reasons for variation include differences in case-load size and in levels of patient contact between members of community mental health teams, or differences in length of stay in hospital which cannot be explained in clinical terms. Adopting simple 'national average' prices for each cluster would fail to take account of the complexity of these differences, particularly when it is borne in mind that it is harder to define the range of interventions associated with the pathway of care for the treatment of someone with psychosis than it is, say, for someone needing a hip replacement or the removal of a cataract.

When acute PbR was introduced, fears about the impact of too sudden a move towards national average prices, and the potential financial destabilisation which might result for both commissioners and providers, led to a 3-year period during which an extra £700 million was allocated to smooth the transition on both sides. There is very little prospect of such an arrangement being repeated for the introduction of PbR in mental health or indeed any other sector of care in the current economic climate.

Instead, it was decided to use the clusters as the basis for calculating local costings, recognising that the variations these revealed would encompass both legitimate and unjustifiable causes, and that they could form the basis of a discussion leading to a more sophisticated understanding, while protecting both providers and commissioners from sudden and unsustainable shifts in prices and cost pressures. This is sometimes referred to as being the use of clusters as 'currencies' rather than tariffs, the currency being a consistent way of calculating what the local cost is, thus allowing for comparison, rather than a tariff, which is a standard set price. Much work has been done allocating patients to clusters using the adapted HoNOS tool, but except among those most closely involved with the subject, the principles of PbR in mental health are often confused with the very different set of incentives created by acute PbR.

The sometimes perverse set of incentives in acute PbR has become an increasingly fundamental strategic problem for the NHS. Across all care groups, but particularly in relation to older people and those with long-term conditions, the strategy for care now being espoused is very similar to that which has been at the heart of mental healthcare for the last 20 or 30 years: the aim is to look after people in their own homes wherever possible, intervene early and prevent relapse, and wherever possible to reduce the default reliance on admission to hospital as the normal pattern of care. Current funding mechanisms, however, are such that they create incentives for doing the opposite. They reward doing more of what we say we want to do less of, while they afford no incentive to any of those sectors of care which we need to stimulate to do more, whether that be mental healthcare, community health services or general practice. Accordingly, the new authorities responsible for payment mechanisms, NHS England and Monitor, the provider regulator, have commenced a far-reaching review of payment mechanisms, and the term 'payment by results' has been dropped from the lexicon, 'payment systems' being preferred instead. Some have interpreted this as meaning that mental health PbR has been abandoned, but in fact it looks as though it will continue to be supported as the basis for the development of more local payment arrangements, wherever possible with a focus on the achievement of better outcomes for patients. The real need is to find a means of translating some of the principles which have underpinned the development of mental health PbR into the funding mechanisms for non-elective acute hospital care.

Productivity in healthcare

Measuring productivity in healthcare is a vexed issue, and many of the indicators used are primitive, highly selective or very general. Overall life expectancy has improved very dramatically by comparison with historical trends in the last 40 years for example, but the extent to which that can be attributed to better productivity within healthcare, as opposed to wider social and economic factors, is questionable. Nevertheless, for the individual provider trust, but perhaps most importantly for each local system of care, an understanding of productivity is crucial.

It is important not to confuse productivity with cost. For example, if a ward with a cost per bed day that is 5% higher than a comparator nevertheless achieves an average length of stay 10% shorter, it is more productive, and the additional investment is worthwhile. That is one of the attractions of any funding system which, rather than being geared to managing within a fixed budget whatever the amount of work undertaken, instead allows the benefits of effective investment to be more clearly delineated and realised. It is also important not to look at productivity purely in the context of individual components of the service – to assess it properly one must look across what Porter & Teisberg (2006) call the 'whole cycle of care'. An ostensibly very efficient in-patient service might, for example, discharge patients very rapidly, but lead to a high readmission rate, which overall would cost more. Paradoxically, a larger number of readmissions would increase the apparent throughput and, when taken in isolation, might make the service appear more efficient. For a proper understanding of efficiency it is necessary to look across the whole range of services which might be involved in caring for a particular patient, including those provided by other agencies. Indeed, it is commonly the case that other bodies – voluntary sector organisations for example – can provide an element of service more cost-effectively and more productively than a trust itself, and so it is in the interests of more efficient and productive healthcare that such activities are subcontracted.

As described earlier in this chapter, expectations of the scale of productivity improvement have increased significantly in recent years. Back in 2002, the Wanless report assumed improvements in productivity of between 1.5% and 3% per year in the three scenarios it constructed for the future of the NHS (Wanless, 2002). Recently the expectation has been of an annual improvement of up to 4%, and arguably that can be achieved only if the contribution and value brought by patients themselves and their carers are taken into account, and if those parties are engaged as part of a collective endeavour. This approach shares common ground with the principles of the 'recovery model' in mental health services, and it requires much clearer recognition of the immense time, effort, knowledge and value brought to care in all its forms by individual service users and their informal carers. That may well not be a bad thing in its own right, but it

79

is also possibly the only means to reconcile the ever-growing demand and the potential to offer more effective care through advances in science with the constraints of the wider economic situation.

The revolution in digital technology, in its application to healthcare, offers some exciting new means of developing that opportunity. Eric Topol, MD, in his thought-provoking book *The Creative Destruction of Medicine*, observes that:

> 'the ability to digitally define the essential characteristics of each individual – the high-definition human – sets up a unique era of medicine... Medicine today relies on the median, whereas in the imminent future it can and will be anchored to the individual. The median will ultimately not be the message in medicine. Beyond the advances in technology, for that to happen, individuals – consumers – will need to step up and lead the way' (Topol, 2012: p. 18).

Electronic health records genuinely shared between practitioners and patients, remote monitoring and self-reporting, virtually delivered psychological therapies, personalised medicine derived from full genome sequencing and the revolution in the availability of information and apps directly to consumers will transform healthcare as we know it, will profoundly challenge many established patterns of care delivery and will require providers to adapt and engage with service users to make care a joint endeavour. If we can, then we also stand the best chance of improving our productivity sufficiently to meet the efficiency improvement requirements of the age.

Outcome-based funding and value-based healthcare

One of the models now emerging to try to achieve efficiency improvement is 'outcome-based' commissioning. At the time of writing it remains experimental, but essentially it combines the principles of Porter's 'value-based healthcare' with the use of PbR clusters to define the needs and extent of the population served, with the gradual adoption of better measures of the degree to which the system of care achieves the outcomes service users themselves desire. The model has already been used on a small scale for contracting drug and alcohol services, where outcomes have often been defined in terms of reduction of illicit substance misuse or offending behaviour. In such cases the sanction of the criminal justice system creates an element of coercion, which means that the outcomes can be defined for the service users, rather than by them. There must be the strong caveat therefore than in translating the model to the much wider realm of the rest of healthcare it is important to ensure that patients are not put in a position where they are being obliged to achieve certain outcomes in order to satisfy the requirements of the contract and the resource distribution system, rather than because they have real meaning for them. The best measure of whether outcomes really have been achieved will probably involve asking patients directly whether it worked for them rather than by counting pre-set contractual indicators.

Accounting for resources

Because the resources used across the NHS are provided by taxpayers there are of course systems to ensure that there can be proper accountability for their use. Trust boards have statutory duties for the effective management of their finances, and if a board does not respond to its responsibilities in that regard, it will attract the attention of regulators, and, *in extremis*, be replaced by one that will.

In addition to the overall responsibility upon boards, there are specific duties placed upon the chief executive and finance director of each trust. Every NHS chief executive is also the 'accountable officer' for the trust – accountable, that is, to Parliament (through the Public Accounts Committee) for the use of public money in their organisation. That accountability extends not just to probity – tackling fraud, corruption and extravagance – but also to ensuring that resources are used efficiently and effectively, and not exceeded. 'Accountable officer' status is conferred like a licence, and if trust chief executives are deemed not to have discharged their responsibilities properly, they can have that status withdrawn, which effectively prevents them from continuing in such a role at that or at any other trust. Finance directors have a professional duty to the accounting body of which they are a member (and they must be a qualified accountant to hold the office) to ensure that the financial position of the organisation is properly represented. It is possible for either a chief executive or a finance director to be placed in a position where the board of their organisation will not act as they consider it should to tackle the financial problems facing it. In such circumstances, they both have a duty (and to some extent powers) to make sure that their advice is clearly minuted and communicated to the Department of Health.

The majority of NHS trusts are now foundation trusts, and their position is essentially similar, although they do have more flexibility to manage their finances over time. The ultimate recourse is to their regulator, Monitor, and a key measure is a foundation trust's EBITDA (earnings before interest, taxation, depreciation and amortisation), which is essentially a test of whether its underlying position is one of making or losing money on its operations in relation to its income. Foundation trusts, precisely because their finances are independent of the rest of the NHS, are also much more exposed to the requirements to manage their cash. In real life, we are all familiar with the need to manage a cash flow – to make sure that we do not run out of money before the end of the month – and with the need from time to time to borrow cash to manage large investments or projects. When the NHS functioned more as an organisation and less as a 'market', one part of the system was able to rely on another for borrowing and so cash management was historically less at the forefront of consideration. However, as each component organisation becomes more autonomous then cash management becomes a real issue if trusts are to be able to pay their suppliers and their staff. For that reason, foundation trusts are expected either to hold substantial cash reserves or to have the facility to borrow cash if necessary to continue to function; it is therefore all the more important to anticipate and correct financial problems. If the underlying position of the trust is such that it costs more for it to conduct its operations than it recoups in income, then it will sooner or later run out of cash, even though one-off items, like the sale of property, mean that it breaks even in a given year. It then needs to take fundamental corrective action.

Trust boards have the help of internal and external auditors to give them a proper grasp of their financial standing and of the reliability of their financial systems. For foundation trusts external auditors are appointed by the council of governors – the equivalent of the shareholders' meeting for a PLC (public limited company) – and both the auditors and the council of governors must approve the trust's annual accounts. Trust boards are required to establish an audit subcommittee, to which auditors can bring their reports and give advice, and also to publish an annual 'audit letter' from the external auditors, advising the board of its financial standing. External auditors also have the power to produce a report 'in the public interest' if they are sufficiently concerned about the position of an organisation.

The other aspect of resources which boards must consider is capital investment in maintaining or rebuilding the infrastructure of their organisation, which can include equipment and information technology as well as buildings. That can be funded from cash which has been generated in previous years and earmarked for the purpose, by borrowing, or by various models of public/private partnership such as the Private Finance Initiative (PFI). Under a PFI, a consortium of builders and lenders finances and constructs a facility (and perhaps continues to maintain and service it); in exchange, the trust pays a charge over a long period of time, typically 25–30 years. Whichever approach is adopted, it helps to illustrate the overriding consideration in looking at any form of capital investment: what is the value that it brings? Can the costs of the capital be afforded, whether they are represented as capital charges (the costs of depreciation and an interest payment charge to the Treasury on traditional NHS capital investment), PFI charges, or the cost of borrowing capital commercially? Is there the flexibility to cope with changing circumstances?

Does mental health get the resources it requires?

This, despite the obvious temptation, is not an easy question to answer. Some international comparisons tend to suggest that mental health services in the UK do relatively well, at least in terms of the percentage of total health expenditure devoted to mental health (around 12%). In terms of overall health expenditure (as a percentage of GDP), however, the UK tends to be more in the middle of the range of high-income countries. Moreover, the definition of the scope of mental health resources is critical to the validity of such calculations. Some systems will count expenditure on dementia as part of neurology, and resources used for the care of offenders with mental disorders, clearly part of the mental health system in the UK, can be counted as part of the criminal justice system in some countries. In the USA the federal penitentiary system is the single largest provider of in-patient psychiatric care. There are other key boundaries that can make all the difference, depending on where they are set, often very specific to national cultures, for example between healthcare, social welfare and benefits expenditure, housing and education. It is quite possible, therefore, that the rather positive picture of the UK in mental health investment when compared with other countries is in fact relatively overstated because a lot is included which would be differently classified elsewhere.

This brings us to perhaps the most important point of all in considering the allocation and use of resources in mental health services. Mental health is generally considered just from the standpoint of overall health expenditure, and it is a commonplace that it tends to come low down the list of health priorities. If one looks instead at expenditure on mental health promotion and care as an investment, then the 'payback' is not limited merely to improvement in health outcomes for individuals and populations (although there is very strong evidence that a great many more people would benefit from psychiatric care than ever actually receive it), but extends to wider social benefits. Viewed thus, mental healthcare brings an important contribution and value to a number of wider, high-priority government agendas.

Taken even more broadly, this has led to mental health being drawn directly into the heart of considerations previously the main province of economists. In his book *Happiness*, Professor Richard Layard explores the limits of equating changes in the happiness of a society with changes in its purchasing power, the traditional approach in economics, and turns instead to better ways of understanding, ordering and achieving society's priorities, drawing specifically on psychology and neuroscience, as well as sociology and philosophy (Layard, 2005). If we were to take happiness seriously, he concludes, then we should:

'spend more on tackling the problem of mental illness. This is the greatest source of misery in the West, and the fortunate should ensure a better deal for those who suffer. Psychiatry should be a top branch of medicine, not one of the least prestigious'.

Conclusions

Improvements in educational attainment, greater social cohesion, reduced levels of offending and addiction, wider participation in work and greater personal independence are all areas in which good mental health services can make a difference. They are all areas which are ripe for further development by viewing care as a joint endeavour between practitioners, service users and carers. That is where the most fruitful discussion of resources and mental health will be in the next few years. The past habit of simply struggling to attract as big a share of the health pot as possible will serve us poorly in a world in which productivity and effectiveness will count for much more. When good mental health services are viewed in their wider social context, beyond the traditional confines of health expenditure, and their benefits can be demonstrated, there is a strong case for investment.

References

Davis K, Stremikis K, Squires D, Schoen C (2014) *Mirror, Mirror on the Wall, 2014 Update: How the US Health Care System Compares Internationally.* Commonwealth Fund.

Enthoven AC (1985) *Reflections on the Management of the National Health Service.* Nuffield Provincial Hospitals Trust.

Layard R (2005) *Happiness: Lessons from a New Science.* Allen Lane.

Porter ME, Teisberg EO (2006) *Redefining Healthcare: Creating Value-Based Competition on Results.* Harvard Business School Press.

Topol E (2012) *The Creative Destruction of Medicine: How the Digital Revolution Will Create Better Health Care.* Basic Books.

Wanless D (2002) *Securing Our Future Health: Taking a Long Term View.* Her Majesty's Treasury.

CHAPTER 6

The development of community care policies in England

Koravangattu Valsraj and Graham Thornicroft

Mental health services have been in a process of transformation in England since the start of the 21st century. The main aim of this chapter is to highlight the development and content of current community care policies in English adult mental health. The chapter focuses on the building blocks of government policy and guidance for mental health services. We shall present a brief overview of the recent policy and legal changes that constitute milestones in the development of community (and hospital) care (Table 6.1).

The NHS and Community Care Act 1990

This 1990 Act was the culmination of a series of reports, as indicated in Table 6.1. One of these was the 1985 authoritative review of community care provisions produced by the House of Commons Social Services Select Committee, under the chairmanship of Renée Short (hence it was called the 'Short report'); it made 101 recommendations, and concluded with the message that community care 'cannot be and should not be done on the cheap'. The NHS and Community Care Act aimed to bring greater coordination to the provision of community care by the health and social services. The Act required local social services and health authorities to jointly agree community care plans which clearly indicated the local implementation of needs-based, individual care plans for long-term, severely ill and vulnerable psychiatric patients. The key objectives of the Community Care Act are listed in Box 6.1.

A key role defined in the Act was that of the *care manager*. 'Care management' needs a special word of clarification. The term was introduced in 1991 as a variation of the term 'case manager', which had been used for the previous decade in the USA. 'Care manager' described the role of qualified social workers who assessed the needs of service users and who then purchased care services from other providers. It was different from the role of Health Service 'key workers', who assessed needs and then also

Table 6.1   Milestones in the development of community care policy

Year	Policy development
1975	Department of Health white paper *Better Services for the Mentally Ill*
1983	Mental Health Act
1985	House of Commons Social Services Select Committee report on community care
1986	Audit Commission report *Making a Reality of Community Care*
1988	Report by Sir Roy Griffiths, *Community Care: Agenda for Action*
1990	National Health Service and Community Care Act
1990	Department of Health publishes guidance on the Care Programme Approach
1992	Department of Health publishes *Health of the Nation*, in which mental health is a key area
1994	Ritchie report into the case of Christopher Clunis
1994	House of Commons Health Select Committee report *Better Off in the Community* ('Short report')
1994	Introduction of supervision registers
1995	Seito Trust report, *Learning the Lessons*
1995	Mental Health (Patients in the Community) Act introduces supervised discharge
1999	National Service Framework for Mental Health and NHS Plan
2000–2003	Policy Implementation Guidelines on various services from the Department of Health, including: early intervention; home treatment; crisis intervention; community mental health teams; suicide prevention strategies; women's mental health; black and ethnic minority mental health
2005	Mental Capacity Act
2007	Mental Health Act 2007 – amendment of the Mental Health Act 1983 with the introduction of supervised community treatment
2008	*Refocusing the Care Programme Approach*
2009	*New Horizons: A shared vision for mental health*
2011	*No Health Without Mental Health: A cross-government mental health outcomes strategy for people of all ages*
2013	*Whole-Person Care: From rhetoric to reality – achieving parity between physical and mental health*
2014	*Closing the Gap: Priorities for essential change in mental health*

provided care. The Act made the following statutory requirements of care managers:

'Where it appears to a local authority that any person for whom they may provide or arrange for the provision of community care services may be in need of any such services, the authority (a) shall carry out an assessment of his needs for those services and (b) having regard to the results of that assessment, shall then decide whether his needs call for the provision by them of any such services'.

Box 6.1 Key objectives of the NHS and Community Care Act 1990

- To promote the development of domiciliary, day and respite services
- To enable people to live in their own homes wherever feasible and sensible
- To promote the development of a flourishing independent sector alongside good-quality public services
- To coordinate social care through the 'care manager'
- To make proper assessment of need
- To provide services on the basis of needs assessments
- To clarify the responsibilities of agencies and so make it easier to hold them to account for their performance
- To secure better value for taxpayers' money by introducing a new funding structure for social care
- To ensure that service providers make practical support for carers a high priority

---

This distinction is now less clear cut as many social workers are members of community mental health teams as 'care coordinators', a term that was introduced in the 1999 revision of the Care Programme Approach (CPA), and this role effectively replaces the roles previously referred to as 'case manager' and 'key worker'.

The Care Programme Approach 1991

The CPA is guidance the government instructed mental health and social services to implement in 1991 (Department of Health, 1991). The CPA is still a central part of the government's mental health policy, and was brought in following concern that, after discharge, many service users did not have a named member of staff to contact, nor was there a defined care plan.

The CPA is the central process to be applied to adults in contact with specialist mental health and social care services. The aim is to achieve an integrated approach across health and social services. The key guiding principles in developing the CPA were the following: to specify an approach focused on the service user, appropriate to the needs of the individual; to provide a framework to prevent service users falling through the net; to recognise the role of carers and the support they need; to facilitate the movement of service users through the healthcare system according to need and service availability; to put into effect the full integration of health and social services; to ensure service users have a copy of their care plan; and to include risk assessment and crisis contingencies in care planning.

In 2000 the three 'levels' of the CPA were simplified into two types of CPA (Department of Health, 2000a): 'standard' and 'enhanced' (Box 6.2). With the publication in 2008 of the guidance *Refocusing the Care Programme Approach* (Department of Health, 2008) which became effective in October

---

Box 6.2 The two 'levels' of Care Programme Approach (2000, and revised in 2008): standard and enhanced

Standard CPA

- requires the support or intervention of one agency or discipline
- applies to people more able to self-manage their mental health problems
- applies to people with an informal support network
- applies to individuals who pose little danger to themselves or others
- applies to those more likely to maintain contact with services
- requires no specific CPA paperwork

Enhanced CPA

- automatically applies to all service users who fulfil the criteria for section 117 of the Mental Health Act 1983 for after-care (i.e. patients who have been detained in hospital under sections 3, 37, 37/41,47/49 and 48/49 of the Mental Health Act 1983) and who have a diagnosis of severe and enduring mental illness
- has a requirement for multi-agency involvement and coordination
- applies to individuals with a history of repeated relapse of their illness due to a breakdown in their medical and/or social care in the community
- applies to individuals with severe social dysfunction, or major housing difficulties, as a consequence of their illness
- applies to people with a history of serious suicide risk, or self-harm, severe self-neglect, violence, or dangerousness to others consequent on their illness.

These patients will:

- receive a written copy of their care plan
- have a care coordinator allocated with clear responsibilities and tasks agreed in the care programme
- have regular reviews for as long as this is deemed appropriate

---

2008 these two levels of CPA were abolished, and in their place came a single system of CPA. The aim was to reduce bureaucracy by removing people on 'standard' CPA from the formal CPA system (so they became 'non-CPA'). This was to enable a 'refocusing' of care onto those with higher levels of need and complexity, and to establish national competencies for the role of the care coordinator, to embed it into the CPA system as a specialist skill.

The guidance highlighted personalised mental healthcare, a whole-systems approach and improvement of quality. The principal aims were: to embed an integrated care pathway approach into service delivery; to improve information sharing between agencies; to provide for protocols and arrangements for working between different assessment and planning systems; to improve local shared provider agreements; to provide for commissioning of a range of services to meet service users' and carers' needs; and to ensure multi-agency local area agreements between health and social care commissioners facilitated planning across agencies. The hope was that a more authoritative and competent cohort of care coordinators, working closely and effectively with partners from a range of agencies, would drive through improvements in care for those people remaining under the CPA system (Goodwin *et al*, 2010).

Importance of the Care Programme Approach

The CPA represents a managed process of care, which remains the cornerstone of policy for adults with severe mental illness. The limitations of the CPA need to be recognised, however. Firstly, it does not in itself contribute to the active therapeutic content of direct face-to-face treatment and support. Secondly, there remain considerable local variations in how far the CPA has been implemented.

The importance of the CPA is that it is designed to target resources to those who need them most, to ensure that vulnerable people do continue to receive the care they need, and to coordinate the delivery of such care (Bindman *et al*, 1999).

Supervised discharge

Supervised discharge was introduced in 1996 following the implementation of the Mental Health (Patients in the Community) Act 1995. It amended the Mental Health Act 1983 to provide a legal framework for the supervision of after-care in the community. Supervised discharge applies to the limited number of patients who, after being detained in hospital for treatment under the Mental Health Act 1983, need formal supervision in the community to ensure that they receive suitable after-care. It reflects the principles of the CPA and is intended to be operated as part of the CPA for the patients concerned. Supervision is for 6 months and is renewable in the first instance for 6 months, and later for periods of up to 1 year (Bindman *et al*, 2000).

The 1996 NHS Executive report on 24-hour nursed care

The report on 24-hour nursed care focused on the needs of the 'new long stay' group (NHS Executive, 1996). Numbering an estimated 5000 or more in England and Wales, these people include many who respond only partially to acute treatment and who remain with substantial disability. They usually require transfer to longer-term high-intensity treatment and support, without which they often remain for too long in acute psychiatric beds. The NHS Executive report made it clear that when service users require facilities which offer 24-hour nursing care, this is an NHS responsibility, as it was in the days when many more long-stay wards in psychiatric institutions were provided.

The likely client group for this service are people who are severely socially disabled by mental illness, and many similar service users in

---

Box 6.3   The client group for 24-hour nursed care

The provision of 24-hour nursed care is for people with severe and enduring mental illness who need:

- daily mental state monitoring
- frequent monitoring of risk
- supervision of medication
- assistance with self-care and daily living
- support to access with day care/rehabilitation
- skilled management of challenging behaviour
- active support in the evening and at weekends.

---

previous decades would have become long-term in-patients in psychiatric institutions (see Box 6.3). These services require each local area to have a residential care strategy, which is carefully coordinated and costed by health and social service purchasers.

National Service Framework for Mental Health, 1999

A central element of current policy is the National Service Framework for Mental Health (NSFMH), which includes health promotion, primary care services, local mental health and social care services, the treatment of substance misuse, and more specialised mental health services, including all forensic mental health services. The Framework therefore encompasses a wide range of services, those provided both by local authorities and by health authorities, and it draws upon a review of the vast array of relevant evidence, including related information from other countries (Thornicroft, 2000).

The NSFMH is a strategic blueprint for services for adults of working age. It is both mandatory, in being a clear statement of what services must seek to achieve in relation to the given standards and performance indicators, and permissive, in that it allows considerable local flexibility to customise the services the Framework requires (Department of Health, 1999).

The stated aims of the NSFMH are:

- to help drive up quality
- to remove the wide and unacceptable variations in provision
- to set national standards and define service models for promoting mental health and treating mental illness
- to put in place underpinning programmes to support local delivery
- to establish milestones and a specific group of high-level performance indicators against which progress within agreed time scales will be measured.

Before drafting and publishing the NSFMH, the Department of Health established an external reference group (ERG) to offer advice on its content.

Core values and principles

The ERG established a consensus on the fundamental values that should be used to guide practical service developments, namely that services should:

- show openness and honesty
- demonstrate respect and offer courtesy
- be allocated fairly and provided equitably
- be proportional to needs
- be open to learning and change.

Upon this foundation, services should also be guided by the following core fundamental principles, that users can expect services:

- meaningfully to involve users and their carers
- to deliver high-quality treatment and care which is effective and acceptable
- to be non-discriminatory
- to be accessible
- to help when and where services are needed
- to promote user safety and the safety of their carers, staff and the wider public
- to offer choices which promote independence
- to be well coordinated between all staff and agencies
- to empower and support their staff
- to deliver continuity of care as long as needed
- to be accountable to the public, users and carers.

National standards

In the NSFMH, seven standards were set, in five areas:
- mental health promotion (standard 1)
- primary care and access to services (standards 2 and 3)
- effective services for people with severe mental illness (standards 4 and 5)
- caring about carers (standard 6)
- preventing suicide (standard 7).

Standard 1. Mental health promotion

Health and social services should:

- promote mental health for all, working with individuals and communities
- combat discrimination against individuals and groups with mental health problems, and promote their social inclusion.

91

Standard 2. Primary care and access to services

Any service user who contacts their primary healthcare team with a common mental health problem should:

- have their mental health needs identified and assessed
- be offered effective treatments, including referral to specialist services for further assessment, treatment and care if they require it.

Standard 3. Primary care and access to services

Any individual with a common mental health problem should:

- be able to make contact round the clock with the local services necessary to meet their needs and be able to receive adequate care
- be able to use telephone support for first-level advice and referral on to specialist helplines or to local services.

Standard 4. Severe mental illness

All mental health service users on CPA should:

- receive care which optimises engagement, anticipates or prevents a crisis, and reduces risk
- have a copy of a written care plan which:
  - includes the action to be taken in a crisis by the service user, their carer, and their care coordinator
  - advises their GP how they should respond if the service user needs additional help
  - is regularly reviewed by their care coordinator
  - allows the service user to be able to access services 24 hours a day, 365 days a week.

Standard 5. Severe mental illness

Each service user who is assessed as requiring a period of care away from their home should have:

- timely access to an appropriate hospital bed or alternative bed or place, which is:
  - in the least restrictive environment consistent with the need to protect them and the public
  - as close to home as possible
- a copy of a written after-care plan agreed on discharge, which sets out the care and rehabilitation to be provided, identifies the care coordinator and specifies the action to be taken in a crisis.

Standard 6. Caring about carers

All individuals who provide regular and substantial care for a person on CPA should:

- have an assessment of their caring, physical and mental health needs, repeated on at least an annual basis

- have their own written care plan that is given to them and implemented in discussion with them.

Standard 7. Preventing suicide

Local health and social care communities should prevent suicides by:

- promoting mental health for all, working with individuals and communities (standard 1)
- delivering high-quality primary mental healthcare (standard 2)
- ensuring that anyone with a mental health problem can contact local services via the primary care team, a helpline or an accident and emergency department (standard 3)
- ensuring that individuals with severe mental illness have a care plan which meets their specific needs, including access to services round the clock (standard 4)
- providing safe hospital accommodation for individuals who need it (standard 5)
- enabling individuals caring for someone with severe mental illness to receive the support which they need to continue to care (standard 6).

The NHS Plan, 1999

The creation of the NHS in 1948 was a seminal event. No longer would wealth determine access to healthcare. The NHS was an extraordinary act of emancipation. For that reason, the NHS retains, in its essential values, huge public support. But its funding did not keep pace with the healthcare systems of comparable countries. So urgent was the need for extra money for the NHS that many of the failures of the system were masked or considered secondary. The Labour government of the day decided to make a historic commitment to a sustained increase in NHS spending. Over 5 years this amounted to an increase of a third in real terms, to bring health spending up to the European Union average. Money had to be accompanied by modernisation, investment and reform (Department of Health, 2000*b*)

In relation to mental health, the NHS Plan added more specific detail than the NSFMH in describing what services should be provided in each local area. It required the provision of teams for early intervention, assertive outreach and crisis resolution.

Mental Health Amendment Act 2007

This amendment of the Mental Health Act 1983 enabled the introduction of supervised community treatment, through community treatment orders (CTOs), which became available in England and Wales in 2008. The provision of supervised discharge was repealed when CTOs were introduced in November 2008, by section 17(A–G) of the amended Mental Health Act 2007. The Code of Practice uses the term 'supervised community treatment';

in the Act those subject to CTOs are called 'community patients'. The nearest equivalent in the past was supervised discharge (after-care under supervision) under section 25(A–J) of the Mental Health Act 1983.

The Oxford Community Treatment Order Evaluation Trial (OCTET) published its findings in the *Lancet* in 2013. The conclusion was that in well-coordinated mental health services the imposition of compulsory supervision does not reduce the rate of readmission of psychotic patients and the trial found no reduction in overall hospital admission support that might justify the significant curtailment of patients' personal liberty (Burns *et al*, 2013).

New Horizons, 2009

The NSFMH was a 10-year plan and it ended in 2009. In 2009 the Department of Health produced the New Horizons cross-government programme of action with the twin aims of improving the mental health and well-being of the population and improving the quality and accessibility of services for people with poor mental health. Following the change of government in 2010, New Horizons was superseded by No Health Without Mental Health.

No Health Without Mental Health, 2011

This was another cross-government initiative, 'a mental health outcomes strategy for people of all ages'. No Health Without Mental Health incorporated six objectives for better mental health for the population:

- more people will have good mental health
- more people with mental health problems will recover
- more people with mental health problems will have good physical health
- more people will have a positive experience of care and support
- fewer people will suffer avoidable harm
- fewer people will experience stigma and discrimination.

Whole-person care and parity of esteem

Whole-Person Care: From Rhetoric to Reality (Achieving Parity Between Mental and Physical Health) was a report published by the Royal College of Psychiatrists (2013) following a request to advise the Ministerial Advisory Group on Mental Health Strategy on how to achieve parity of esteem between mental and physical health in practice, and to develop a definition for 'parity of esteem'.

Mental health does not receive the same attention as physical health. People with mental health problems frequently experience stigma and discrimination, not only in the wider community but also from services.

This is exemplified in part by lower treatment rates for mental health conditions and an under-funding of mental healthcare relative to the scale and impact of mental health problems.

There is an ambition for the NHS to put mental health on a par with physical health. However, the concept of parity in this context is not always well understood. In this report, an expert working group defines 'parity of esteem' in detail, and examines why parity between mental and physical health does not currently exist and how it might be achieved in practice.

This was followed up by *Closing the Gap: Priorities for Essential Change in Mental Health* (2014), a government policy document for England that set out the principle of 'parity of esteem': that services for people with mental disorders should be on a par with those for people with mental disorders. The policy specifies 25 aspects of mental healthcare and support where government – along with health and social care leaders, academics and a range of representative organisations – expect to see tangible changes.

The 5-year forward view for mental health

In March 2015, the independent Mental Health Taskforce brought together health and care leaders, people using services and experts in the field to create a 5-year forward view for mental health for the NHS in England. This national strategy, which covers care and support for people of all ages, was published in February 2016 and signifies for the first time that there has been a strategic approach to improving mental health outcomes across the health and care system, in partnership with the health arm's-length bodies.

When drafting the 5-year forward view the Taskforce was responsible for ensuring that there was cross-system commitment and alignment when developing actions within the national strategy and that continued partnership, working effectively and meaningfully, will enable the strategy to be delivered.

The 5-year forward view is NHS England's commitment to the biggest transformation of mental healthcare across the NHS in a generation, pledging to help more than a million extra people and investing more than £1 billion a year by 2020/21. This investment is in addition to the previously announced new funding for children, young people and perinatal care.

The report (Mental Health Taskforce, 2015) proposes a three-pronged approach to improving care:

- through prevention
- through the expansion of mental healthcare, such as 7-day access for people in a crisis
- integrated physical and mental healthcare.

The key areas are summarised below.

- By 2020, new funding should increase access to evidence-based psychological therapies to reach 25% of need, helping 600000 more people to access care. Combined with investing to double the reach of individual placement and support for people with severe mental illness, this should support a total of 29 000 more people to find and stay in work each year by 2020.

- By 2020, at least 280 000 more people living with severe mental health problems should have improved support for their physical health.
- The £1.4 billion (over 5 years) committed for children's and young people's mental health should be invested to ensure that by 2020 at least 70 000 more children and young people have access to high-quality care. The Taskforce endorses the recommendations in the *Future in Mind* report in 2015.
- New funding should be made available so by 2020/21 crisis resolution and home treatment teams (CRHTTs) can offer intensive home treatment as an alternative to acute in-patient admission in each part of England.
- New funding should ensure that by 2020/21 no acute hospital is without all-age mental health liaison services in emergency departments and in-patient wards, and at least half of acute hospitals meet the 'core 24' service standard.
- New funding should be invested to support at least 30 000 more women each year to access evidence-based specialist mental health care in the perinatal period.
- To reduce suicides by 10% by 2020 all areas should have multi-agency suicide prevention plans in place by 2017 that are reviewed annually.
- The practice of sending people out of area for acute in-patient care due to local acute bed pressures are to be eliminated entirely by no later than 2020/21. The report also states that clinical standards, including maximum waiting times for NICE-recommended care, should be developed and rolled out as soon as funding allows.
- The NHS must make significant improvements in mental health research and kick-start a 'data revolution' to ensure transparency on spending and the quality of care that people receive.

Appendix. Key national guidelines, acts and documents that have influenced community care

- The NHS Plan National Service Framework for Adult Mental Health Services
- National Service Framework for Older People
- National Service Framework for Children
- The Journey to Recovery: The Government's Vision for Mental Health Care
- Cases for Change: A Review of the Foundations of Mental Health Policy and Practice 1997–2002

- Positive Approaches to the Integration of Health and Social Care in Mental Health Services: Briefing for Directors of Social Services on the Integration of Mental Health Services
- Refocusing the Care Programme Approach
- New Horizons – A Shared Vision for Mental Health
- No Health Without Mental Health – A Cross-Government Mental Health Outcomes Strategy For People Of All Ages (https://www.gov.uk/government/uploads/system/uploads/attachment_data/file/213761/dh_124058.pdf)
- Whole-Person Care: From Rhetoric To Reality – Achieving Parity Between Physical and Mental Health (Royal College of Psychiatrists, Occasional Paper 88, March 2013; http://www.rcpsych.ac.uk/files/pdfversion/OP88xx.pdf)
- NHS and Community Care Act
- The Five Year Forward View for Mental Health (February 2016)
- Mental Health Policy Implementation Guide: Community Mental Health Teams

References

Bindman J, Beck A, Glover G, *et al* (1999) Evaluating mental health policy in England. *Care Programme Approach and supervision registers. British Journal of Psychiatry*, **175**: 327–30.

Bindman J, Beck A, Thornicroft G, *et al* (2000) Psychiatric patients at greatest risk and in greatest need. *Impact of the supervision register policy. British Journal of Psychiatry*, **177**: 33–7.

Burns T, Rugkasa J, Molodynski A, *et al* (2013) Community treatment orders for patients with psychosis (OCTET): a randomised controlled trial. *Lancet*, **381**: 1627–33.

Department of Health (1991) *The Care Programme Approach*. Department of Health.

Department of Health (1999) *National Service Framework for Mental Health: Modern Standards and Service Models*. Department of Health.

Department of Health (2000a) *The Revised Care Programme Approach*. Department of Health.

Department of Health (2000b) *The NHS Plan: A Plan for Investment, a Plan for Reform*. TSO.

Department of Health (2001) Crisis resolution/home treatment teams. In *The Mental Health Policy Implementation Guide*. Department of Health.

Department of Health (2002) *Community Mental Health Teams: Policy Implementation Guidance*. Department of Health.

Department of Health (2008) *Refocusing the Care Programme Approach*. Department of Health.

Goodwin N, Lawton-Smith S (2010) Integrating care for people with mental illness: the Care Programme Approach in England and its implications for long-term conditions management. *International Journal of Integrated Care*, **10**: e040.

Mental Health Taskforce (2015) *The Five-Year Forward View for Mental Health*. NHS England.

NHS Executive (1996) *Commissioning 24 Hour Nursed Care for People with Severe and Enduring Mental Illness*. Department of Health.

Thornicroft G (2000) National Service Framework for Mental Health. *Psychiatric Bulletin*, **24**: 203–6.

CHAPTER 7

Psychiatry management and legislation in Northern Ireland

Edward Noble

Structure and administration

Northern Ireland is a province of some 1.8 million people comprising the six north-eastern counties of Ireland. It was formed in 1921 by remaining in the United Kingdom after the partition of the island created the Republic of Ireland. It remains part of the UK, although powers have been devolved. Following the 1998 Good Friday Agreement, the Northern Ireland Assembly was formed, with limited self-governing powers that include health and social services. The Assembly has been suspended on a number of occasions due to a lack of political agreement. During these times, government functions have been the responsibility of a Minister of State, who has control over a number of varied departments within the province and who reports to the Secretary of State for Northern Ireland (a UK cabinet minister). At present, the Northern Ireland political institutions are in operation and are responsible for legislation of transferred matters. These are matters that are not 'reserved' or 'excepted' – matters that remain under Westminster. Reserved matters are transferred to the Assembly based on competence.

Northern Ireland is the only part of the UK with a land border. It would appear reasonable for all Ireland mental health services to secure economies of scale and offer specialisms not readily available in a small population and to allow integrated care across the border. With few exceptions progress towards such rational provision has been faltering.

During periods of direct rule from Westminster, legislation affecting only the province is most often passed through an Order in Council and without a full debate in parliament. It is then called an Order rather than an Act. The current mental health legislation is the Mental Health (Northern Ireland) Order, 1986. A draft Mental Capacity Bill has been formulated. This work was a result of the Bamford review (Bamford, 2004). In 2002 the Northern Ireland government commissioned a review of 'learning disability'

The author has updated and revised this chapter based on that written by the late Graeme McDonald for the third edition of *Management for Psychiatrists*.

and mental health law, policy and services. This was the Bamford review. The review made ambitious recommendations for services in Northern Ireland. These included the development of mental health and capacity law. The current bill is the first of its kind, in that it will subsume mental health law into a single piece of capacity legislation with no differentiation between physical and mental health. At present progress is slow and there is understandable anxiety about the wide effects of the change in legislation and the colossal training needs and service demands that will emerge.

Health and social care in Northern Ireland cost the taxpayer around £4 billion a year. The budget expected for 2015–2016, although a monetary increase, still represents a cut in spending when altered for inflation. The Department of Health, Social Services and Public Safety argues that healthcare in the other UK jurisdictions remains in a less difficult financial environment. The province has higher rates of all-cause disability and socioeconomic deprivation than other parts of the UK. The emotional burdens of prolonged civil disturbance add to the demand on services.

A key distinctive aspect is the administrative unity of health and social services at all levels. It is a matter of debate whether this administrative cohesion leads to any greater service unity than elsewhere.

In previous editions of this book it has been remarked that in comparison with other parts of the UK Northern Ireland has an administratively heavy management structure. The Review of Public Administration 2007 set out to address this. However, in the recently published report *The Right Time, The Right Place* it was still said that Northern Ireland is relatively small to justify its intricately designed health and social care management structure (Donaldson *et al*, 2014).

It remains the case that the Department of Health, Social Services and Public Safety mirrors health departments elsewhere in the UK. It is administratively managed by a Permanent Secretary and medically led by the Chief Medical Officer of the province. Following the Review of Public Administration it is a smaller department than before and mainly provides policy support to the minister. There is a Health and Social Care Board which replaces the previous four, with five local commissioning groups, a Public Health Agency (which has a statutory role in approving the Health and Social Care Board's commissioning plans) and several other statutory bodies. There are six trusts in Northern Ireland, reduced from 18. Five are health and social care trusts and the sixth is the Ambulance Service of Northern Ireland. Mental healthcare is delivered through each of the five trusts: there is no separate mental health trust in Northern Ireland.

Healthcare in Northern Ireland continues to develop. There have been many reviews of the provision of health and social care and administration. The most recent have been *Transforming Your Care* (Compton, 2011) and *The Right Time, The Right Place* (Donaldson *et al*, 2014). *Transforming Your Care* poses a challenge for the current healthcare system in that it proposes a 'shift left': that is, funding that would traditionally be used for hospital-based care should instead be used to develop care within the community, which should be more efficient. It is arguable that mental health services are already ahead of this, as this had been the message of the earlier Bamford review that directed that the number of psychiatric beds be reduced.

Psychiatric care

The practice of psychiatry in Northern Ireland has evolved. Our services have moved away from the traditional sector-based psychiatry towards the formation of specialist teams. However, it may be that this functionalisation has come at a cost and that some services are beginning to consider a move away from functionalisation. As mentioned, the Bamford review has changed the landscape of mental healthcare in Northern Ireland. Long-stay beds have been closed and it is an aim that no one should have a hospital as their permanent address. This is providing some challenges, as community-based services have not fully evolved to meet the needs of some small groups of patients. Many trusts have, or are going to build, new mental health in-patient units on the same site as the general hospitals, although some asylum sites remain.

The workforce structure is similar to that found elsewhere in the UK. 'New Deal' provisions apply to trainees. There is a local contract for consultants that reflects the principles found elsewhere in terms of time, value and salary progression. However, local arrangements for clinical excellence awards restrict availability more than in mainland Britain.

The psychiatric workforce is largely drawn from local graduates who have trained locally. There is at present one university medical school, based in Belfast. Academic psychiatry posts in the university are only in general adult psychiatry. This insularity carries both risks and benefits. There have been relatively few unfilled consultant jobs. The narrow job market means that trainees in psychiatry take significant risks if they train in a smaller specialty as there are no guarantees that a job will become available at the end of training. Equally, trusts may find it difficult to recruit candidates to a specific job when no local trainee has been prepared for that job.

Education and training

Psychiatric training in the province is carried out under the aegis of the Postgraduate Medical Education and Training Board (PMETB). It is delivered as a province-wide scheme with local devolution at basic specialist level.

The Northern Ireland Medical and Dental Training Agency (NIMDTA) is an autonomous agency managed by the postgraduate dean, who is also the chief executive. The agency has a management board with a lay chair and includes a majority of lay members. Each large specialty has a training committee responsible for specialist training, from foundation years to completion of specialist training. The head of school for psychiatry coordinates training, which is led by a basic specialist training programme director (TPD) and higher training TPDs in each of the psychiatric disciplines. Each trust has educational supervisors and representation on the training board equivalent to previous College tutors. The training committee is keen to encourage the involvement of all doctors in psychiatry in training, practice development and management.

Legislation

The statutory basis for mental healthcare in the province is the Mental Health (Northern Ireland) Order, 1986. This allows for the detention of patients with mental disorder, their compulsory treatment, reception into guardianship, treatment of offenders with mental disorder and review by tribunals. The Order is supported by a code of practice and by rules for mental health review tribunals.

Mental disorder is defined as mental illness, mental handicap and any other disorder or disability of mind. The Order contains specific provisions that prevent compulsory admission of patients by reason only of personality disorder, substance misuse, sexual deviancy or immoral behaviour.

Action under the Order is triggered where a person suffers from a mental disorder of a nature *or* degree which warrants detention in a hospital *and* failure to so detain him or her would create a substantial likelihood of serious physical harm to him- or herself or to another person. This criterion of 'serious physical harm' – with no mention of welfare – and the specific exclusion of personality disorder make the conditions for detention the narrowest in the UK.

Compulsory admission to hospital follows an application by a patient's nearest relative (defined according to a hierarchy) or an approved social worker and is founded upon a medical recommendation which should usually be given by a medical practitioner who has had previous clinical knowledge of the patient. It is preferable that this is the patient's general practitioner. Only in exceptional circumstances should a doctor who is on the staff of the receiving hospital give the medical recommendation. It is not expected that the recommending doctor will be a psychiatrist or a general practitioner with specific training in psychiatry.

On admission, the patient will immediately be examined by a doctor. Consultants (approved under part II of the Order) may detain patients, in the first instance, for up to 7 days for assessment. Should a doctor not approved under part II examine the patient on admission, the initial period for assessment will be 48 hours. Further examination and report by a consultant psychiatrist may extend the period of assessment to a maximum total of 14 days.

Voluntary patients may be detained in hospital for up to 6 hours by an experienced nurse and 48 hours by a registered medical practitioner in order to allow an application for assessment to be made.

At any point during the period of assessment the patient may be detained for treatment. In order to proceed to detention for treatment, a part II approved consultant, usually the responsible medical officer, must report that the patient suffers from mental illness or severe mental impairment.

The definition of severe mental impairment has caused much controversy in recent years. Challenges mounted through the Northern Ireland Mental Health Review Tribunal sought to define the category in terms of measured intelligence quotient (IQ). Those mounting the challenges have suggested that patients with an IQ of greater than 55 should not be detained under the category of severe mental impairment.

In practice, consultant psychiatrists in intellectual disability viewed the legislative definition of severe mental impairment as a broad concept measuring patients' global functioning. The Royal College of Psychiatrists has produced a consensus statement reflecting the views of the profession locally that IQ measurement of itself is not the definition of severity of impairment and that evidence to tribunals should include factors which might cause a global estimate of impairment to be substantially different from measured IQ. At present, the outcomes of tribunal hearings continue to show that those who drew up the 1986 Order did not foresee this debate.

Reception into guardianship requires recommendations by two medical practitioners, one of whom should be a consultant psychiatrist, and an approved social worker. An application may be made on the grounds that a patient suffers from mental illness or severe mental handicap and it is necessary in the interests of the welfare of the patient that he or she should be so received. Guardianship allows the receiving trust to require the patient to reside at a specified place, to attend for treatment and to allow access to his or her residence at any time to any medical practitioner or approved social worker. It is most commonly used by intellectual disability services and has proven a valuable protection for those at risk of exploitation and abuse. There is no real sanction against patients who are disinclined to facilitate the trust's legal powers under guardianship.

Patients, or in some circumstances their relatives, may apply to the Mental Health Review Tribunal for discharge from hospital or guardianship at prescribed intervals. Treating trusts are obliged to refer patients to the Tribunal. A Tribunal hearing has a legal member, who presides, a medical member (experienced consultant psychiatrist) and a lay member (recruited by open advertisement), supported by a civil service secretariat. The Northern Ireland Mental Health Review Tribunal has consistently taken the view that it is for the treating trust to prove that the patient should remain detained or subject to guardianship.

The medical member of a Tribunal review performs an examination of the patient and reports the findings. Representatives of patients have questioned the apparent dual role of the medical member in both giving evidence and decision-making. It is presently believed to be compliant with European human rights legislation, providing the content of the examination is disclosed to both parties.

The Order defines three groups of treatments for the purposes of consent. Treatments that require the patient's consent and a second opinion are psychosurgery and the implantation of sex hormones. Treatments requiring either the patient's documented valid consent or a second opinion include electroconvulsive therapy (ECT) and the administration of medicines by any means but only after 3 months of such treatment. All other treatments may be administered to detained patients without either their consent or a second opinion. Treatment provided urgently to save life, to prevent deterioration or to prevent danger to the patient or others is exempt from the consent provisions.

The courts may, on conviction, order treatment in hospital with or without restriction. The Department of Justice, on receipt of reports by two medical practitioners, can also direct the transfer of sentenced or remand prisoners who suffer from mental disorder to a psychiatric hospital. In practice, such transfer directions are likely to take effect to the medium-secure unit at Knockbracken Healthcare Park on the south-eastern outskirts of Belfast.

Previous editions described how the Mental Health Commission for Northern Ireland had statutory responsibility to keep under review the care and treatment of patients. In discharging this duty it held Tribunal reviews, scrutinised legal forms, made announced and unannounced visits and enquired into cases where it believed there to be evidence of ill-treatment or deficiency of care. The Commission appointed medical members by interview following open advertisement; these medical members would be the medical members for Tribunal hearings and for second opinions for treatment under the Mental Health Order, as described above. Then, under the Health and Social Care Reform (Northern Ireland) Act 2009 the functions of the Mental Health Commission were transferred to the Regulation and Quality Improvement Authority (RQIA).

Several problems are evident with current mental health legislation. Patient groups have expressed concern that an apparently large proportion of patients who apply to the Tribunal find themselves regarded as having voluntary status before the hearing takes place. There is also the so-called 'Bournewood gap': this describes the position of patients who are not detained but who are not able to leave hospital; they are not covered by the Mental Health Order and as such are denied the protection of being able to apply to the Tribunal. The only capacity provisions in the legislation relate to property, finance and consent.

Future developments

Health and social care trusts continue to work to meet the challenges outlined by the Bamford review. Mental healthcare will continue to develop and the number of mental health in-patient beds is likely to continue to fall. The community care infrastructure will continue to need to develop to better support patients in the community and to reduce the need for admission to hospital. The role of psychiatric liaison services is gaining momentum. There is likely to be increased development of these services. We eagerly await the development of our capacity legislation but it is understandable that anxieties remain about the challenges this will present to services.

References

Bamford D (2004) *The Review of Mental Health and Learning Disability (Northern Ireland). A Strategic Framework for Adult Mental Health Services. Consultation Report.* Department of Health Social Services and Public Safety.

Compton J (2011) *Transforming Your Care. A Review of Health and Social Care in Northern Ireland.* Department of Health Social Services and Public Safety.

Donaldson L, Rutter P, Henderson M (2014) *The Right Time, the Right Place. An Expert Examination of the Application of Health and Social Care Governance Arrangements for Ensuring the Quality of Care Provision in Northern Ireland.* Department of Health Social Services and Public Safety.

CHAPTER 8

Mental health services in Scotland

Alastair Cook

In 1999 responsibility for all aspects of health policy and the organisation and management of the NHS in Scotland were devolved to the then newly formed Scottish Parliament. Since that time there has been a divergence of approach to healthcare policy and organisation between Scotland and the other jurisdictions of the UK. Some differences of approach and resourcing stretch back for far longer than this but the devolution of all responsibility for health to the Scottish Parliament in 1999 has allowed the divergence to become more marked. This chapter describes some of the main differences in organisational structures, regulation and management that have an impact on the way mental health services function and thus on the way the jobs of those working in them as psychiatrists are shaped.

The NHS in Scotland

The Scottish government is responsible for all matters relating to health policy and healthcare delivery in Scotland. The funding available for this is directly transferred to the Scottish government and forms part of a block grant, the amount of which is determined by the Treasury using what is known as the Barnett formula. In 2013/14 the budget for NHS Scotland amounted to £11.8 billion (of a total block grant allocated to Scotland of around £28 billion).

Legal responsibility for the delivery of healthcare in Scotland lies with the Scottish ministers and is framed in legislation through the National Health Service (Scotland) Act 1978. That Act opens with the statement: 'It is the duty of the Scottish Ministers to promote the improvement of the physical and mental health of the people of Scotland'. The minister in the Scottish government with lead responsibility for health is the Cabinet Secretary for Health and Sport, Scotland's equivalent to the Minister for Health. Responsibility for mental health and well-being tends to fall into the remit of a junior minister, the Minister for Mental Health.

The Scottish government manages health through the Scottish Government Health Directorates (SGHD), Scotland's equivalent of the Department of Health. The Directorates that make up the SGHD are headed by a director general who also holds the position of chief executive of NHS Scotland.

The Health Directorates are as follows:

- Finance, eHealth and Pharmaceuticals
- Health Workforce and Performance
- Chief Nursing Officer, Patients, Public and Health Professions
- Chief Medical Officer – Public Health and Sport
- Health and Social Care Integration
- Children and Families.

The directors of each of these directorates form a health management board that has responsibility for the running of the service. The mental health division sits within the Health and Social Care Integration Directorate.

The primary responsibility of the SGHD is to Scottish ministers and the civil service roles of the directorates include ensuring that ministers are briefed, parliamentary questions are responded to and the various parliamentary committees are serviced. The directorate teams also, however, have close linkages with local health boards and NHS staff are regularly seconded or transferred to the government departments where their specialist knowledge and expertise are needed and valued.

The SGHD sets policy across all aspects of health and social care. The directorates set targets and ensure the accountability of health boards to the Scottish ministers. The SGHD also has a role in developing staff governance, including working with employers (NHS boards) and unions to negotiate terms and conditions of service.

Health boards

There are 22 health boards in Scotland made up of 14 'territorial' boards responsible for an area of the country, 7 special health boards and 1 public health body that is responsible for a range of supporting and national activities.

The territorial boards are responsible for public health, well-being and service provision in their areas. The organisations vary hugely in size and scope. The largest, NHS Greater Glasgow and Clyde, covers a population of over 1.2 million, and has an annual budget in the region of £3.2 billion. This contrasts with smaller boards, such as the three island boards, Orkney, Shetland and Western Isles, each of which has a population below 30 000 and a budget in the region of £50 million.

The special health boards include NHS Education Scotland (NES) and Healthcare Improvement Scotland (HIS), both of which will be covered below. Another special board of particular relevance is the State Hospitals Board for Scotland, which is responsible for the State Hospital at Carstairs, South Lanarkshire, a high-secure forensic mental health facility that serves Scotland and Northern Ireland. NHS24 provides 24-hour access to healthcare advice and also serves as a host for services such as telephone counselling and electronic cognitive–behavioural therapy (e-CBT) services. The other special boards are the Scottish Ambulance Service, NHS Health Scotland (health improvement), the National Waiting Times Centre (elective surgery) and National Services Scotland (support services).

All the boards are headed by a board of directors, executive and non-executive, and they are directly accountable for their performance to the Cabinet Secretary. The chairs of boards and non-executive directors are selected through a public appointments process but then agreed by the Cabinet Secretary. Non-executive directors will usually include representatives of the local authorities. There are 32 local authorities in Scotland, mapping to the 14 territorial health boards. Some smaller boards have the same boundaries as their local authorities but many boards contain more than one local authority area, with Greater Glasgow and Clyde containing six.

The executive director team is headed by a chief executive, and will always include a board medical director and a director of nursing, midwifery and allied health professionals. Directors of finance, human resources and planning are usually present, as are directors with responsibility for operational areas of the service.

The territorial boards have a wide range of responsibility. Many have multiple acute hospitals and they all have mental health services; they are also responsible for primary care services and public health. The range of services means that boards in Scotland have developed quite differently from trusts in England. The benefits that should follow from the ability to take a whole-system approach are numerous, but can be offset by the fact that the business of boards is so wide-ranging that it is difficult for them to focus on the detail of some smaller services.

Boards operate through a series of operating divisions and committees. In most boards the acute services are managed through an acute operating division. Until 2016 community and primary care services were managed through community health partnerships (CHPs). These were created in the 2004 amendment to the NHS (Scotland) Act, and mental health and intellectual disability services were managed or hosted within CHPs. From 1 April 2016 the Public Bodies (Joint Working) (Scotland) Act 2014 introduced integrated health and social care partnerships across Scotland. Partnerships will take both operational and strategic control of mental health services.

Local development plans and HEAT targets

Health boards produce and agree a local development plan (LDP) with the Scottish government each year. The LDP sets out the work plan for the board in the year to come. The structure of the LDP varies from time to time but includes 'single outcome agreements', joint objectives that are shared with the local authorities covered by the board. It also includes detailed trajectories for how the various targets (outlined below) will be met. The LDP also covers finance, workforce and progress against other strategic programmes.

Boards are set targets on an annual basis and must detail in the LDP how they intend to achieve these. Targets in Scotland are grouped under the headings 'Health', 'Efficiency', 'Access' and 'Treatment', hence the acronym HEAT. The value or otherwise of targets as a driver for service improvement is as controversial in Scotland as it is in the rest of the UK. In recent years the Scottish government has moved many of its 'targets' to become 'standards' that boards are expected to sustain as opposed to targets that must be achieved.

Until 2006 boards were not formally set targets that were directly applicable to mental health services. There was concern that the lack of targets could actually disadvantage mental health services in the recognition of their priority at board level, so since that time the Scottish government has tried, with varying degrees of success, to set targets that are designed to ensure boards give appropriate attention to mental health services.

As an example, in 2014/15 the targets that boards had to meet that were directly relevant to mental health were as follows:

- To deliver faster access to mental health services by delivering 26 weeks' referral to treatment for specialist child and adolescent mental health services (CAMHS) from March 2013, reducing to 18 weeks from December 2014; and 18 weeks' referral to treatment for psychological therapies from December 2014.
- To deliver expected rates of dementia diagnosis and by 2015/16 for all people newly diagnosed with dementia to have a minimum of a year's worth of post-diagnostic support coordinated by a link worker, including a person-centred support plan.

Standards included:

- 90% of clients will wait no longer than 3 weeks from referral received to appropriate drug or alcohol treatment that supports their recovery.
- NHS boards and alcohol and drug partnerships (ADPs) will sustain and embed alcohol brief interventions (ABI) in the three priority settings (primary care, accident and emergency, antenatal), in accordance with the Scottish Intercollegiate Guidelines Network (SIGN) Guideline 74. In addition, they will continue to develop delivery of alcohol brief interventions in wider settings.

As well as the directly relevant targets and standards, mental health services are expected to contribute to other general targets and standards, such as meeting financial requirements, reducing greenhouse gas emissions and managing sickness absence in staff, as well as contributing to clinical targets that are set across the health system, including reductions in delayed discharges, reducing emergency in-patient days for people aged over 75 and of course ensuring that 98% of patients leave the emergency department within 4 hours.

Policy context: '2020 Vision', the 'Quality Strategy' and the Scottish Patient Safety Programme

As well as targets and standards, health boards are also guided by numerous policy documents and national programmes (see 'Useful links' at the end of the chapter). The policy context within mental health is covered in more detail below, but overarching health policy in Scotland is largely driven by the 2020 Vision for Health and Social Care. The policy document states:

> 'Our vision is that by 2020 everyone is able to live longer healthier lives at home, or in a homely setting. We will have a healthcare system where we have integrated health and social care, a focus on prevention, anticipation and supported self management. When hospital treatment is required, and cannot be provided in a community setting, day case treatment will be the norm. Whatever the setting, care will be provided to the highest standards of quality and safety, with the person at the centre of all decisions. There will be a focus on ensuring that people get back into their home or community environment as soon as appropriate, with minimal risk of re-admission'.

The other key driver of healthcare policy in Scotland is the Healthcare Quality Strategy for NHS Scotland. Published in 2010, the Quality Strategy sets out three 'quality ambitions', which are normally shortened to: person centred, safe and effective. In full, they are:

* Mutually beneficial partnerships between patients, their families and those delivering healthcare services which respect individual needs and values and which demonstrate compassion, continuity, clear communication and shared decision-making.
* There will be no avoidable injury or harm to people from the healthcare they receive, and an appropriate, clean and safe environment will be provided for the delivery of healthcare services at all times.
* The most appropriate treatments, interventions, support and services will be provided at the right time to everyone who will benefit, and wasteful or harmful variation will be eradicated.

These ambitions are at the centre of the objectives of all health boards in Scotland and all other policy is set in the context of this, with most boards declaring themselves to be 'quality-driven' organisations.

One unique programme in Scotland that has influence across the health spectrum is worthy of note here. The Scottish Patient Safety Programme (SPSP) aims systematically to improve the safety and reliability of hospital care throughout Scotland. By building capacity and capability in the improvement methodology, the aim is to develop a sustainable infrastructure for continuous quality improvement. Scotland was the first country to take this strategic, national approach to improving patient safety. The aim of the SPSP is to reduce adverse events by 30% and mortality by 15%, improving everyday practice. The Programme aims to do this while recognising the complexities involved in delivering modern healthcare and the need to standardise an approach to making care safer.

In its initial stages, from 2007, the Programme largely focused on acute care, but since 2009 it has moved into other areas, including maternity care and, more recently, primary care. The SPSP – Mental Health was launched in 2012 and is described in more detail below.

The board medical director

In contrast to the position in England, where medically trained chief executives are not uncommon, doctors in leadership and management positions in Scotland are mostly but not exclusively within a clear medical leadership framework. The Chief Medical Officer is the senior doctor in Scotland, and has a leadership role across the profession. Within health boards the key leadership role is that of the board medical director.

In Scotland, the board medical director is the responsible officer for revalidation purposes, making revalidation recommendations to the General Medical Council (GMC) for all non-training-grade doctors employed by their organisation, in primary and secondary care. The board medical director of NES is the responsible officer for all training-grade doctors in Scotland.

Board medical directors usually carry a portfolio that will include clinical governance, quality improvement and patient safety, medical staffing and workforce planning, as well as differing degrees of operational responsibility for the management of the doctors in the organisation. Most boards have a medical leadership structure that includes divisional and/or associate medical directors with responsibility for different parts of the organisation. In most of the medium and large boards, the senior medical leadership role in mental health services sits with an associate medical director.

The board structure in Scotland means that boards have a role both as commissioners and as providers of all services in their local area. This requires board medical directors to develop an understanding of services across primary care, acute hospital care and mental health services and to report on all of these to the board regularly.

Medical education and training

The Medical Act, which establishes the GMC as regulator of the profession, is UK legislation that applies in Scotland. This gives the GMC the same responsibility in Scotland as elsewhere for the regulation of medical education and training at undergraduate and postgraduate level, as well as its other duties.

Scotland has five undergraduate medical schools, which produce approximately 850 new medical graduates each year. Postgraduate training for doctors and all other healthcare professionals is managed by NES, which was formed in 2002 to provide a single leadership focus for all healthcare education in Scotland. The UK Tooke report (Modernising Medical Careers Inquiry, 2008) suggested NES was an example of good practice and it became the blueprint for what is now Health Education England.

NES originally contained four distinct medical deaneries, based around the four larger medical schools (Glasgow, Edinburgh, Aberdeen and Dundee). Each deanery provided reports to the GMC and had developed training programmes at core and higher level in all the major specialties. Since 2014, NES has been a single deanery for regulatory purposes, although it is committed to retaining its regional focus, training programmes in major specialties in each region and has retained, for now at least, four postgraduate deans.

Health boards are local educational providers and medical education and training at board level are led by a director of medical education (DME). The DME is responsible for the quality management of training across undergraduate and postgraduate placements, in hospitals and in the community, including general practice.

NES has a well-developed advisory structure that involves specialty training boards (STBs), which cover broad specialty areas in medicine. The STB for Mental Health brings together representatives from each region and psychiatric specialty and service, including trainee representatives, as well as representatives of the Royal College of Psychiatrists and the British Medical Association (BMA). The STBs provide advice to NES and through them to the SGHDs on workforce numbers, recruitment and retention and on quality improvement of training in Scotland.

NES and the Scottish NHS were contributors, along with the rest of the UK services, to the Greenaway report, *Securing the Future of Excellent Patient Care* (Greenaway, 2013), and it is expected that reforms resulting from implementation of that report will apply equally in Scotland as they do in the rest of the UK.

Mental health service provision

Other than the State Hospital, NHS mental health services in Scotland are managed by the 14 territorial health boards. Within those boards, primary and community care services are managed through health and social care partnerships (HSCPs), formed following the enactment of the Public Bodies (Joint Working) (Scotland) Bill 2014. Most services involving secondary care and therefore psychiatrists in Scotland have been retained within full NHS control as part of the HSCPs. In every board area the mental health services manage all or nearly all secondary care services for mental health, intellectual disability and addictions.

111

Most Scottish health boards (excluding two of the island boards) have dedicated in-patient provision for adult and old age psychiatry and variable models for managing in-patient provision for children and young people, forensic care, intellectual disability, rehabilitation and other subspecialist provision. There is a mix of dedicated psychiatric hospitals and psychiatric units on general hospital sites, largely dependent on how organisations have developed within the different boards. Some boards have moved towards split working for consultants in in-patient or community jobs but many have retained a sector-based model, with consultants working both in hospitals and in the community.

Most acute hospital services have liaison psychiatry support to a greater or lesser extent. Liaison services tend to be better developed in the largest boards, which have direct links with medical schools.

Community services are generally based around the model of a community mental health team (CMHT). The CMHT model in Scotland varies from board to board, with some adult teams following a path of specialisation into assertive outreach or crisis resolution/home treatment teams, while others have retained a more generic approach, usually with some form of primary/secondary care split. Psychological therapy services are generally managed within the same service, with variable degrees of integration into local CMHT models.

As well as adult CMHTs, most boards will have multidisciplinary or multi-agency community teams working in old age mental health, addiction, child and adolescent mental health, forensic services, medical psychotherapy and intellectual disability services.

In summary, much of the mental health service provision in Scotland would look very familiar to a psychiatrist working elsewhere in the UK. The major difference is the lack of commissioning and the fact that almost all secondary care service provision is directly managed by the local NHS board in partnership with local authorities.

Policy

Mental health policy in Scotland is set by the Scottish government. The Mental Health Strategy for Scotland 2012–2015 brought together a strategy for service development and delivery and a strategy for mental health improvement. This unified strategy superseded two previous overarching policy documents, *Delivering for Mental Health* (2006) and *Towards a Mentally Flourishing Scotland* (2008). A new Strategy for 2016 onwards is due to be published later in 2016.

There have been a number of key policy initiatives over the time of these documents that have shaped mental health services and also increased the profile of mental health improvement initiatives. Notable examples include:

- work to reduce the stigma of mental illness, including the 'See Me' campaign and the Scottish Mental Health Arts and Film Festival

- improved access to telephone support, managed through NHS24 and including 'Breathing Space' and 'Living Life' guided self-help and telephone CBT
- coordinated action between health services, local authorities and the voluntary sector to reduce suicide, including the 'Choose Life' initiative, targets and standards for NHS boards and a suicide prevention strategy launched late in 2013
- a dementia strategy for Scotland, now in its second iteration
- workforce developments leading to improvements in access to CAMHS and psychological therapies.

The 2012–2015 strategy built on the successes of the previous years and aligned mental health with the goals set out in the 2020 Vision and Quality Strategy described above. The 2016 strategy is likely to continue this pattern.

A good example of the linkage of new initiatives to wider strategic goals has been the development of the SPSP – Mental Health. This sits within the wider SPSP, which aims to reduce avoidable harm in healthcare settings. All boards in Scotland are participants in the Programme, with in-patient wards working on one of four areas: improving risk assessment and management, restraint and seclusion, medicines management or communication at transitions. All participating wards also contribute to work on leadership and culture. Learning is shared nationally through the Programme's website and regular online meetings, as well as through national meetings for participants. Data are collected from all participating wards and will in due course allow a national overview of progress that can be evidenced by improved outcomes.

Regulation

Healthcare Improvement Scotland (HIS) is a special NHS board set up to monitor and regulate the NHS and the independent healthcare sector in Scotland. Its stated purpose is to support healthcare providers in Scotland to deliver high-quality, evidence-based, safe, effective and person-centred care; and to scrutinise those services to provide public assurance about the quality and safety of that care.

HIS's work in mental health includes hosting the SPSP – Mental Health described above, and leading a national development programme for integrated care pathways. HIS also supports a suicide review team, which receives reports on every completed suicide of those who have been in contact with mental health services in the 12 months preceding their death. HIS also runs inspection programmes that currently focus on healthcare environments and older people's care but will conduct reviews and inspections where these are triggered by concerns.

The Mental Welfare Commission for Scotland (MWC) was established as part of the Mental Health (Scotland) Act 1960 and has retained its role as an independent organisation working to safeguard the rights and interests of people with a mental disorder since that time. The MWC has responsibility for monitoring the use of the Mental Health Act in Scotland and it regularly visits services, providing advice, support and sometimes making recommendations for changes. The MWC also visits individual patients subject to compulsory treatment or guardianship and will make recommendations for changes in care plans or treatment if these are thought to be indicated. Commission visitors meet annually with senior health board officials to discuss the year's activities in their board and receive updates on progress against any recommendations made. In the event of a serious incident or a possible deficiency in care, the MWC has the power to investigate, report and make recommendations. MWC reports are published and all boards will review the recommendations within them to assess their applicability to their own service.

As well as its regulatory role, the MWC can be a valuable source of advice for psychiatrists and other healthcare professionals, particularly on matters relating to the application of the legislation. The MWC also has a role in promoting good practice, and shaping and influencing mental healthcare policy through its links with the Scottish government.

Mental health legislation in Scotland

Legislation relating to mental health, incapacity and adult support and protection is fully devolved to the Scottish Parliament and while many of the principles are similar to their equivalents in the rest of the UK, the administration and practical application of the legislation will differ considerably.

A description of the different powers and the interrelationship between these pieces of legislation is beyond the scope of this chapter. The MWC website is probably the best source of material for those who require further information.

Mental Health (Care and Treatment) (Scotland) Act 2003

This came into force in 2005 and was widely regarded as a good example of mental health legislation. The Act is based on the application of principles, which include informing the person, encouraging patient participation and taking account of patients' views. They emphasise the importance of benefit, using the least restrictive option, and include a principle of reciprocity. The Act moved civil procedures under mental health law from the court system into a newly created Mental Health Tribunal for Scotland.

The Act created the role of an 'approved medical practitioner' (AMP) and only an AMP can perform certain duties. A psychiatrist wishing to act as an AMP must undergo training and be named on a list that is maintained by health boards on behalf of the Scottish government. To become an

AMP, psychiatrists must have obtained membership of the Royal College of Psychiatrists or have 4 years of experience in psychiatry and the support of their medical director. Psychiatrists who meet these criteria still need to complete AMP training before they are legally able to undertake duties as an AMP.

Adults With Incapacity (Scotland) Act 2000

This provides a legal framework for financial and welfare interventions for adults who lack capacity. It is also built on a clear set of principles, including benefit, least restrictive option and taking account of the views of the person and carers as far as possible. The Act defines incapacity as being incapable of acting, or making decisions, or retaining the memory of decisions.

Adult Support and Protection (Scotland) Act 2007

This seeks to protect and benefit adults at risk of being harmed. The Act requires councils and a range of public bodies to work together to support and protect adults who are unable to safeguard themselves, their property and their rights. It provides a range of measures which they can use. The public bodies are required to work together to take steps to decide whether someone is an adult at risk of harm, balancing the need to intervene with an adult's right to live as independently as possible.

The Royal College of Psychiatrists in Scotland

The UK College established an office in Scotland in 1994 to support the activities of an increasingly active Scottish Division. With devolution in 1999, the need for a separate Scottish office became greater, as the Scottish Parliament began to develop mental health legislation and policy and as services in Scotland began to differ more from those in the rest of the UK.

The Royal College of Psychiatrists in Scotland (RCPsychiS) mirrors much of the College organisation at UK level, with faculties and interest groups, all of which organise and run active academic programmes. There is a particularly active medical managers group attended by associate medical directors and clinical directors from all the health boards; it is also attended by officials from the Mental Health Department of the Scottish government. In this way RCPsychiS facilitates close linkages between the policy generated by government and the services being delivered by psychiatrists at ground level. This is one of the advantages of working in a system that is small enough to allow key leaders from around the country to meet regularly.

RCPsychiS is also very active in trying to influence the political agenda. The College is a regular attendee at party conferences, in cross-party groups in the Scottish Parliament, and at meetings with MPs and with other organisations and groups that are influential in the mental health field in Scotland. RCPsychiS is part of the Academy of Medical Royal Colleges and Faculties in Scotland and as such plays a part in the wider leadership of the medical profession in Scotland.

As with the rest of the UK, involvement with College activity in Scotland is frequently a starting point for those who subsequently go on to accept leadership and management roles. Scotland sends six representatives (core and higher trainees from three regions) to the UK College Psychiatric Trainees Committee and all are invited to meetings of the executive committee of RCPsychiS and encouraged to participate in the wider work of the College.

Leadership and management opportunities in Scotland

NHS Scotland has a leadership framework, supported by a National Leadership Unit, hosted by NES; NES and the leadership unit deliver a range of modules and courses that are targeted at all levels within Scotland.

All trainees working towards the Certificate of Completion of Training (CCT) in all specialties are encouraged to access NES's Leadership and Management Programme (LaMP). Many Colleges offer leadership events and courses, including one for higher trainees in psychiatry organised by RCPsychiS. NES also hosts 'clinical leadership fellow' posts that allow trainees to be out of programme in a leadership role for a year.

Consultants with an interest can apply for courses supported by the National Leadership Unit or access resources available through their local boards. The Faculty of Medical Leadership and Management is active in Scotland as in the rest of the UK and many doctors access its conferences, events and online resources.

For those psychiatrists who take up a management role, the RCPsychiS medical managers group can provide a source of information, support and advice.

Summary

The system in Scotland is different in many ways from that in the rest of the UK but most doctors transferring between the countries would quickly adapt to those differences. The smaller size of the healthcare system in Scotland gives both advantages, in that it is relatively easy to bring leaders together, and disadvantages, in that there are fewer posts at senior level. The importance of trainee and consultant psychiatrists developing as leaders and managers and using those skills to advance the cause of improving mental health and well-being is recognised just as much in Scotland as it is in the rest of the UK.

References

Greenaway D (2013) *Securing the Future of Excellent Patient Care*. Shape of Training. Available at http://www.shapeoftraining.co.uk/static/documents/content/Shape_of_training_FINAL_Report.pdf_53977887.pdf (accessed May 2016).

Modernising Medical Careers Inquiry (2008) *Aspiring to Excellence* (Tooke report). Available at http://www.asit.org/assets/documents/MMC_FINAL_REPORT_REVD_4jan.pdf (accessed May 2016).

Useful links

NHSScotland 2020 Local Delivery Plan Guidance
http://www.scotland.gov.uk/Publications/2013/11/4395

The Healthcare Quality Strategy for NHS Scotland
http://www.scotland.gov.uk/Publications/2010/05/10102307

A Route Map to the 2020 Vision for Health and Social Care
http://www.scotland.gov.uk/Resource/0042/00423188.pdf

The Scottish Patient Safety Programme
http://www.scottishpatientsafetyprogramme.scot.nhs.uk

Mental Health Strategy for Scotland: 2012–2015
http://www.gov.scot/Publications/2012/08/9714/0

Delivering for Mental Health
http://www.gov.scot/Publications/2006/11/30164829/0

Towards a Mentally Flourishing Scotland
http://www.scotland.gov.uk/Resource/Doc/271822/0081031.pdf

Scottish Government: Suicide Prevention Strategy 2013–2016
http://www.gov.scot/Publications/2013/12/7616

CHAPTER 9

Mental health services in Wales: policy, legislation and governance

Rob Poole and Manel Tippett

Welsh devolution

The process of devolution in Wales has been described as 'cautious' by Welsh politicians and their English counterparts. Devolution has been far more rapid in Scotland and Northern Ireland, primarily because of historical differences; for example, prior to devolution they had separate legal systems, whereas Wales was fully subsumed into 'England and Wales'. However, in recent years Welsh politics, policy and legislation have diverged from England at an increasing pace. Wales has obtained significant legislative and financial powers, but it remains far from autonomous. Welsh mental health services operate in conditions that in some respects are similar to or the same as those in England, but which in other respects are very different.

Under the Government of Wales Act 1998, a new National Assembly for Wales ('the Assembly') with 60 Assembly Members (AMs) was established as the legislative arm of government. The Assembly was given secondary legislative powers in 20 'conferred areas', including health and health services. At first, the Welsh Assembly government was a committee of the Assembly. In law it had no executive power. It had only those powers that the Assembly as a whole voted to delegate to ministers. The Government of Wales Act 2006 gave the Assembly limited primary law-making powers on some matters in specific areas. These laws were known as 'Assembly measures', and they required the approval of the UK Parliament in the form of Legislative Consent Orders. The same Act also formally recognised a division between the Assembly and the Welsh Assembly government, creating an executive branch of government that is now called the Welsh Government. A referendum in 2011 gave the National Assembly further primary law-making powers. These are known as 'Acts of the Assembly', and they become law without UK parliamentary approval. However, many areas of domestic policy continue to be legislated across England and Wales by the UK Parliament.

The Wales Act 2014 granted further powers over some taxes and in relation to housing debt. The system of conferred areas has caused confusion over what is, and what is not, under the authority of the Welsh Government. In place of this system of devolved powers, the UK government plans to move to a system of exemptions. It proposes a list of 'reservations' – areas that will remain under the authority of Westminster, all other powers being devolved. Scotland and Northern Ireland have a similar system, but there has been opposition within the Welsh Assembly to the finer details of the Bill, as many AMs believe that it will reduce the Assembly's powers.

The health portfolio in Wales is held by the Minister for Health and Social Care, supported by the Welsh Government's Health and Social Services Directorate. As part of the remit, the minister is responsible for the provision of services to people in Wales who are mentally ill. The Health and Social Care Committee at the Welsh Assembly undertakes inquiries and scrutinises Welsh Government performance and Welsh legislation on health-related matters. The Welsh Assembly has cross-party groups that hold broad remits. Many are relevant to psychiatry, including mental health, autism, dementia, eating disorders, neurological conditions, older people and ageing.

Up to 2016, four political parties have been represented within the Assembly: Welsh Labour, Welsh Liberal Democrats, Plaid Cymru and the Welsh Conservatives. All parties apart from the Welsh Conservatives have been proponents of devolution to varying degrees. However, Welsh Labour has had unrivalled influence on its realisation. Not only is Welsh Labour the largest political party in Wales, it is also the most successful in electoral terms. Welsh Labour has won the largest share of the popular vote at every Welsh Assembly election since 1999. It has led the Assembly since its inception, albeit sometimes in coalition. Although it would be wrong to construe this as a political monoculture, the consequence has been that Welsh Labour has enjoyed a high degree of control over policy formation and implementation within the devolved areas, including in public health and health services.

In May 2016, UK Independence Party (UKIP) AMs were elected for the first time. The party is opposed to devolution. It is too soon to know what impact they will have on Welsh health policy.

The management and governance structure of the NHS in Wales

Regular restructuring and reorganisation are fixed features of the NHS across the UK. However, over the past 20 years Wales has experienced a particularly large number of structural changes in the management and governance of health services. Between 1996 and 2010, NHS Wales underwent four major reconfigurations of organisations and services providing healthcare, resulting in a constant state of instability in terms of planning, commissioning and funding of services.

In 1996, eight district health authorities and eight family health authorities merged to form five new health authorities, which acted as purchasers and contract negotiators of health services. The providers of acute care were almost exclusively NHS trusts in Wales, although there was some cross-border provision in England. As in England, long-stay psychiatric beds were increasingly provided in independent-sector facilities. In 1999, 22 local health boards were created, ostensibly to bring together health professionals, local government and the voluntary sector in order to improve integration of health and social care services. Each local health board was coterminous with one of the 22 unitary local authorities in Wales. In April 2003, the health authorities were abolished. Their responsibilities were divided between the local health boards and the National Assembly. Just 6 years later, in October 2009, there was a root-and-branch reconfiguration of the NHS in Wales. Twenty-two local health boards and 13 NHS trusts were reorganised to create seven new local health boards.

Although the terminology of 'local health boards' was retained, the new organisations are much larger and more complex than old local health boards. The new organisations are generally known as health boards, and we shall use this term here for clarity. They are responsible for both planning and delivering all NHS healthcare services within their geographical boundaries. Anticipating economies of scale, management infrastructure was reduced. The division between commissioning and providing was abolished, except with respect to highly specialised and tertiary services. The Welsh Health Specialist Services Committee (WHSSC) now commissions such services centrally, which in mental health includes medium- and high-security services, and gender dysphoria and eating disorder services.

With respect to exposure to market pressures, Welsh services have moved in exactly the opposite direction to England, where foundation trusts proliferate and increasingly compete with non-NHS organisations to provide services. The health boards' main roles are: corporate and clinical governance; securing and providing primary and community care health services; securing secondary care services; improving the health of communities; partnership; public engagement; and provision of services.

In Wales, there are no separate NHS mental health organisations analogous to English mental health and social care trusts. In 1999, community and mental health services across Wales were absorbed into generic NHS trusts that delivered acute, community and mental health services. More recently, health boards have been responsible for delivering mental health services in primary and secondary care through close collaboration with local authorities (a health board may provide services to a geographical area containing up to nine local authorities). In keeping with UK national trends, there has been a general move of mental health services from the hospital setting and into the community, although this tended to occur later and more slowly in Wales than in England. Wales put increased resources into crisis resolution, home treatment and assertive outreach services while reducing the number of in-patient beds both for adults and for children. As in England, enthusiasm for specialist teams has waned, but in Wales this has been influenced by the demands of the Mental Health Measure (see below).

Challenges faced by the NHS in Wales

Wales receives a sum of money from the UK government to run public services. Under the Barnett formula, introduced in 1980, funds for Wales are allocated on the basis of a rudimentary formula linked to English per capita expenditure. Thus changes to programmes in England result in changes in budget for Wales, calculated on the basis of population size and not population need (House of Commons, 1998). The money is allocated as a lump sum. The devolved administration is responsible for determining how these funds are distributed according to priorities that it sets.

Wales (and indeed the other Celtic jurisdictions) benefited from this arrangement in the early 2000s when there was persistent growth in the UK economy. The Assembly inherited a £2.5 billion budget for the NHS in 1999. This grew by 50%, to £3.8 billion, within 2 years (see http://www.wales.nhs.uk/news/599). This allowed the Welsh Government to introduce initiatives such as free prescriptions and free parking in hospitals. The economic depression following the banking crisis of 2007 has led to reductions in public expenditure in England that have resulted in reductions of £1.7 billion in the overall budget for Wales, and this trend is unlikely to change in the foreseeable future. However, Welsh Labour has made a strong commitment to protecting the NHS, which has been relatively spared from budget reductions. Since 2008, the budget for NHS expenditure has remained at around £6 billion, and the Welsh Government promised an additional £570 million to be allocated to the NHS over the three years 2013–2016 (see http://www.bbc.co.uk/news/uk-wales-24450817).

The NHS in Wales is nevertheless facing major financial pressures, necessitating a change in priorities and in patterns of service delivery. *Together for Health* was the Welsh Government's 5-year strategy for the NHS in Wales. It aimed to address financial problems and other pressures, including a growing elderly population, changes in clinical practice, enduring health inequalities, an increase in the number of people with chronic illnesses and poor organisational performance (Welsh Government, 2011: p. 1). The main plans outlined in the strategy were:[1]

- service modernisation, including specialist 'centres of excellence' and providing more care close to home
- addressing health inequalities

---

1. See http://wales.gov.uk/topics/health/publications/health/reports/together/?lang=en.

- better information technology systems and an information strategy to improve care for patients
- improving quality of care
- workforce development
- instigating a 'compact with the public'
- a changed financial regime.

It was intended that the strategy would modernise the NHS in Wales and improve the health of the country by giving better access to improved and safer services.

In 2011, the NHS in Wales responded to the strategy by commissioning Marcus Longley, Professor of Applied Health Policy and Director of the Welsh Institute for Health and Social Care, to review the state of the NHS. The purpose was to determine what factors were influencing changes in service provision, and to provide possible solutions. Some of the main findings of the review (Longley, 2012) were that:

- the current configuration of hospital services does not deliver the best outcomes for patients uniformly across Wales
- service quality needs to be improved if Wales is to have services comparable to the best healthcare systems in the world
- unless action is taken quickly, the shortage of medical staff in some services is likely to lead to the unplanned closure of those services
- the increasing specialisation of some types of services means that centralising expert clinical staff leads to better patient outcomes in these specialties
- the nature of healthcare means that many hospital services are interdependent and outcomes for patients could be improved if certain types of services were brought together onto one site
- the impact of longer travelling distances as a result of centralisation can be lessened by boosting pre-hospital care, using telemedicine more widely and effectively, and providing better transport links.

Following the publication of the review, the Welsh Government required local health boards to draft individual programmes to describe how they planned to meet the objectives that had been set out. The approach that was favoured by the authors of the report and supported by the Minister for Health and Social Care was: centralisation of specialist services; concentrating resources on fewer but better facilities in a reduced number of locations; and developing and extending community services. The Welsh National Specialist Advisory Group on Mental Health and the Royal College of Psychiatrists in Wales emphasised that health board reconfiguration plans must take into account and support other plans for change and modernisation of mental health services.

As in other areas of the UK, the NHS in Wales is facing a recruitment and retention crisis across a number of medical disciplines. Many areas are affected by a low uptake of training and consultant posts. This is a particular concern in psychiatry. In Wales, regions that are relatively far from urban areas have particular problems. Marcus Longley wrote in his report:

> 'There are now acute pressures on medical staffing in paediatrics, emergency medicine, core surgical training and psychiatry, and more generally in some of the more remote parts of Wales. A 'perfect storm' has developed, with more doctors in our hospitals, but actually less availability in comparison with the demand for their services.' (Longley, 2012: p. 3)

Mental health policy and legislation

Together for mental health

In 2012, the Welsh Government published its new mental health strategy for Wales, *Together for Mental Health*, in conjunction with its overall strategy, *Together for Health*. The strategy was devised through a collaborative approach with third-sector organisations and gained cross-party support, which reflects uniformity in the views of the political parties in Wales regarding mental health provision. Unlike previous mental health strategies, *Together for Mental Health* encompasses all ages in order to promote better mental health and well-being in the population as a whole. It addresses the needs of people with mental health problems and impairments regardless of age, sexual orientation, marital status, gender and so on. The strategy will be overseen by an implementation panel, the National Partnership Board, led by the Welsh Government, with representation from service users and carers, professional groups and the voluntary sector.

Stakeholder comments on the strategy have been published and show that many commended the Welsh Government and the political parties for their unanimous support for improvement in services for people with mental health conditions. However, many commented that the strategy has outcomes that were too numerous, too broad and too 'high level', making implementation very difficult to monitor effectively. The Royal College of Psychiatrists in Wales was concerned that the outcomes were too ambitious and that lines of accountability were unclear. Welsh mental health policy has shown these weaknesses before, which the College believes have contributed to a lack of progress in the development of service despite sincere good intentions.

The Mental Health (Wales) Measure

Together for Mental Health was drafted against the backdrop of the imminent implementation of the Mental Health (Wales) Measure 2010. The Measure was pioneering legislation in two senses. It was the first Welsh Measure to be made law, and it is unique in international mental health law in establishing positive legal rights for service users and obligations on service providers that, for the most part, are not directly related to detention or compulsory treatment. Like the mental health strategy, the Measure gained cross-party support. Its content was heavily influenced by the mental health charities and voluntary organisations. The Measure passed through the Assembly and received royal assent in 2010. It was implemented in stages through 2012.

The Measure places statutory duties on local mental health partners (health boards and local authorities) to meet the needs of people in primary care and secondary mental healthcare. It aims to ensure more efficient services in primary care, particularly timely assessment and referral. It prescribes the style of services for patients in secondary care ('relevant patients') to give them greater ownership of their treatment and recovery. The Measure sets out a right of 'relevant patients' to re-refer themselves back into the services after discharge without the need for the involvement of their general practitioner. Finally, the Measure extends advocacy services under the Mental Health Act 1983 to all 'relevant patients', effectively to nearly all situations where the Mental Health Act is used. Like the mental health strategy, the Measure prescribes a holistic approach in planning care for the patient and it places an emphasis on personal ownership of recovery.

The Measure places a new set of responsibilities and statutory duties on psychiatrists working in Wales. Part 2 of the Measure states that care coordinators must complete care and treatment plans for all relevant patients. These plans must be reviewed at regular intervals. Care and treatment plans replace the Care Programme Approach (and unified assessments for those with intellectual disability). Mental health charities in Wales lobbied heavily that there should be a strong emphasis on a holistic approach. They were instrumental in devising the care and treatment plans, so that they cover eight areas of the patient's life:

- accommodation
- education and training
- finance and money
- medical and other forms of treatment
- parenting or caring responsibilities
- personal care and physical well-being
- social, cultural and spiritual concerns
- work and occupation.

They were keen for there to be a requirement to cover all eight areas. After a public consultation, and in the light of a range of concerns raised by the healthcare professions, it was decided that at least one area must be covered in all cases.

The Royal College of Psychiatrists in Wales expressed concerns regarding the implications of the legislation throughout the drafting and consultation processes. Legislating for good clinical practice made many psychiatrists uneasy. There were concerns that the good intentions of the Measure would be difficult to deliver and that there could be unintended adverse consequences. The College surveyed its members in Wales and over 120 responded. They reported that organisational fear of legal action where new care and treatment planning requirements were not met had resulted in an inappropriate movement of staff and patients from mental health services into primary care teams. They reported reluctance among many health professionals to take on the role of care coordinator, the role falling disproportionately upon psychiatrists. General adult psychiatrists reported reduced patient contact to cope with the burden of new paperwork.

In December 2013, the Welsh Government published its first annual report on the Together for Mental Health strategy, which briefly claimed success in the uptake of care and treatment planning and that positive feedback had been received from patients about the new process of treatment planning. This provoked many other mental health organisations to raise their own concerns about the Measure. They complained that there was too much emphasis on meeting targets for completing care and treatment plans and too little emphasis on monitoring the impact on patient outcomes. They shared the concern that patients were being systematically moved to primary care services.

The Welsh Government had a statutory duty to review the Measure. The final report was published in December 2015, based on evidence presented from a variety of sources (Welsh Government, 2015). The report proposed legal and implementation changes to the Measure, which would: extend Part 3 (a right of reassessment on patient request) to children and young people; broaden the definition of care coordinator to include a wider range of health professionals (such as paediatric nurses and counsellors); expand the list of health professionals able to conduct primary care mental health assessments; introduce the systematic monitoring of access to psychological therapies; and re-evaluate the content of care and treatment plans to reflect the needs of specific groups. The report recommended that a working group oversee the implementation of its recommendations.

Some psychiatrists feel that the Measure has negatively affected patient care. It is unclear whether these are short-term transitional problems or whether there are going to be permanent difficulties. If so, these may be difficult to resolve because of the statutory nature of the Measure.

Scrutiny of services and influencing policy

With devolution, Wales has seen the establishment of several bodies whose remit is to scrutinise and influence policy and legislative decision-making. Official inspection and regulatory bodies, charitable and third-sector organisations, and professional organisations, including the medical Royal Colleges, have become lobbying groups with direct involvement with Welsh Government officials and policy-makers. Most of these began as regional offices of their parent organisations, usually based in London. Over the years they have gained increased autonomy in recognition of the changing political climate and increasing differences between Wales and England.

The NHS in Wales is inspected and regulated by two main bodies: Health Inspectorate Wales (HIW) and the Wales Audit Office (WAO). The remit of both HIW and the WAO is to report on the quality of service provision to the National Assembly for Wales, and both are intended to work independently of government.

HIW is part of the Welsh Government and works on behalf of Welsh ministers. A significant element of HIW's work is to provide regular review of the use of the Mental Health Act. HIW also oversees the 'deprivation of liberty' safeguards. HIW takes the role of external scrutiny of investigation of homicides committed by people under the care of the mental health and intellectual disability services. In 2014, HIW's role was reviewed by the National Assembly's Health and Social Care Committee, which looked into its functions, responsibilities, accountabilities and relationships. The Committee reported back a number of recommendations for improvement (Health and Social Care Committee, 2014).

The WAO is led by the Auditor General for Wales, who reports to the Assembly's Public Accounts Committee. The WAO conducts detailed value-for-money investigations into government expenditure, providing bespoke pieces of work culminating in reports presented to the National Assembly's Public Accounts Committee.

There have been a number of national reports concerning mental health services. In 2005, the WAO conducted a baseline review of adult mental health services and reported on four main areas where services were failing (Auditor General for Wales, 2005). It identified: significant gaps in key elements of service delivery, which were said to be preventing full implementation of the Welsh National Service Framework for Mental Health (as in many other matters, Wales had its own National Service Framework); the need for greater integration and coordination of adult mental health services across different agencies and care sectors; wide variation in the approach to empowering and engaging service users and carers; and planning and commissioning arrangements that did not fully support the development of whole-system models of care.

In 2011, the WAO conducted a follow-up review and concluded that although there had been much improvement in the areas of concern, more progress was required to ensure that mental health services met the needs of the patients (Auditor General for Wales, 2011). It concluded that:

- Since 2005, there had been important improvements in adult mental health services in many parts of Wales, although progress had been variable and some service gaps and inequalities remained.
- The Welsh Government, NHS bodies and councils had had mixed success in addressing barriers to change.
- The new health boards, supported by the national programme for mental health, needed to sustain improvement during a period of financial restraint.

In November 2009, the WAO and HIW published a joint report, *Services for Children and Young People with Emotional and Mental Health Needs*. Their investigation focused on prevention and early intervention for those with less severe problems, on specialist community services, and on in-patient and residential services. The report concluded that there were failings in all three areas, and it explained that the barriers to improvement were far-reaching, including fundamental weaknesses in service development, workforce challenges in child and adolescent mental health services (CAMHS) and poor performance management processes (Auditor General for Wales & Healthcare Inspectorate Wales, 2009). In December 2013, they published a follow-up report, *Child and Adolescent Mental Health Services: Follow-Up Review of Safety Issues,* and concluded that, although improvements had been made since the publication of the initial investigation, 'children and young people continue to be put at risk due to inappropriate admissions to adult mental health wards, problems with sharing information and acting upon safeguarding duties, and unsafe discharge practices' (Auditor General for Wales & Healthcare Inspectorate Wales, 2013: para. 5).

In response to this, in 2014 the Children, Young People and Education Committee at the Welsh Assembly held an inquiry into CAMHS. A report was published in November 2014 with findings but no recommendations. The Health and Social Services Minister promised a programme for change, using the expertise of Professor Dame Sue Bailey, former President of the Royal College of Psychiatrists, which would address the issues raised in the inquiry (Children, Young People and Education Committee, 2014). The programme, known as Together for Children and Young People (T4C&YP), was launched in February 2015. There have been tangible changes, such as investment in services for young people (up to the age of 25) with a first episode of psychosis.

The third sector has a powerful voice in Wales. Historically, Welsh voluntary groups and charities have been a cornerstone of community life. As healthcare has relocated to the community against the background of current financial pressures, their political influence has increased. The Welsh Government increasingly relies on the expertise of these groups.

Hafal, Gofal and Mind Cymru are the three main mental health charities in Wales. Hafal and Gofal provide services for those suffering from mental health conditions. Hafal focuses only on those with severe and enduring mental illness. Mind Cymru supports affiliate groups around Wales. These organisations, along with smaller mental health charities, form the Wales Alliance for Mental Health. This came into existence in 1994 to address the issues raised by Welsh devolution. The Alliance set up and now runs the National Assembly's cross-party group on mental health. Membership of the group is restricted to those in the Alliance. However, interested parties are often invited to attend and contribute to discussions.

Despite the relatively strong political power of the third sector, this often fails to translate into a strong voice for patients at the local level.

The main charities in the third sector are all service providers, either as individual organisations or through their federated structures. This raises doubts as to how truly representative they can be of service users and carers, owing to conflicts of interest. Unlike England, Northern Ireland and Scotland, in Wales there is no independent service user organisation. This lack of representation is problematic. The Welsh Government has set up the Service User and Carer Forum, with representatives drawn from each of the health boards' partnership boards. Representatives sit on the National Partnership Board of Wales to ensure the service user and carer voice is heard.

Since devolution, particularly since the most recent referendum, in May 2011, there has been an emphasis within the larger UK medical Royal Colleges on increasing the public profile of their Welsh organisations. This has occurred in recognition of the changes brought about by devolution and the increasing differences in English and Welsh policy and legislation. As a result, the medical Royal Colleges in Wales have a greater political and legislative role than previously. They have increased their influence with the Welsh Government and the National Assembly by engaging directly with political parties and government officials, by becoming involved in public consultations, and by attending and holding high-profile events. Welsh branches of the medical Royal Colleges enjoy varying degrees of autonomy. Although they are less separate than some of their counterparts in the other Celtic nations, it is clear that they are moving in the same direction.

The medical colleges in Wales form the Academy of Medical Royal Colleges Wales (AMRCW, or the Academy). The ARMCW was established in 1999 as a non-statutory committee with an advisory function by the Welsh Government, which provided funding until April 2014. Since 1 April 2016, the AMRCW has been completely dependent upon the financial support of its constituent Royal Colleges. The AMRCW has been seen to be less effective than its English counterpart, partly because of difficulties in harnessing joint working across the range of medical specialties and subspecialties, many of which are represented in small numbers in Wales. The future of the AMRCW is unclear.

The Welsh Government is starting to develop its own approach to public health, which is to be expected, given the apparent permanent Welsh Labour majority in the Assembly. For example, there is a strong commitment to introduce minimum unit pricing of alcohol in Wales, if this proves to be legally possible. This stands in contrast to the Westminster government's abandonment of the policy in the face of concerted lobbying by commercial interest groups.

Conclusions

This summary of the situation of mental health services in Wales in 2016 is not exhaustive, nor could it be. As is clear, many aspects of service provision, organisational structure, governance and law are in a state of rapid change. In our judgement, the overall position is mixed.

In the 20th century, Welsh mental health services showed even greater inertia than those in England. Deinstitutionalisation came slowly and late. The National Service Framework for Mental Health of 1999 provoked rapid change in England, in part because implementation was linked to the formation of mental health trusts and a substantial increase in financial resources. The Welsh National Service Framework lacked these drivers and had much less impact. The Care Programme Approach was not used anywhere in Wales until 2002, and it was never fully adopted. The recent influence of the third sector in forming policy has not been matched by service user and carer involvement in service planning, and advocacy services remain scarce. There is no doubt that frustration among service users, carers and policy-makers over slow progress was a major factor in the development of the Mental Health Measure, which must now be acted upon because it is statute. There is concern among psychiatrists that the Measure may distort priorities while reifying the solutions identified when it was enacted. The Measure is essentially a significant experiment in the use of law to change professional behaviour and patterns of service delivery, and there is considerable international interest in its success or failure.

If Wales lagged behind England in the past, it is now protected from the effects of the Health and Social Care Act 2012 that have caused such disruption, cost and conflict in England. The commitment of the Welsh Government to integrated health and social care services, if it continues, is likely to prove an important strength for services in the years to come. On the other hand, the traditional industries of Wales closed in the 1980s, and the post-2008 economic depression has hit Wales hard. The link between mental health problems and economic hardship is well established (Poole *et al*, 2014). The combined effects of reorganisation, the Measure and rising poverty place considerable pressure on services.

The Assembly held its sixth election on May 2016. Although they still have the largest number of seats, Welsh Labour's hegemony appears to be over. The presence of new UKIP AMs is likely to lead to a sharp change in the debate about health in Wales. Although we are cautiously optimistic about the general direction of Welsh policy and priorities on mental health, we believe that it is likely that 2016 will come to be seen as a watershed year for Welsh health services.

References

Auditor General for Wales (2005) *Adult Mental Health Services in Wales: A Baseline Review of Service Provision*. Wales Audit Office.

Auditor General for Wales (2011) *Child and Adolescent Mental Health Services: Follow-up Review of Safety Issues*. Wales Audit Office.

Auditor General for Wales, Healthcare Inspectorate Wales (2009) *Services for Children and Young People with Emotional and Mental Health Needs*. Wales Audit Office.

Auditor General for Wales, Healthcare Inspectorate Wales (2013) *Child and Adolescent Mental Health Services: Follow-up Review of Safety Issues*. Wales Audit Office.

Children, Young People and Education Committee (2014) *Inquiry into Child and Adolescent Mental Health Services*. National Assembly for Wales.

Health and Social Care Committee (2014) *The Work of Healthcare Inspectorate Wales*. National Assembly for Wales.

House of Commons (1998) *The Barnett Formula*. Research Paper 98/8. House of Commons.

Longley M (2012) *The Best Configuration of Hospital Services for Wales: A Review of the Evidence*. National Assembly for Wales.

Poole R, Robinson CA, Higgo R (2014) *Mental Health and Poverty*. Cambridge University Press.

Welsh Government (2011) *Together for Health*. National Assembly for Wales.

Welsh Government (2013) *Duty to Review Inception Report: Post Legislative Assessment of the Mental Health (Wales) Measure 2010*. National Assembly for Wales.

Welsh Government (2015) *The Duty to Review Final Report: Post-legislative Assessment of the Mental Health (Wales) Measure 2010*. National Assembly for Wales.

CHAPTER 10

The Mental Capacity Act – an update

Jonathan Waite

Since the last edition of this book was published in 2007 there have been many developments in the way the Mental Capacity Act 2005 (MCA) is used in England and Wales. This chapter will consider the recent post-legislative scrutiny of the Act by a Select Committee of the House of Lords, together with some of the most significant case law affecting the interpretation of the Act. The 2006 United Nations (UN) Convention on the Rights of People with Disabilities may also have a significant impact on mental health law (Kelly, 2014).

The MCA is not generally popular with health professionals. It is a subject which demands mandatory retraining. It appears to many to have created barriers which impede the smooth delivery of care and to have caused rifts between patients and families, doctors and social workers. It even sometimes brings lawyers into clinical situations. There was a period between the Mental Health Act 1983 (MHA) coming into force and the implementation of the Mental Capacity Act (MCA), in 2007, when there was no statute law on incapacity, but this was not a golden era and decision-making was even trickier then.

The MCA has been subject to a comprehensive review by a Select Committee of the House of Lords. The Committee felt (House of Lords, 2014) that the Act was well drafted and still relevant, but that it was not being used as it was intended. It had not become 'embedded' in practice. The Committee found that despite the Act, professional practice had not changed; doctors were still acting paternalistically and social workers used the Act to maintain their customary aversion to risk. The Committee did acknowledge (para. 128) that alone among the medical Royal Colleges, the Royal College of Psychiatrists regarded the Act as a priority. The Committee concluded that the principles of the Act to maximise autonomy and support decision-making by people with intellectual and cognitive impairments were not being put into practice.

The UN Convention also lays stress on the importance of supporting people with disabilities to make their own decisions. The UN Committee on the Rights of Persons with Disabilities (2013) recommended that governments should take active steps to phase out substitute decision-makers (such as deputies and attorneys) and replace them with a system of supported decision-making. The House of Lords declined to rule on whether the MCA is compatible with the UN Convention, but emphasised that implementing the Act properly would be a significant step towards achieving compliance with the Convention.

Key concepts of the Act

Section 1. Principles

The following principles apply for the purposes of the Act.

- A person must be assumed to have capacity unless it is established that he or she lacks capacity.
- A person is not be treated as unable to make a decision unless all practicable steps to help him or her to do so have been taken without success.
- A person is not be treated as unable to make a decision merely because he or she makes an unwise decision.
- An act done, or a decision made, under this Act for or on behalf of a person who lacks capacity must be done, or made, in his or her best interests.
- Before the act is done, or the decision is made, regard must be had to whether the purpose for which it is needed can be as effectively achieved in a way that is less restrictive of the person's rights and freedom of action.

The Act refers to a person who may lack capacity as 'P'. Chapters 3 and 4 of the MCA *Code of Practice* (Ministry of Justice, 2007) give examples of how P's capacity to make decisions can be enhanced. When making capacity assessments practitioners should document the steps they have taken to maximise P's capacity. Independent mental capacity advocates (IMCAs) have a statutory role and as a result of their training they are often in a good position to support P in the decision-making process. There is a certain irony that if P has capacity as a result of the IMCA's efforts, P then (having capacity) becomes ineligible for an IMCA!

Having a severe mental disorder does not mean that patients lack capacity to make crucial decisions for themselves. For example, in a recent High Court case (*Re SB* [2013]) the patient was suffering from severe depression. The professionals who were responsible for care were unanimous in their view that she lacked capacity to consent to an abortion, but the judge found that:

> 'even if aspects of the decision making are influenced by paranoid thoughts in relation to her husband and her mother, she is nevertheless able to describe and genuinely holds, a range of rational reasons for her decision' (para. 44).

Sections 2 and 3. Capacity

Section 2. People who lack capacity

For the purposes of the Act, a person lacks capacity in relation to a matter if at the material time he or she is unable to make a decision for him- or herself in relation to the matter because of an impairment of, or a disturbance in the functioning of, the mind or brain. It does not matter whether the impairment or disturbance is permanent or temporary.

A lack of capacity cannot be established merely by reference to:

- a person's age or appearance, or
- 'a condition of his, or an aspect of his behaviour, which might lead others to make unjustified assumptions about his capacity'.

In proceedings under the Act any question of whether a person lacks capacity is decided on the balance of probabilities.

No power which a person ('D') may exercise under the Act in relation to a person who lacks capacity, or where D reasonably thinks that a person lacks capacity, is exercisable in relation to a person under 16.

Section 3. Inability to make decisions

For the purposes of section 2, a person is unable to make a decision for him- or herself if he or she is unable:

- to understand the information relevant to the decision
- to retain that information
- to use or weigh that information as part of the process of making the decision
- to communicate the decision (whether by talking, using sign language or any other means).

The fact that a person is able to retain the information relevant to a decision for a short period only does not prevent him or her from being regarded as able to make the decision.

The information relevant to a decision includes information about the reasonably foreseeable consequences of deciding one way or the other, or failing to make the decision.

Sections 2 and 3 are often considered together as the 'two-stage test of capacity' (Ministry of Justice, 2007: para. 4.10, p. 44). In this approach the practitioner first assesses whether P has a disorder of mind or brain and then whether P is able to make the relevant decision by applying the section 3 tests. However, in a Court of Appeal case (*PC v City of York Council* [2013]) it was emphasised that 'Section 2(1) is the single test, albeit that it falls to be interpreted by applying the more detailed description given around it in ss 2 and 3' (para. 56). The judge stated:

> 'There is, however, a danger in structuring the decision by looking to s 2(1) primarily as requiring a finding of mental impairment and nothing more and

in considering s 2(1) first before then going on to look at s 3(1) as requiring a finding of inability to make a decision. The danger is that the strength of the causative nexus between mental impairment and inability to decide is watered down' (para. 58).

In other words, a decision in P's best interests can be made only if P lacks capacity to make that decision for him- or herself as a result of the mental disorder.

Section 4. Best interests

The MCA makes it clear that capacity to make a decision is time and decision specific. In reality, many patients' capacity does fluctuate over time and it may be practicably impossible to comply with the full aspirations of the Act to support decision-making on every occasion when this is likely to be required. This means that determination of what is in P's best interests is the crucial aspect of the decision-making process. If the decision is genuinely in P's interests when P lacks capacity, it is likely to be the decision P would make if P had capacity.

Section 4 does not define 'best interests' but does give guidance on the process which has to be undertaken to ascertain P's best interests. Essentially, the practitioner is required to consider a number of key questions (for full details see Ministry of Justice, 2007: ch. 5):

- Is the person likely to regain capacity, and when?
- How can we maximise their participation in the process of decision-making?
- What are the past and present wishes of the person? What are his or her beliefs and values? Are there other relevant factors?
- What are the views of carers and other nominated or appointed persons?

In practice there are usually a number of options as to what course of action to follow. The courts have considered possible mechanisms of establishing the optimal outcome, and there are no hard and fast rules, but:

'the weight to be attached to P's wishes and feelings will always be case-specific and fact-specific. ...One cannot, as it were, attribute any particular a priori weight or importance to P's wishes and feelings; it all depends, it must depend, upon the individual circumstances of the particular case.' (*ITW v Z* [2009] para. 35)

In considering how much weight to give to P's wishes and feelings, the following factors are relevant:

- the degree of P's incapacity, for the nearer to the borderline the more weight must in principle be attached to P's wishes and feelings
- the strength and consistency of the views being expressed by P
- the possible impact on P of knowledge that his or her wishes and feelings are not being given effect

Table 10.1 Example of a 'best interests' balance sheet: choice of residence for P

Potential decision	Advantages	Disadvantages
Return to own home	P's preferred option Easy to implement Familiar surroundings	Has previously failed P may not allow carers to visit Neighbours are hostile to P's return
Move to care home	Ensures 24-hour care and supervision Home able to offer bed now	P's least favoured option Most intrusive on P's freedoms Funding may not be available
Move to sheltered accommodation	Allows a better prospect of continuing support and supervision than return home P keen to retain a degree of autonomy	P's furniture and belongings will not be suitable for potentially available property Not clear that P would be able to manage without 24-hour supervision

- the extent to which P's wishes and feelings are, or are not, rational, sensible, responsible and pragmatically capable of sensible implementation in the particular circumstances
- crucially, the extent to which P's wishes and feelings, if given effect, can properly be accommodated within the court's overall assessment of what is in her or his best interests.

The Court of Protection now advocates a 'balance sheet' approach to the determination of best interests (*Re A* [2000]). This technique can easily be used in clinical practice and can be helpful in resolving disputes between care providers or between professionals and families. A hypothetical example of such a balance sheet is presented in Table 10.1.

Deprivation of liberty

The 'deprivation of liberty' safeguards (DoLS) were introduced after the ruling of the European Court of Human Rights in the *Bournewood* case, which concerned the *de facto* detention of a compliant incapacitated person. They had been controversial even prior to their implementation (House of Lords, 2014: para. 254). They were reviewed by the House of Commons Health Committee (2013). The Committee stated:

'The evidence the Committee heard regarding the application of DoLS revealed a profoundly depressing and complacent approach to the matter. There is extreme variation in their use and we are concerned that some of the most vulnerable members of society may be exposed to abuse because the legislation has failed to implement controls to properly protect them.'

The Lords Select Committee was equally scathing (House of Lords, 2014):

'The provisions are poorly drafted, overly complex and bear no relationship to the language and ethos of the MCA. The safeguards are not well understood and are poorly implemented.

The only appropriate recommendation in the face of such criticism is to start again.'

To compound the problem for psychiatrists, the courts have displayed some inappropriate thinking in their rulings as to what constitutes a deprivation of liberty; the leading judgments seemed to imply that if a placement was in P's best interests then this could not be a deprivation of liberty (*P&Q v Surrey CC* [2011]) or that people with disability were not entitled to the same rights as people without (*P v Cheshire West and Chester Council* [2011]). These cases have been reconsidered by the Supreme Court (*P&Q v Surrey CC*; *P v Cheshire West and Chester Council* [2014]) and there is now a much clearer picture of what constitutes deprivation of liberty. Giving the leading judgment, Lady Hale (who was responsible for writing the first Draft Mental Capacity Bill) stated (para. 46):

'If it would be a deprivation of my liberty to be obliged to live in a particular place, subject to constant monitoring and control, only allowed out with close supervision, and unable to move away without permission even if such an opportunity became available, then it must also be a deprivation of the liberty of a disabled person. The fact that my living arrangements are comfortable, and indeed make my life as enjoyable as it could possibly be, should make no difference. A gilded cage is still a cage.'

The Department of Health has confirmed that it accepts this ruling. Its guidance in a circular of 28 March 2014 states that:

'There is deprivation of liberty where the person is under continuous supervision and control and is not free to leave, and the person lacks capacity to consent to these arrangements. The person's compliance or lack of objection, the reason or purpose behind a particular placement and the relative normality of the placement are not relevant.'

Deprivation of liberty can occur in domestic settings where the state is responsible for imposing such arrangements; however, the DoLS mechanism applies only in hospitals and registered care homes. Deprivation of liberty in domestic settings can be authorised only by application to the Court of Protection.

Deprivation of liberty in hospitals (not only mental health units) can also be authorised under the MHA. The interface between the MHA and the MCA causes many difficulties (Clare *et al*, 2013). The relevant part of the MCA (schedule 1A) is extraordinarily opaquely drafted; the senior judge who has had to rule on its interpretation described the process as feeling 'as if you have been in a washing machine and spin-dryer' (House of Lords, 2014: para. 271).

Essentially, DoLS should not be used to detain a person who is mentally ill in hospital in whole or in part for the treatment of mental disorder where the patient is objecting (Mental Capacity Act 2005, Schedule 1A). This can cause grave difficulties for patients in acute trusts who require treatment for mental disorder to which they object, who are too physically ill to be transferred to a mental health unit where their care can be provided under the supervision of an approved clinician.

In 2009 (*GJ v The Foundation Trust*) Charles J ruled that in general the Mental Health Act has primacy where it applies. Revisiting the DoLS eligibility criteria in 2013 (*AM v SLAM Foundation Trust*) he revised his opinion and suggested that in some circumstances where the MHA did apply, authorisation under DoLS might afford a less restrictive alternative to detention under the MHA.

Conclusion

The aspirations of the MCA to confirm the statutory rights of people who may lack capacity and transform their lives by assisting them to make decisions and take risks for themselves has not been fulfilled. This has been the result of a failure of health and social care practitioners to embed its principles in their practice. Psychiatrists will have an important role to play in achieving the implementation of the MCA sought by Parliament.

The Supreme Court judgement on DoLS is likely to result in many more compliant incapacitated people in hospitals and care homes coming under statutory safeguards. This may cause significant problems with resources until a more satisfactory scheme of legal protection is devised.

References

Clare ICH, Redley M, Keeling A, *et al* (2013) *Understanding the Interface Between the Mental Capacity Act's Deprivation of Liberty Safeguards (MCA-DoLS) and the Mental Health Act (MHA)*. Intellectual and Developmental Disabilities Research Group. Available at https://www.researchgate.net/publication/258867517_UNDERSTANDING_THE_INTERFACE_BETWEEN_THE_MENTAL_CAPACITY_ACT%27S_DEPRIVATION_OF_LIBERTY_SAFEGUARDS_MCA-DOLS_AND_THE_MENTAL_HEALTH_ACT_MHA (accessed 22 March 2016).

House of Commons Health Committee (2013) *Post-legislative Scrutiny of the Mental Health Act 2007* (HC584). TSO.

House of Lords (2014) *Mental Capacity Act 2005: Post-legislative Scrutiny* (HL Paper 139). TSO.

Kelly BD (2014) An end to psychiatric detention? Implications of the United Convention on the Rights of Persons with Disabilities. *British Journal of Psychiatry*, **204**: 174–5.

Ministry of Justice (2007) *Mental Capacity Act 2005: Code of Practice*. TSO.

UN Committee on the Rights of Persons with Disabilities (2013) *General comment on Article 12: Equal recognition before the law* (UN CRPD/C/11/4). United Nations.

Cases

AM v SLAM Foundation Trust [2013] UKUT 365 (AAC) MHLO 80
GJ v The Foundation Trust [2009] EWHC 2972 (Fam)
ITW v Z [2009] EWHC 2525 (Fam)

P v Cheshire West and Chester Council [2011] EWCA Civ 1257

P&Q v Surrey CC [2011] EWCA Civ 190

P&Q v Surrey CC; P v Cheshire West and Cheshire Council [2014] UKSC Civ 19

PC v City of York Council [2013] EWCA Civ 478

Re A [2000] 1 FLR 549 at 560 per Thorpe LJ

Re SB (A patient: capacity to consent to termination) [2013] EWHC 1417 (COP)

Part II
Changes and conflicts

CHAPTER 11

Medical leadership skills: what is needed to be a successful leader?

Alex Till, Antonio Ventriglio and Dinesh Bhugra

Clinical leadership is central to service planning, delivery, evaluation and improvement. To deliver sustainable high-quality healthcare it is vital that doctors, by virtue of their training, determine resource requirements and allocation to ensure resources are used efficiently and efficaciously. While at present societal determinants dictate that policy-makers and government ultimately govern this, as a profession, we must not revoke our responsibility for it. With increasing economic pressures and an overwhelming increase in the demand for healthcare, it has never been more important for doctors to uphold their professional values and highlight to policy-makers, based on clinical evidence, what is needed and where priorities must lie, to ensure that equitable healthcare of the highest possible standard is delivered to patients, who deserve no less.

Historically, this has been challenged within the UK by recurrent governmental reforms of the healthcare system. The lack of direction in service delivery resulting from this, compounded by a series of high-profile healthcare tragedies across the country, not excluding mental health, has challenged one of the principles that lies at the heart of every doctor's practice, 'to do no harm' (Department of Health, 2012; Francis, 2013; Keogh, 2013). It could be argued that both the lay and the professional perception of healthcare professionals and the healthcare service as a whole has worsened, and that the trust placed in professionals to look after patients, indeed, to provide even the very basics of care, has been irreparably damaged.

It is clear that questions as to our professionalism must be answered and that we must now, more than ever, demonstrate that, as doctors, we value patients as being at the centre of healthcare delivery and strive for the highest quality of healthcare in everything we do, by upholding and developing our leadership responsibilities.

Professionalism

The Charter on Medical Professionalism, published simultaneously in the UK and USA in 2002, was an attempt to restore the profession's reputation.

The Charter outlines values, behaviours and relationships that underpin the essential components of professionalism through what it terms the *fundamentals* which doctors must uphold and the *commitments* they must have (Medical Professionalism Project, 2002).

Fundamentals

Incorporated as a fundamental principle is 'primacy of patient welfare', whereby the dedication to altruism is outlined, and how as doctors we must not let external factors compromise this. Another is 'patient autonomy', whereby the importance of being honest and respecting our patients' decisions must be upheld. Finally there is 'social justice', whereby doctors have a key role in ensuring the just distribution of finite resources in the face of seemingly infinite demand.

Commitments

The Charter lists ten commitments it considers are essential components of being a good medical professional (Medical Professionalism Project, 2002). These can be summarised as follows:

1 *Professional competence.* Keeping up to date and maintaining competence in all clinical matters and skills are important. The experience and skills needed for the delivery of high-quality care must be maintained and developed in line with changing practice and the evidence base. This includes lifelong learning to sustain knowledge and skills.
2 *Honesty with patients.* As far as possible, clinical decisions should be made jointly by doctor and patient, with both parties sharing responsibility for health. Being honest with patients about their condition, potential outcomes and adverse events in medical care, through an equitable relationship, is vital to achieve this goal, as is sharing the lessons learnt from failures when they occur.
3 *Patient confidentiality.* Patient confidentiality is of paramount importance, although certain cultures and settings may carry different emphases. Doctors should be mindful of ensuring that confidentiality is strictly upheld in relation to patient information, particularly with the increasing use of computer-based systems and social media.
4 *Maintaining appropriate relations with patients.* The doctor must ensure that the vulnerability of patients is not exploited for personal gain, particularly sexual or financial. This is especially important within psychiatry.
5 *Improving quality of care.* The doctor must take responsibility and be actively involved in quality improvement of healthcare systems, individuals and institutions within healthcare. This must take into account evidence but also the role of the resources, both financial and human, needed to deliver this.

6 *Improving access to care.* The doctor must ensure that throughout society there is equitable access to an adequate standard of healthcare. Healthcare must include the promotion of public health and preventive medicine.

7 *Just distribution of finite resources.* Based on evidence and the literature, the doctor must take responsibility for the cost-effective, efficient and efficacious allocation of resources and avoid providing superfluous services.

8 *Scientific knowledge.* The doctor must ensure that scientific evidence and technology are appropriately used clinically, while promoting an active involvement in research.

9 *Maintaining trust by managing conflicts of interest.* Doctors must ensure that their professional responsibilities are not compromised by personal gains and any conflicts of interest are declared openly. This is particularly relevant within the National Health Service, where much of the provision is being privatised – any financial gains should be declared.

10 *Professional responsibilities.* The medical profession must ensure self-regulation and collaboration with other stakeholders to maximise the quality of patient care.

While these recommendations do not guarantee professionalism, combined with specific guidance from the Royal College of Physicians, the Royal College of Psychiatrists and the General Medical Council, a 'gold standard' is provided, setting out what the professional bodies expect of doctors in daily clinical practice. Doctors should then reflect on and assess their own personal values, behaviours and relationships against this and consider whether they are upholding what is expected of them as medical professionals.

Leadership

Embedded throughout almost all tragedies within healthcare, an unacceptable standard of medical leadership and management can be found. The reasons for this are many and include a lack of interest by clinicians and also increased bureaucracy, which detracts from direct patient care. While it is possible to consider these incidents as 'special cause variation' it is clear that there are ongoing concerns related not only to service delivery but also to service improvement.

Of course, leadership and the importance of its development have been recognised for some time. Tooke (2008: p. 90) stated that 'The doctor's frequent role as head of the healthcare team and commander of considerable clinical resources requires that greater attention is paid to management and leadership skills regardless of specialism'. However, it was not until the conclusion of Sir Robert Francis's and Sir Bruce Keogh's reviews that a fresh emphasis was placed on the development of trainees' leadership skills. It is now increasingly recognised that trainees are arguably the best placed to act as the 'eyes and ears' within healthcare organisations, as they are on the 'shopfloor' 24 hours a day, 7 days a week, and that rather than being considered the leaders of tomorrow, they should in fact be considered the clinical leaders we need today (Francis, 2013; Keogh, 2013).

These reports and their recommendations should be studied carefully. Embedding the lessons learnt into the culture of every healthcare organisation is vital to minimise the probability of recurrence, if not eliminate it altogether. The disempowerment, alienation and failure to engage trainees, some of the brightest people in any country, is a defining weakness in our healthcare organisations. Like all specialties, we within mental health must rapidly overcome this to harness these powerful agents for change and utilise this currently untapped resource of energy, creativity and ideas (King's Fund, 2011, 2012).

It is worth recalling at this point that in a study of the top 100 hospitals in the USA, Goodall (2011) found that there was a strong association between successful hospitals and their chief executive officers being physicians by background.

Who is a leader?

A leader is someone who sets direction for an organisation by setting out its mission, its goals, vision and purpose. The leader's task is to build commitment through motivation, teamwork and spirit, and to confront challenges through innovation, change and turbulence (Tappen *et al*, 2004). Leadership is about seeing what is needed and making it happen, recognising the bond between improvement and change, managing the threats, disturbances and disruptions. Leadership requires a certain set of skills (Bhugra *et al*, 2013).

Leaders have to be clearly differentiated from managers. In order to understand and develop leadership skills at any level, one must be aware of the definitions and distinctions between management and leadership. Individuals interested in taking on such a role also need to be aware of what the needs of patients and the healthcare systems are. Regrettably, 'management' and 'leadership', as terms, are often used interchangeably but these tasks need two distinct, but overlapping, skill sets. Leaders lead, and their key role is to develop the right strategic vision and a clear purpose for the organisation which can be translated into action by the managers, who are responsible for orchestrating people and resources to deliver that strategic vision. However, often in clinical settings there may be such a degree of overlap that management roles may be confused with leadership roles; while it can be argued that they are embedded within each other, it is crucial that a degree of clarity exists between the two.

Table 11.1 is modified from Bennis (1998) and Kotter (1998) and provides a differentiation between the two roles.

Table 11.1 Leadership versus management

Leadership	Management
Sets direction by creating a vision, developing a strategy and empowering followers to seize opportunities and adapt to change	Sustains efficient, effective and reliable systems through administration and control
Deals with uncertainty and disagreement by making connections and conversations, promoting diversity	Deals with certainty and agreement
Innovates with an eye on the horizon, developing a long-range vision	Task-oriented, with a short-range vision; copes with complexity and arranges resources; a classic good soldier
Does the right thing	Does things right

What qualities and characteristics do leaders have?

Inspiring and enabling individuals to realise the collective vision, because they want to follow, is the core essence of leadership. This, however, is not easily accomplished and requires multiple qualities and characteristics to be expressed by the psychiatrist. These can be considered at three distinct levels, or domains: the personal, the interpersonal and the organisational (Bhugra, 2011). The following characteristics are not a comprehensive list but highlight various aspects of leadership that can be seen as helpful in understanding what makes a successful leader.

The personal

Within this domain there are certain personality traits and qualities that are a core part of the individual's personality. Leaders need not only energy, passion and a high level of commitment but also vision and courage. With the skills necessary to create and communicate their vision clearly, they can establish the same within their followers. A similarly attractive quality for followers is a leader who remains open minded to suggestions from others and who maintains an innovative attitude for improvement, yet is decisive when facing uncertainty and ambiguity in clinical settings or within the healthcare system as a whole. Translating practical wisdom gained through experience is an important and effective component of this; leaders must, however, also maintain humility with wisdom (called *phronesis* in Greek) to maintain their integrity and respect.

Central to all of the above is emotional intelligence, a construct of understanding oneself and others through a combination of self-awareness, social awareness, self-management and relationship management (Goleman, 1995).

145

The interpersonal

At the heart of good leadership is an ability to communicate, empower and inspire followers. Leaders should enable others to reach higher levels of personal and professional development, leading to effective agreement in the vision and mission of the organisation. They should be able to articulate and convey that vision to the organisation or team so that they are clear about the vision and potential outcomes. Critical at all levels of leadership is building effective team working, whereby all members work collaboratively to deliver an effective, efficacious and efficient service. Leaders should work in partnership with their followers, command respect and embrace diversity, in both strategy and personnel, yet not be afraid to hold to account those who do not deliver. Maintaining the political nous and a broader perspective on potential allies and impediments is essential for this.

Furthermore, good leaders understand that, in order to function effectively, they must be aware of their deficiencies and surround themselves with people who address these needs. They establish the support networks where they can formally or informally discuss decisions, seek advice and direction, and make decisions in a safe place.

The organisational

Clinicians have multiple roles and responsibilities extending beyond the delivery of high-quality patient care; this is embodied within the professional standards and responsibilities outlined in the Charter on Medical Professionalism (see above). As clinicians, we are responsible to patients, their employers, trainees and society at large, along with other stakeholders such as policy-makers. It is therefore imperative that clinicians remain cognisant not only of the existing internal organisational policies and values but also the external healthcare policies and the broader contexts and challenges that underpin and drive these. Leaders must constantly maintain the ability to broadly scan the horizon and identify healthcare policies that could influence clinical practice, so that they can combat potential conflicts and reduce the risk that these may bring to their patients and their organisation.

It could be argued that, within the medical profession, psychiatrists are best placed to be good leaders because they are used to dealing with complexity and uncertainty with patients on a daily basis and are expected to overcome them. They make diagnoses and clinical management plans and may predict potential problems and courses of illnesses, and doing so, using the biopsychosocial model, naturally provides psychiatrists with a greater insight and understanding of how to manage complexity, ambiguity and change. Translating this into a leadership setting, psychiatrists, as leaders, should be able to do much the same (Bhugra, 2011).

What styles of leadership are available?

While it would be a challenge for an individual to have all these qualities, this does not mean that one cannot be a good leader without them. Furthermore, it is important to remember that the leadership qualities and characteristics that work in one organisation may not work in another; this is largely determined by the organisational culture and leadership style adopted. For example, it is often said that a hierarchical, 'command and control' structure predominates within the NHS. This stems from a culture whereby with rising seniority one gains 'legitimate' power, which precipitates an authoritarian or 'autocratic' leadership style. With this in place, there is a tendency for leaders to feel that they do not need to achieve consensus or agreement. The resultant controlling, closed-minded and power-oriented approach demoralises staff and creates fear within the organisation, to the extent that the culture becomes pathological, with staff being frightened of reporting errors and admitting mistakes (Edmondson, 1996; Bass, 2008). It is exactly this type of leadership that may predispose organisations to problems such as those identified by Francis (2013) and Keogh (2013). As very cogently argued by Berwick (2013), this rhetoric of blame must be avoided.

Contrastingly, transformational leadership is increasingly valued and seen to embody the essence of clinical leadership (NHS Confederation & Nuffield Trust, 1999); this comprises four key domains, commonly known as the four 'I's (Table 11.2). Transformational leaders value the development of 'followership' and use the four 'I's to engage and work with followers. The role of followers in psychiatry is complex, in that there is a wide array of specialists within the different teams that are responsible for delivering patient care. It is critical, especially from a clinician's standpoint, that leaders do not see their followers as inferior to them but, even as leaders, they are among equals. Sivers (2010) suggests that 'early followers' are perhaps more important to the success of leaders than the leaders

Table 11.2 Transformational leadership – the four 'I's

'I'	Characteristics
Individualised consideration	Provision of personal attention, ideally through mentoring and coaching, to meet followers' needs
Intellectual stimulation	Active encouragement of innovation and improvement from followers
Inspirational motivation	Articulation of a clear vision which challenges and engages followers
Idealised influence	This is role-modelled through the trust and respect established from followers

Adapted from Bass (2008)

themselves. Thus, a key task for leaders is to be available and visible. They must also ensure that they can empower, encourage and support their followers. Mentoring is key for this and, delivered effectively, these domains help both the leader and the follower to rise to higher levels of productivity (Bass, 2008; Allio, 2013).

The relationship between leaders and their followers is extremely important, although often it may be complex and unclear. At times leaders must lead from the front, whereas at others leaders may, like a shepherd, need to lead from behind. Leaders can also shepherd values. Good leaders will adapt their approaches in response to the context and needs of their followers.

There are different styles of leadership and different theories used to explain these leadership styles. Some of the better-known styles and approaches are described in Table 11.3.

Table 11.3 Leadership styles

Style	Characteristics
Autocratic	Leaders who are seen as autocratic are controlling and closed-minded. They may make unilateral decisions and expect others to carry out these tasks unconditionally and without challenge. Such an approach may work while dealing with a crisis but carries high risk, generates low morale and makes followers afraid to question or challenge the leader
Democratic	Often seen in membership organisations, such leaders encourage consensus, creativity, contribution and collaboration but may find it difficult to make quick and prompt decisions, leading to a paralysis in the organisation
Laissez-faire	Laid-back approach to leadership where leaders let the followers get on and decide, and leaders may sit and watch. The problem with such an approach is there may be chaos and unclear, ineffective and ineffectual options and little may be achieved
Visionary	Leaders have a clear vision about what they want to achieve and how they are going to go about it using clear, masterly communication to mobilise their followers towards a predetermined and almost united vision. This may be valuable in engaging and enabling followers but may require detailed guidance and understanding
Coaching	Leaders focus on developing followers by discussing, supporting and motivating them and ensuring that their own and organisational visions match
Pace-setting	Leaders demand high standards of not only themselves but also others and can set the pace, which their followers may or may not be able to match. Although such an approach can produce effective and timely results and a highly competent team, unless supported thoroughly the followers may find this hard to achieve and as a result both morale and confidence can be affected

How does one develop leadership skills?

All doctors have a responsibility to develop their leadership skills. As such, it is important that trainees and early-career psychiatrists understand and have opportunities to develop these skills, in order to fill the leadership positions and potential roles they will be expected to occupy as their career progresses. There has been an ongoing debate within the field of leadership studies, especially in relation to business, as to whether the ability of an individual to lead is 'trait based' (suggesting that certain individuals have an inherent leadership ability) or 'process based' (suggesting that leadership is observable and can be learnt) (Daft, 2005; Yukl, 2006). While this debate continues apace, there is little doubt that certain individuals, with inherent personality traits, are more suited to leadership than others. This is, however, not to say that certain skills, such as communication and teamwork, cannot be learnt. Given the right training, in the right environment, all individuals can develop their leadership potential, albeit that some may naturally flourish more than others.

To optimise the ability to harness the potential within the broadest range of trainees possible, it is clear that we must utilise a variety of techniques to engage learners. Leadership training and learning courses may offer certain opportunities to explore one's personal style and understand one's own personal strengths and weaknesses. Equally, it is important that individuals set time aside, within a safe environment, for their vertical leadership development (Petrie, 2015).

Considering this, one must look towards the literature and evidence-based models or frameworks that help trainees pursue a journey of self-development. The advantage of encouraging trainees to consider these frameworks, as opposed to set definitions, is their dynamism and ability to guide individuals towards developing the key behaviours required to lead effectively and their ability to identify where trainees attention should be focused, rather than simply being statements of what should be provided.

Frameworks for competency in medical leadership

The NHS Institute for Innovation and Improvement & Academy of Medical Royal Colleges (2010) developed the Medical Leadership Competency Framework, later refined to the Leadership Framework (NHS Institute for Innovation and Improvement, 2011), which outlines seven domains (Fig. 11.1), each with four key elements, considered to be essential to leading what should be at the centre of our attention, delivering services to patients. Within each domain, the four key elements are further refined into competencies expected at the various levels of training (undergraduate, postgraduate and post-certification).

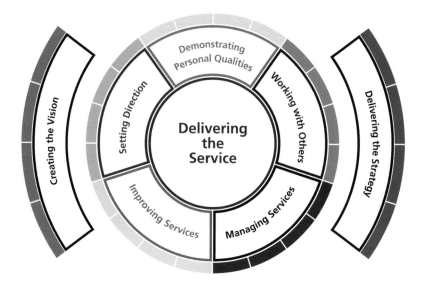

Fig. 11.1 The Leadership Framework. (The Leadership Framework and associated graphics are © NHS Leadership Academy, 2011. All rights reserved.)

Within the Healthcare Leadership Model, nine 'leadership dimensions' (with the accompanying graphic) are described as the behaviours to be developed:

1 Inspiring a shared purpose
2 Leading with care
3 Evaluating information
4 Connecting our service
5 Sharing the vision
6 Engaging the team
7 Holding to account
8 Developing capability
9 Influencing results

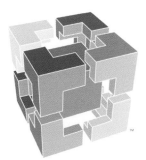

The benefit of this model is the emphasis on the fact that all healthcare professionals have a responsibility and, more importantly, the capability to lead. Rather than focusing on the competencies expected at any particular hierarchical position, reflective questions are asked for learners to consider the level of leadership behaviour that they currently exhibit and to categorise this as 'essential', 'proficient', 'strong' or 'exemplary'. This reinforces the view that within healthcare we all have the power to lead, we are all responsible for reducing risks to patient safety, and we all can act as powerful agents for change to improve patient care.

Table 11.4 Elements of High-Impact Leadership

Elements	Characteristics
Mental models	*Philosophies to adopt throughout the organisation*
1	Considering individuals and families as partners in their care
2	Continually aiming to reduce operating costs in order to compete on value while improving outcomes, quality and safety
3.	Reorganising services to address new payment systems
4	Valuing everyone within the healthcare organisation as an 'improver'
Behaviours	*Behaviours to adopt and embed in the organisation*
1	Person-centred care
2	Front-line engagement with both providers and recipients of care
3	Relentless focus on the organisation's vision and strategy
4	Transparency of both positive and negative aspects of the organisation and healthcare provided
5	Boundaryless thinking and collaboration across services involved in a patient's pathway of care
Framework	*Critical domains where leadership efforts should be targeted*

IHI High-Impact Leadership Framework

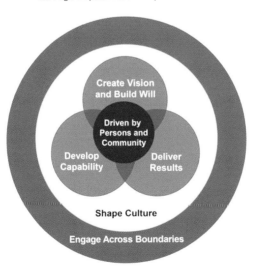

Fig. 11.2 The High-Impact Leadership Framework. (Source: Swensen S, Pugh M, McMullan C, Kabcenell A. *High-Impact Leadership: Improve Care, Improve the Health of Populations, and Reduce Costs*. IHI White Paper. Cambridge, Massachusetts: Institute for Healthcare Improvement; 2013. Available at ihi.org.)

Meanwhile, in the USA, Swensen *et al* (2013), on behalf of the Institute for Healthcare Improvement (IHI), developed what they term 'High-Impact Leadership' (Fig. 11.2). This comprises mental models, behaviours and a framework (Table 11.4) that they consider vital to achieving the 'triple aim' – the IHI's goals to improve the patient experience of care, to improve the health of populations and to reduce the cost of care (Berwick *et al*, 2008).

Quality improvement

Trainees want to give more than is currently expected of them and not only contribute to 'delivering the service' but progress beyond this basic requirement to lead to improvements in patient care and outcomes through systemic change (Bagnall, 2012). Carefully implemented in the right way, this approach can and will encourage doctors to think of themselves as leaders because they can see where improvements are needed and work with their teams to achieve them (Turnbull, 2011).

When we consider the techniques needed for practical implementation, there are many well-studied examples arising from business models. These include: 'Lean' methodology (focusing on waste reduction, flow and value), 'Six Sigma' (focusing on product improvement and reducing 'defects') and the 'Model for Improvement' (focusing on continuous 'Plan, Do, Study, Act' (PDSA) cycles, which test improvements). For trainees within healthcare systems perhaps the 'Model for Improvement' is most powerful.

The Model for Improvement was developed by the Associates in Process Improvement (Langley *et al*, 2009). It provides a clear and simple formula for trainees to begin quality improvement projects. This approach provides an attractive and effective introduction to quality improvement and encourages interest in leadership development (Till *et al*, 2015).

If understood and implemented effectively the power of trailing small-scale change through PDSA cycles within the workplace, measuring the improvements delivered to patients and seeing this practically on a daily basis will allow trainees to understand and realise their potential to act as powerful agents for change and be encouraged to lead these towards larger, more sustainable systems-based improvements.

Harnessed in the right way, this positive feedback loop can build a cycle of continuous leadership development, engage trainees with wider organisational objectives, develop a broader focus on patient safety and embed quality-improvement science into the culture of healthcare organisations (Berwick, 2013).

The future

Training and engaging leaders in any organisation, but especially one related to healthcare, is of major benefit to that organisation.

Traditional autocratic leadership styles within healthcare may be effective in some settings but overall negatively impact on team morale, stifle the development of trainees and create a culture that, in relation to patient safety, should be considered pathological.

A collective leadership approach, with a transformational leadership style, should be adopted within healthcare to nurture trainees as followers and the clinical leaders we need to deliver a high-quality healthcare service. To deliver this effectively, trainees require mentoring, time for reflection and an understanding of evidence-based leadership models; they need to consider their own leadership qualities, strengths and weaknesses.

The institutions themselves, as well as trainees, must take on this responsibility to nurture leadership talent. It must be delivered early within doctors' postgraduate education and continue throughout their careers.

Leadership development can no longer remain a minority interest and should be seen as a longitudinal key component of training, which, rather than occurring in isolation, should be integrated naturally within trainees' clinical experience, through systems of quality improvement.

References

Allio R (2013) Leaders and leadership – many theories, but what advice is reliable? *Strategy and Leadership*, **41**: 4–14.

Bagnall P (2012) *Facilitators and Barriers to Leadership and Quality Improvement. The King's Fund Junior Doctor Project*. King's Fund.

Bass BM (2008) *The Bass Handbook of Leadership: Theory, Research, and Managerial Applications* (4th edition). Free Press.

Bennis W (1998) *On Becoming a Leader*. Arrow.

Berwick DM (2013) *A Promise to Learn – A Commitment to Act: Improving the Safety of Patients in England. National Advisory Group Report on the Safety of Patients in England*. Department of Health.

Berwick DM, Nolan TW, Whittington J (2008) The triple aim: care, health, and cost. *Health Affairs*, **27**: 759-69.

Bhugra D (2011) What makes a medical leader? *Advances in Psychiatric Treatment*, **17**: 160–1.

Bhugra D, Gupta S, Ruiz P (2013) What is leadership? In *Leadership in Psychiatry* (eds D Bhugra, R Ruiz, S Gupta): 1–12. Wiley-Blackwell.

Daft RL (2005) *The Leadership Experience* (3rd edition). Thomson/South-Western.

Department of Health (2012) *Transforming Care: A National Response to Winterbourne View Hospital: Department of Health Review Final Report*. Department of Health.

Edmondson A (1996) Learning from mistakes is easier said than done: group and organizational influences on the detection and correction of human error. *Journal of Applied Behavioural Science*, **32**. 5 28.

Francis R (2013) *Report of the Mid Staffordshire NHS Foundation Trust Public Inquiry. Executive Summary* (HC 947). TSO.

Goleman D (1995) *Emotional Intelligence*. Bantam Books.

Goodall A (2011) *Physician-Leaders and Hospital Performance: Is There an Association?* IZA Discussion Paper No. 5830. IZA (Institute for the Study of Labour).

Keogh B (2013) *Review into the Quality of Care and Treatment Provided by 14 Hospital Trusts in England: Overview Report*. Department of Health.

King's Fund (2011) *The Future and Leadership Management in the NHS: No More Heroes*. King's Fund.

King's Fund (2012) *Leadership and Engagement for Improvement in the NHS: Together We Can.* King's Fund.

Kotter J (1998) *What Leaders Really Do.* Harvard Business Review on Leadership. Harvard Business School Press.

Langley GL, Nolan KM, Nolan TW, *et al* (2009) *The Improvement Guide: A Practical Approach to Enhancing Organizational Performance* (2nd edition). Jossey-Bass.

Medical Professionalism Project (2002) Medical professionalism in the new millennium: a physicians' charter. *Lancet,* **359**: 520–2.

NHS Confederation & Nuffield Trust (1999) *The Modern Values of Leadership and Management in the NHS.* NHS Confederation.

NHS Institute for Innovation and Improvement (2011) *Leadership Framework.* NHS Institute for Innovation and Improvement.

NHS Institute for Innovation and Improvement & Academy of Medical Royal Colleges (2010) *Medical Leadership Competency Framework* (3rd edition). NHS Institute for Innovation and Improvement.

Petrie N (2015) *The How-To of Vertical Leadership Development – Part 2: 30 Experts, 3 Conditions, and 15 Approaches.* Centre for Creative Leadership.

Sivers D (2010) Leadership lessons from dancing guy. Technology Entertainment Design (TED) Conference, February.

Swensen S, Pugh M, McMullan C, *et al* (2013) *High-Impact Leadership: Improve Care, Improve the Health of Populations, and Reduce Costs.* IHI White Paper. Institute for Healthcare Improvement.

Tappen R, Weiss S, Withehead D (2004) *Essentials of Nursing Leadership and Management* (3rd edition). FA Davis.

Till A, Banerjee J, McKimm J (2015) Supporting the engagement of doctors in training in quality improvement and patient safety. *British Journal of Hospital Medicine,* **76**: 166–9.

Tooke J (2008) *Aspiring to Excellence: Final Report of the Independent Enquiry into Modernising Medical Careers.* Aldridge Press.

Turnbull JK (2011) *Leadership in Context: Lessons from New Leadership Theory and Current Leadership Development Practice.* King's Fund.

Yukl G (2006) *Leadership in Organizations* (6th edition). Pearson-Prentice Hall.

CHAPTER 12

Understanding systems

Amit Malik and Kate Jefferies

Clinical medicine, and especially psychiatry, cannot be practised in isolation. Psychiatrists operate within the internal systems of their employing organisations and the external systems within which those organisations exist. It is, therefore, important that psychiatrists understand the context within which they practise. It is even more crucial that medical managers not only understand the systems but are also able to leverage this understanding to bring about service improvements, within omnipresent resource constraints, to maximise quality of care for their patients.

This chapter is set out as a checklist of areas that psychiatrists should seek an understanding of if they are to operate effectively within the complex healthcare environment. The lead author (A.M.) has covered some of these issues, especially in relation to finances and operations, in a recent publication (Malik *et al*, 2015) but has outlined them here as well for completeness. The work of relevant opinion leaders from the world of business and healthcare management has been contextualised to mental health services using the authors' experience and knowledge of working in and managing such services in the UK. The overall aim is to provide the reader with a comprehensive coverage of areas to consider while managing mental health services.

The level of detail that readers need to be aware of will depend on the type of organisation they practise in, as well as their formal and informal extra-clinical activities, both within and external to their employing organisation. Key questions are listed throughout the chapter, which we would suggest readers seek the answers to, to increase their understanding of their own services. These key questions could also be used as the basis for a reflective learning journal. The chapter also indicates why these areas are important and how understanding them could help the psychiatrist in service improvement. Psychiatrists need to develop good working relationships with operational managers and work alongside them to gain better understanding of and enhance the healthcare service they provide.

Since political devolution in 1999, there has been increasing divergence between the healthcare systems of the four component countries of the UK. While each country has a tax-funded, universal healthcare service with similar operating principles and values, there have been differing priorities and policies for healthcare. For the purposes of this chapter, the authors will focus on the English commissioning system. Further information about the devolved nations' healthcare systems can be found in other chapters of this book.

Understanding commissioning objectives

The starting point of any clinical service is to meet the health needs of the local population. Commissioners are responsible for evaluating these needs and developing commissioning intentions based on this public health analysis. More often than not, this is the point where clinical managers can most effectively affect service delivery. Having a close working relationship with your local commissioners is critical to ensure that clinical knowledge (demographic changes, developments in the evidence base, learning from current services, etc.) can guide them to make the most effective commissioning decisions. Commissioning objectives are usually translated into detailed service specifications that form the basis of services. In the case of existing contracts, these service specifications are negotiated with providers through annual contract review meetings. For new contracts, the services are put out to tender through a formal procurement process. Good service specifications support outcomes-based rather than process-based commissioning, as this allows providers to innovate services to deliver similar or better outcomes more efficiently.

Key questions

- Who is commissioning (paying for) the service?
- Are there opportunities to have clinical input in the development of commissioning intentions?
- Are there avenues to influence internal and external discussions regarding service specifications?
- Are there obvious gaps in services, resources or expertise in delivering a proposed service specification?

Understanding the role of regulators

In addition to understanding the commissioning landscape, the medical manager needs to be fully conversant with the requirements of the healthcare regulators. The regulatory authorities differ in the four countries of the UK. Regulation in England comprises two main elements (Table 12.1).

Table 12.1 The two main elements of healthcare regulation in England

Role	Organisation
Regulation of quality and safety of healthcare	Care Quality Commission
Regulation of the healthcare market	Monitor

Key questions
- What are the domains of assessment used by the Care Quality Commission?
- What areas of clinical care require improvement in your organisation?

Understanding key performance indicators

The providers and commissioners usually agree on 'key performance indicators' (KPIs), which are derived from the service specification and are rooted in either evidence or best practice. They could also be derived from areas where a provider's performance has lagged in the past, or areas that are new strategic priorities for the commissioners. The KPIs usually comprise a combination of quality (e.g. suicide rates, in-patient falls, MRSA infections, patient feedback), performance (e.g. activity, waiting times) and organisational indicators (e.g. staff training, staff turnover) and if agreed on constructively can generate focus in provider performance and strengthen the commissioner–provider collaboration. These KPIs are then monitored on a regular basis at an organisational level and reviewed with the commissioners at contract meetings. Achieving KPIs often has positive consequences, for example under the Commissioning for Quality and Innovation (CQUIN) payments framework, while non-achievement usually has negative consequences, for example in the form of financial penalties. Therefore, it behoves medical managers to apprise themselves of the KPIs that are relevant to their service and ensure that these are met, thereby helping to ensure the long-term viability of the service.

Key questions
- What are the commissioner and organisational KPIs for the organisation?
- Which of these KPIs are relevant for your service?
- How is your service performing on these KPIs?
- What are the commercial and regulatory consequences of your service not delivering on these KPIs?

Understanding financial modelling of the service

At the most basic level, clinical services receive income to provide care to patients and incur costs to deliver those services. The income could be given as a lump sum to provide care to a defined population; it could be capitated (i.e. a fixed amount per time period per patient) or it could be on a fee-for-service basis (Malik *et al*, 2015). Increasingly, commissioners are making attempts to commission based on outcomes and although this still remains a challenge in mental health services, certain services, such as psychological therapies, are beginning to see the advent of outcome-based commissioning, with, for example, some of their compensation being based on the percentage of patients returning to full-time employment. It is important that medical managers fully understand the range of income sources that fund their service and factor this information into difficult decisions regarding service transformations.

On the other side, costs are incurred to deliver services. In mental health services, the most significant costs relate to people (Malik *et al*, 2015). Some staffing groups cost a lot more than others. However, managerial temptations to reduce high-cost staff are not always valid and a thorough cost–benefit analysis of each post should always be undertaken when vacancies arise, or when setting up a new service or redesigning existing services. It is critical that medical managers understand the cost drivers within their services so that they can make informed decisions when it comes to developing cost improvement programmes, which, at least within the English healthcare system, have been an annual requirement for some years.

Medical managers should always be on the lookout for, and ready to apply for, any additional *ad hoc* funding that might become available for new initiatives. These monies not only may enhance patient care but may also indirectly reduce demand on already commissioned pathways. However, caution should also be exhibited, to ensure that *ad hoc* programmes are well defined and deliverable and do not increase the demands on core commissioned services.

Key questions

- What are the various sources of income that make up the funding for my service?
- What are all the cost drivers for my service?
- Can I influence any of the cost drivers to contribute to a cost improvement programme?
- Is my service generating a surplus or a loss?
- How is the surplus (if any) being utilised?

Understanding allocation of resources

Most mental health organisations in England are still funded through a block contract. Therefore, a service's funding for the following year is largely based on its funding for the current year. This system of resource allocation ignores issues of case mix and demographic shift within the population served by the organisation. Often, it falls upon the medical managers to make the case for increased resource allocation for their services, based on hard data collected at an organisational level and contrasting it to other services. In times of stagnant or diminishing budgets, it is not sufficient to demonstrate that one's services are busier than in previous years. To make a valid case for increased funding, one almost always has to demonstrate that one's service is busier than it was in previous years in comparison with other services. As the pie is not growing bigger, more often than not it is a case of getting a bigger share of the pie.

This is less of a challenge in cases of payment-by-result or fee-for-service where services are paid according to performance or activity and can increase their resources using the increased income they generate through their superior performance. The acute sector has been functioning in this way in the UK for some years. However, this is not without its challenges for the health economy – but these are beyond the scope of this chapter.

The funding allocated to a particular service line is then sub-allocated to different teams. In order to undertake this allocation equitably, medical managers and their operational manager colleagues should ensure that they have all the information to make relevant decisions. Before allocating finances through a formal budget-setting process the medical and operational managers should review the population numbers served by each team, and each team's activity numbers and operational efficiency numbers (waiting times, case-load, turnover, etc.), as well as quality factors. If allocation to teams continues to be on a historical basis, then it is not reflecting the changing needs within teams, or encouraging service innovation.

Key questions

- How is the budgetary allocation for my service arrived at?
- What data do I need to obtain to ensure that my service is adequately funded relative to other similar services?
- To whom and how do I communicate the data-set that demonstrates the uniqueness of my service?

Understanding care pathway development and review

Care pathways are variously defined but, broadly:

> 'A clinical pathway explicitly states the goals and key elements of care based on Evidence Based Medicine (EBM) guidelines, best practice and patient expectations by facilitating the communication, coordinating roles and sequencing the activities of the multidisciplinary care team, patients and their relatives; by documenting, monitoring and evaluating variances; and by providing the necessary resources and outcomes.' (De Bleser *et al*, 2006: p. 553)

Therefore, by definition, care pathways should be designed and updated as new evidence emerges. Medical managers should always be questioning the relevance of existing care pathways and asking whether they need to be redesigned or updated. This does not necessarily mean that managers have to be content experts on the evidence base related to the care pathway. Their role is to ensure that the latest evidence base is applied in the most effective and efficient manner by the right professionals and at the right time.

In designing care pathways, due regard should be given to resource allocation within the pathway. For instance, many services create multiple triage steps to ensure that the most expensive resources (such as consultants, senior nurses and psychologists) are prioritised for the patients presenting with the most complex needs. However, experience suggests that in diagnostic groups for whom there is no concrete diagnostic test, it is often more efficient to front-load the assessment process, to clarify diagnosis and management plans at an early stage, than to have less experienced or less well qualified professionals implement these (Christensen *et al*, 2008). This may be relevant to many mental health services (Malik *et al*, 2015).

Key questions

- Are all the care pathways within my service underpinned by the latest evidence base?
- Is there a process in place for regular and timely review of all care pathways?
- Are all care pathways designed to ensure early diagnosis and the development of comprehensive management plans?

Understanding care pathway delivery

Theories of general operations management, derived largely from the manufacturing industry, clarify the relationship between the important concepts of demand, capacity, variability and utilisation. While it is beyond the scope of this chapter to discuss all of these in detail, key areas are touched on in this section. For more details on operational management concepts, interested readers should refer to Hopp & Lovejoy's (2013) volume on hospital operations, which the authors have referred to extensively for the definitions and concepts in this section.

The first step in influencing the operational performance of a service is to understand relevant data describing its current performance. These include very basic quantitative data such as number of staff, referral numbers, case-loads per member of clinical staff and staff sickness rates. The next step is to understand the flow process underlying the care pathway and develop the timelines associated with it. For instance, in considering new referrals to a service, if, on average, referral to triage takes 1 day and triage to allocation takes 3 days, then this information needs to be captured and similar information needs to be recorded for each step of patient flow along the care pathway until the point of disposal (this could be discharge from the service, referral to another service or referral to a follow-up clinic). It is only after this data collection that each step of the process can be analysed and efforts made to improve efficiency at each step to benefit the entire pathway.

Before proceeding further, let us consider a few key definitions.

Definitions of concepts

Capacity

The capacity of a resource is defined as the throughput it can achieve, provided it is never starved of work. For instance, a consultant psychiatrist might have the capacity to see one new patient every 2 hours.

Utilisation

The utilisation of a resource is the long-term fraction of time for which it is busy. This is given by the average arrival rate of work at the station (in a clinical example this could be the arrival of patients at an out-patient setting) divided by the resource capacity over the long term. It is important to understand that as utilisation reaches close to 100%, waiting times and queuing increases exponentially, rather than linearly. If over the long term all clinicians in a team are working at 100% utilisation, then there will always be queuing in the systems.

Bottleneck

Along the flow of the care pathway, the bottleneck in a system is the resource with the highest utilisation. This could be an individual (such as the team psychologist) or a piece of equipment (such as the magnetic resonance scanner).

Demand variability

This refers to scenarios where the demand for services is not uniform with time. Variability can be either synchronised or unsynchronised. Synchronised variability is when the capacity of the service changes in direct relation to the demand. Unsynchronised variability is where the capacity of the service does not change in direct proportion to variations in demand. The variability principle states that the greater the unsynchronised variability in demand for a service, the faster it will reach peak utilisation and lead to queuing and increased waiting times. Therefore, efforts to reduce significant peaks and troughs in referrals can have a similar impact to increasing the capacity of resources.

The other source of variability in the system in the implementation of the care pathway; that is, the patient experience and the duration of treatment and so on can be different from patient to patient. This can further increase the overall variability in the system and have the same impact as reduced capacity.

Key questions

- What is the capacity of the service and of each of its resources?
- What is the utilisation of each of the resources within the service?
- Where are the bottlenecks in the flow (pathway)?
- What is the variability within the service? Is it demand variability or variability in delivery of clinical input?

Application to service-related problems

The diagnosis and resolution of service-related problems can be achieved by combining the basic data on service demographics with the higher-level data around operations, and then benchmarking them internally against other services or externally against other organisations.

Generally, the aim of all services is to see more patients and to see them quicker. While simple ways of increasing capacity or reducing wait times within services are to either reduce workload or increase resources, these are hardly ever practical in real life.

There are, however, other practical ways in which service efficiency can be increased. These might include reduction in demand variability (e.g. by providing general practitioners with consultant psychiatrists' phone numbers), synchronising service capacity to demand (by having a flexible workforce so that more staff are available at known peak times), pooling of resources across teams and specialties, and cross-training of staff to perform a common minimum set of tasks.

Furthermore, care pathways should be simplified and standardised as much as possible, as this will help reduce errors, enhance pathway adherence and effectively improve outcomes and costs. These areas have been discussed in greater detail by Malik *et al* (2015).

Key questions

- Are there ways in which demand variability can be reduced?
- Are there ways in which service capacity can be synchronised as far as possible with demand?
- Are there ways in which service variability can be minimised?
- Are there redundant steps in the pathway that can be removed?
- Are there steps in the pathway that can occur in parallel rather than sequentially?
- What are the key steps affecting quality within the service and are they being protected and enhanced continually?

Understanding the role of service model innovations

Medical managers should continually seek to understand how they can improve their current services. This involves understanding two aspects:

technological and clinical innovations; and service model innovations. The former have briefly been touched on above in the discussion regarding evidence-based reviews of care pathways. The latter relate to innovating service delivery itself by encouraging the clinical team to constantly challenge the existing paradigms of 'This is how we do things here'.

Ramdas, in her seminal paper on service model innovations published in the *Harvard Business Review* (Ramdas *et al*, 2012), provides some food for thought for managers in transforming the service models that underpin care pathway delivery. She outlines four areas, which have been summarised in Table 12.2 with examples relevant to mental health services. Not all examples will be relevant to all services; however, medical managers need to have the awareness and courage to ask these questions in relation to their services and to use the responses to initiate a discussion on service model redesign.

Table 12.2 Service model innovations

Area	Illustrative examples
The structure of the interaction	Some patients will benefit more from receiving therapy in a group format, while in other instances (e.g. making a complex diagnosis) a number of professionals seeing patients simultaneously (or in the same hospital visit) might be more efficient
The service boundary	Co-location of money advice services or metabolic health check services for patients with chronic and severe mental illnesses might improve wider outcomes for this patient group
Allocation of tasks	Getting senior clinicians to transcribe their clinical information electronically might not be the most effective use of their time. Similarly, asking administrative staff to triage clinical telephone calls and messages might be both clinically risky and inefficient
Delivery location	For dementia patients and their carers, would it be more effective and efficient if the psychology team and the magnetic resonance imaging service were co-located with the memory clinic and a phlebotomist was present on site as well?

Understanding service evaluation

The first step in transforming existing services is to understand them both qualitatively and quantitatively. We have outlined the qualitative evaluation of care pathways above. However, to actually understand services quantitatively, one has to fall back on operational science literature from manufacturing. Once again, Hopp & Lovejoy (2013) in their treatise on hospital operations have helpfully outlined four broad areas that should encompass all the metrics requisite to evaluate the performance of a healthcare service or organisation. At an organisational level these metrics are often a combination of those agreed between the payer (commissioner) and provider, or those that the organisation's board has decided, based on the organisation's strategic priorities. The four categories of metrics are operational, clinical, financial and organisational.

Operational metrics

Broadly speaking, this refers to measuring activity, such as the numbers of referrals, admissions, out-patient appointments, waiting times, lengths of stay, time from referral to assessment and treatment (to name but a few).

Clinical metrics

This largely pertains to measuring the quality of clinical pathways, in relation to both process and outcomes. For example, in in-patient units this could include the proportion of patients who received a falls assessment or medication reconciliation on admission (process) or the number of falls or in-patient suicides of detained patients (outcome). Similarly, within the community setting, clinical metrics could include the number of patients who received a copy of their care plan or who had a risk assessment completed (process) or the number of patients who were successfully able to return to work following treatment (outcome).

Additionally, measures of patient experience and patient satisfaction allow organisations to obtain feedback from their patients regarding their performance.

Financial metrics

These metrics largely pertain to the costs of running the service and the income generated by it. Frequently used metrics include over- and under-spend in relation to the budget for a service and the proportion of financial plans (either cost-improvement plans or growth plans) that the service has achieved in the financial year. Additionally, many organisations also measure how their various services are performing in relation to previously set income targets.

Organisational metrics

Finally, there are organisational metrics that include direct measures such as staff satisfaction and indirect measures such as staff sickness. Additionally, services and organisations should also measure the uptake of new knowledge and practices by staff by measuring rates of staff appraisal and attendance at training events, both of which are indirect indicators of organisational learning.

Practical application

Ideally, all the above metrics or indicators are incorporated into an organisational dashboard that sets the performance metrics in relation to benchmarks and then splits the data under the same headings for individual services. Medical managers should work with their operational colleagues to take joint ownership of this dashboard for their service, decide what metrics they will be responsible for and what metrics, if any, should be added that are specific to their service.

In addition to the above, medical managers should ensure that resources are allocated to the collection of the data that feed into the metrics and that clinicians are not asked to expend precious professional energy doing so. Data should be analysed and disseminated to clinicians in a meaningful way. In most instances, the numbers raise questions regarding a particular service rather than providing answers to the challenges it faces. It is then up to medical managers to meet with senior clinicians to collaboratively understand the challenges of failing metrics and come up with action plans to resolve these.

The authors' experience, which is borne out by the work of the Boston Consulting Group (BCG), suggests that making performance data public leads to performance improvement, even though some clinicians might have apprehensions about this initially (Larsen & Lawyer, 2011). However, this relies on the clinical teams having faith in the metrics as well as in their collection methods and, therefore, it is prudent to reiterate the value of developing metrics collaboratively and collecting information in relation to them in a transparent manner.

Finally, in a small number of cases, poor performance metrics are an indicator of poor individual leadership or clinical performance, which needs to be addressed informally and formally, but this is outside the scope of this chapter.

Key questions

- What are the operational, clinical, financial and organisational metrics for the organisation?
- How do these relate to the service I work in?
- Is the data collection, presentation and dissemination being done in the most effective manner?
- Are there other metrics that we should be measuring for our particular service?

Conclusion

This chapter highlights the importance of psychiatrists having a sound understanding of the internal and external system they work within. To be in a position to influence clinical services one must possess the right information. The right information is generally gleaned by seeking answers to well thought out and incisive questions about the clinical services. While the questions set out in this chapter are not an exhaustive list, they are a reasonable starting point. Medical managers should work in collaboration with their operational colleagues to gain a better understanding of the system, share this understanding with their peers and other colleagues, and then collaboratively develop solutions to improve the functioning of clinical services and, ultimately, patient care.

References

Christensen CM, Grossman JH, Hwang J (2008) *The Innovator's Prescription: A Disruptive Solution for Healthcare*. McGraw-Hill.

De Bleser L, Depreitere R, De Waele K, *et al* (2006) Defining pathways. *Journal of Nursing Management*, **14**: 553–63.

Hopp WJ, Lovejoy WS (2013) *Hospital Operations: Principles of High Efficiency Health Care College*. FT Press.

Larsen S, Lawyer P (2011) *Improving Healthcare Value: The Case for Disease Registers*. BCG Perspectives (Boston Consulting Group).

Malik A, Field C, Gorwood P (2015) *Managing Financial Resources in Healthcare Settings*. Oxford University Press.

Ramdas K, Teisberg E, Tucker AL (2012) Four ways to reinvent service delivery. *Harvard Business Review*, December: 98–106.

CHAPTER 13

Working with the team

Frank Holloway and Tom Edwards

This chapter is about teamwork within mental health services. The authors' experience is as adult and rehabilitation psychiatrists with management roles working in England, but the principles are relevant to almost all aspects of psychiatric practice.

It is now a truism that teamwork is an essential component of any safe and effective healthcare organisation (Baker *et al*, 2006; Jenkinson *et al*, 2013; Nancarrow *et al*, 2013). Indeed, effective teamwork is seen as vital for undertaking complex and potentially risky tasks across a wide range of activities, from flying a passenger jet to successfully completing a construction project. Although there is a tendency to think of teams as stable and long-term entities, teamwork is often required when people have little or no knowledge of one another – for example, two pilots newly rostered together to take a flight across the Atlantic Ocean, or when a junior doctor arrives on a ward in an emergency or when agency nursing staff come to work on a ward.

Teamwork is defined in the *New Shorter Oxford English Dictionary* as 'the combined action of a team of players or a group of people especially when effective and efficient' or, alternatively, 'co-operation'. In the organisational literature, teams have been defined as 'social entities embedded in organisations, performing tasks which contribute to the organisation's goals' (West *et al*, 1998: p. 2). Less abstractly, researchers have understood a team to consist of 'two or more individuals, who have specific roles', who 'perform interdependent tasks, are adaptable, and share a common goal' (Baker *et al*, 2006: p. 1578). A concept analysis proposed a more refined definition of teamwork in healthcare: 'a dynamic process involving two or more healthcare professionals with complementary backgrounds and skills, sharing common health goals and exercising concerted physical and mental effort in assessing, planning, or evaluating patient care' (Xyrichis & Ream, 2008: p. 232). These differing definitions share an optimistic view of teamwork.

Mental healthcare has, since the rise of the asylum, always involved people from different backgrounds and with different roles working together in an organisational structure. Samuel Tuke's *Description of the Retreat*, published in 1813, reports in detail the work of key people in the early years of this pioneering asylum, which was set up by the Quaker community in York. Samuel's grandfather, William, was instrumental in the founding of the institution and provided what would now be called strategic direction. George Jepson was the original superintendent, with his later-to-be wife Katherine Allen in charge of female patients. The work of Thomas Fowler, the initial physician to the Retreat, is described in detail by Samuel Tuke, who noted Fowler's 'highly benevolent and unprejudiced mind' and the careful, empirical approach that he adopted towards the 'pharmaceutic means which have failed' (Tuke, 1813: p. 2): only hot baths for melancholia appeared to work, although the authority of the physician was seen as being an effective therapeutic tool. It appears from Samuel Tuke's account that the founding team of this institution worked well together, with considerable mutual respect.

Multidisciplinary working implies that individuals from different professional backgrounds (and increasingly, as the role of the support worker expands, without any professional qualification) come together in the common enterprise of meeting patient and carer need, as well as societal demand. The vast majority of staff in mental health services now acknowledge that they are working within one or more multidisciplinary teams, rather than functioning solely as an independent practitioner ('nurse', doctor', 'occupational therapist', 'social worker', 'welfare benefits advisor', 'support worker') (West *et al*, 2012). They contribute their personal and professional skills to the common enterprise.

Although consultant psychiatrists no longer possess the level of authority and control they once had (or believed they had), within mental health services they continue to play a pivotal role and require a sound understanding of the nature of leadership and how to foster effective team functioning (Jenkinson *et al*, 2013). 'Approved clinicians' are expected to demonstrate specific competencies. The Secretary of State for Health's 'Instructions with respect to the exercise of an approval function in relation to approved clinicians 2015' state that 'competency 7', entitled 'Leadership and Multidisciplinary Team Working', includes 'the ability to lead a multidisciplinary team and to assimilate the (potentially diverse) views of other professionals, patients and carers'. Professionally and personally, one of the worst things that can happen to psychiatrists is to lose the confidence of their teams.

Positives and negatives of teamwork

The generic literature on teamwork identifies many benefits of successful teams. These include: improvements in the confidence, motivation and satisfaction of team members; the value of group discussion in improving the clarity of a group member's ideas and the opportunity for getting new ideas about how to solve a problem; more efficient use of resources;

optimism about achieving a positive outcome; and the ability to respond to change more effectively. Within healthcare, good teamwork has been associated with innovation, improved mental health of staff, better retention and lower staff turnover, and, in acute hospitals, a lower death rate (Borrill *et al*, 2000).

There are, however, some potential drawbacks to teamwork. One is 'social loafing', where a team member contributes little to the overall work of the team. Teams also have a potential for 'groupthink', the development of shared but false assumptions. Effective teams discourage the social loafer and provide internal challenge to false assumptions: the key here is a healthy team culture that both respects and challenges team members.

Even good teams may have members who are performing poorly or behaving badly. Dealing with 'difficult' colleagues is a problem. It can be addressed by support from the team, where difficulties have an understandable cause, and peer pressure. Ultimately it may become a matter for management action. The Royal College of Psychiatrists (2010*a*) provides helpful guidance on this.

There is also an unacknowledged paradox inherent in the current emphasis on teamwork. Referrers, service users, carers, practitioners and the psychotherapy literature all emphasise the importance to the therapeutic outcome of the individual relationship between a practitioner and patient, often sustained over the long term. Even in the contemporary era of 'payment by results', 'care clusters' and 'care pathways', the bedrock of effective mental healthcare lies in the work of each practitioner. Teams are a means of providing structure for and enhancing the quality of this individual work. A particular value of the multidisciplinary team is that it brings together individuals with diverse approaches to understanding mental health problems and a range of professional expertise not available from any single discipline, in a more effective way than referral to a separate service.

Working in a high-functioning team is both enjoyable and professionally rewarding. Trying to work to high standards in a dysfunctional team can be distressing and dispiriting; one of the hardest managerial tasks is to turn around a struggling team or service. Although the vast majority of National Health Service (NHS) staff report that they work within teams, only a minority report working within a team that meets rather minimal criteria for being considered effective (West *et al*, 2012: p. 16).

Failures in care

In the asylum, formal authority was vested in a medical superintendent. In practice, absolute power over the welfare of the patients rested in the hands of senior nurses. Nurses controlled both information flows between the doctors and the patients and the daily routine of care. In the best hospitals doctors, nurses and other staff worked to advance patients' interests – in the worst they colluded in regimes combining financial economy with neglect. A series of scandals resulted in systematic investigation into the determinants of good and bad quality of care within institutions caring for people with a mental illness or intellectual disability, or elderly persons (Martin, 1984). Uniformly, catastrophic failure in care was associated with a team rather than a particular individual. Unacceptably poor-quality care tended to develop where medical and other professional leadership was lacking, training was poor, staff groups worked in isolation and there was no effective external lay or managerial oversight.

Although healthcare has changed enormously in the decades since the hospital scandals of the 1960s and 1970s, the continuing potential for standards of care in facilities providing mental healthcare and care for people with intellectual disability to become unacceptably poor was revealed by the Winterbourne View scandal. Patients in a small hospital for people with intellectual disability who exhibited 'challenging behaviours' experienced psychological and physical abuse, to the extent that 11 members of staff were convicted of a range of offences. The final report on Winterbourne View noted that this was an ostensibly nurse-led facility but that it was in practice reliant on support workers to deliver care (Department of Health, 2012).

Poor care is not confined to mental health and intellectual disability services, as the Francis report into events at Stafford Hospital makes very clear (Francis, 2013). According to Francis, staff teams at the hospital, particularly on wards catering for elderly patients, developed a culture in which unacceptable care was seen as the norm. The root cause identified was the managerial pursuit of financial imperatives, with which some staff acquiesced. Francis made 290 recommendations. These cover broad areas surrounding the governance, regulation, resourcing and leadership of healthcare, as well as training. There is a focus on the quality of front-line nursing and in particular how to embed a 'culture of caring' (recommendation 185). Only in the area of elderly care, where Francis found the abuses were particularly stark, was there a specific recommendation about multidisciplinary working. Recommendation 237 reads:

> 'There needs to be effective teamwork between all the different disciplines and services that together provide the collective care often required by an elderly patient; the contribution of cleaners, maintenance staff, and catering staff also needs to be recognised and valued.'

This recommendation has clear relevance to both community and in-patient mental health services.

A typology of mental health teams

Øvretveit (2001) identified five types of team commonly encountered in mental health services. In a *case manager's team*, people are brought together in an *ad hoc* fashion to organise and coordinate services for a client, as in a multi-agency Care Programme Approach (CPA) meeting. A *network team* allows the exchange of information and referral, for example when primary and secondary care services join together to review shared cases. In a *formal service delivery team*, such as a community mental health team (CMHT) or in-patient ward, a defined range of services is provided for a specific population. *Project teams* are brought together to undertake a defined task in a limited period, for example to review or develop a service or an operational policy. A *management team* will be collectively accountable for service delivery. The effective psychiatrist needs to be able to recognise and operate within all these kinds of teams, and other groupings that come together to achieve shared aims, such as consultants' committees and training committees. This chapter focuses on working within a *formal service delivery team*.

Contemporary mental health services consist of a large number of formal service delivery teams. The names and functions of teams change in accordance with the evidence base, fashion and local taste. At the time of writing, most local adult mental health services have separate community-based teams providing psychological treatments, crisis intervention/home treatment, short-term assessment and treatment, early intervention in psychosis and longer-term care. Liaison teams will work in general hospital settings, including in particular the accident and emergency department. In-patient services will include acute wards, now often differentiated into an immediate-admission ward and a longer-term ward, and a psychiatric intensive care unit. People with more complex problems may be under the care of more specialist teams, for example eating disorders, perinatal psychiatry, rehabilitation and forensic services. People with complex comorbidities (e.g. substance misuse and psychosis) may be under the care of more than one team.

What makes for an effective team?

Readers are likely to have had experience of working in formal service delivery teams that are functioning well, but may also have had less positive experiences. A study of teams providing community rehabilitation and intermediate care (not mental health teams but with an analogous function), identified ten characteristics of a good interdisciplinary team (Nancarrow *et al*, 2013), which they recast as 'team competencies' (Box 13.1). These competencies relate to effective leadership, clarity of goals, team processes and aspects of team staffing.

A large-scale study of CMHTs noted that on average CMHTs report lower levels of resources and organisational support than NHS teams in general: this is plausibly because CMHT staff rarely received praise from more senior management (West *et al*, 2012). However, staff reported 'a strong focus on the needs of clients, a good level of constructive debate, an emphasis on quality and a preparedness to discuss errors and mistakes constructively

---

Box 13.1 Competencies of an effective team

1 Identifies a leader who establishes a clear direction and vision for the team, while listening and providing support and supervision to the team members.
2 Incorporates a set of values that clearly provide direction for the team's service provision; these values should be visible and consistently portrayed.
3 Demonstrates a team culture and interdisciplinary atmosphere of trust where contributions are valued and consensus is fostered.
4 Ensures appropriate processes and infrastructures are in place to uphold the vision of the service (e.g. referral criteria, communications infrastructure).
5 Provides quality patient-focused services with documented outcomes; utilises feedback to improve the quality of care.
6 Utilises communication strategies that promote intra-team communication, collaborative decision-making and effective team processes.
7 Provides sufficient team staffing to integrate an appropriate mix of skills, competencies, and personalities to meet the needs of patients and enhance smooth functioning.
8 Facilitates recruitment of staff who demonstrate interdisciplinary competencies, including team functioning, collaborative leadership, communication and sufficient professional knowledge and experience.
9 Promotes role interdependence while respecting individual roles and autonomy.
10 Facilitates personal development through appropriate training, rewards, recognition and opportunities for career development.

Source: Nancarrow *et al* (2013)

Box 13.2 Recommendations from the Effectiveness of Multi-Professional Team Working in Mental Health Care Study

1 Clarify purpose and functions of community mental health teams
2 Provide good leadership
3 Actively manage team composition and processes
4 Promote inter-team working
5 Ensure reflection and adaptation

Source: West *et al* (2012)

... high levels of trust, safety and support ... good communication and regular meetings ... [and] a strong sense of attachment to the team and its members' (West *et al*, 2012: p. 127). Consistent with other literature and practical experience, West *et al* (2012) found that the more specialised community teams, particularly those providing early intervention in psychosis and assertive outreach, reported a higher level of effectiveness than the generic CMHT, which had a rather poorly defined role.

A number of recommendations emerged from this study (see Box 13.2). These show striking similarities to the findings of Nancarrow *et al* (2013), who used a very different methodology (Box 13.1). West *et al* (2012) include an additional dimension of good functioning – the importance of *inter-team working*. This reflects the highly fragmented structure of contemporary mental health services, which will frequently see patients moving rapidly through a dizzying array of services. During a typical relapse episode, care will be provided for a patient by a CMHT, the psychiatric liaison service, the crisis response/home treatment and/or the approved mental health professional (AMHP) service, one or more acute in-patient wards and then back to the CMHT. If things go less well, the patient may be discharged to yet another team. Hard-pressed teams need to be aware that they are engaged in a common enterprise with other teams, working within a mental health system that should be focused on patient need.

Mental health teams operate in uncertain and unpredictable policy and practice environments, undertake complex tasks and use treatment technologies that are also uncertain and unpredictable. Well over a decade ago, Onyett (2003) noted that an effective team will not only carry out its task-related objectives, but will also cater for the well-being and development of its members and be viable in the long term. Mental health teams require adequate numbers of good-quality staff who have a clear, agreed task and are well managed. Too often, either overall or local management is poor and the task is blurred.

Decision-making

Decision-making processes vary between mental health teams. The 'care pathway' for a service includes a number of obvious key decision points: defining the patient group; accepting a case for assessment; taking an individual onto the case-load or diverting to another service; allocating responsibilities for provision of treatment and care; managing crises that present; reviewing outcomes; and discharge from care. Some teams have little or no control over who comes onto their case-load, for example the acute in-patient ward, while more specialist teams have absolute control over who they take on: these teams tend to have clearer goals, higher prestige and less stressed staff (Johnson *et al*, 2012).

Some professionals in a team may have more control over their case-load by operating a parallel referral pathway. In principle, these decisions are subsumed under the overarching CPA (Department of Health, 2008), within which decisions about specialist mental healthcare are agreed and coordinated. Day-to-day practice is less clear-cut and teams need to develop local agreements (within an operational policy) about how the 'care pathway' is managed.

The CPA process should include all relevant persons in the patient's care, including informal carers and services providing support (Department of

Health, 2008). Where the patient's needs are complex, this may involve a number of individuals and teams coming together to elaborate the care plan and care pathway; this is an example of Øvretveit's *case manager's* team in action. There are specific skills that the chair of a CPA meeting (often the consultant psychiatrist) requires. It is important to obtain consensus on, or 'buy-in' to, the plan that emerges, in order to ensure that everyone understands what has been agreed and to ensure that the meeting has been recorded accurately.

The roles of team members

Members of a multidisciplinary team commonly experience difficulties in defining their roles within the team *vis-à-vis* staff from other disciplines. Increasingly, particularly in community teams, job descriptions emphasise the required competencies over the discipline of the post-holder. Accordingly, there have been repeated attempts over the past three decades to establish a generic mental health worker role. Throughout healthcare, tasks that were traditionally the exclusive province of doctors, such as prescribing medication, have been successfully undertaken by non-medical staff (although evaluation of this delegation of responsibility has focused on relatively routine tasks). The role of the 'responsible clinician' under the Mental Health Act, which replaced the 'responsible medical officer', is now, of course, open to non-doctors.

The dissonance between the so-called 'medical model' and the social work ethos can lead to social workers feeling isolated and devalued. Mental Health Act assessments can be a particular challenge for integrated teams. Many AMHPs feel the independent nature of their role is compromised by working in close proximity to medical colleagues: where this was not the case previously, services are moving towards borough-wide or county-wide AMHP teams that either are stand-alone or draw from locality teams on a rota basis.

Within many mental health teams, a degree of generic working is enthusiastically embraced. However, the specialist skills and conceptual frameworks that individuals with a specific personal and professional background bring with them are also valued. Tyrer (2000) advocated a skill-share model, whereby professionals retained expertise in their core skills but shared them sufficiently with colleagues from other disciplines to enable them to be utilised appropriately.

Management tasks within mental health teams

Øvretveit (2001) set out eight key management tasks for mental health teams: drafting job descriptions; interviewing and appointing staff; induction; assigning work to staff; reviewing work; appraisal and objective-setting; ensuring quality, training and professional development; and engaging in disciplinary procedures. Since the time of that publication, multiple additional responsibilities have been added, particularly in relation to governance, informatics and the legal aspects of mental health, which include highly complex issues in relation to the law on community care. Given the perennial turmoil surrounding mental health services, an important skill for people in leadership roles is the management of change, a topic beyond the scope of this chapter.

Traditionally, professionals within teams worked to line managers in their own profession, all messily responsible for some or all of these management tasks. The allocation of work within a team frequently fell between managerial stools (a good diagnostic test when looking at a service that is struggling is to ask people to identify who has the authority to change things). Management structures for mental health services have evolved rapidly. In the 1980s only 10% of CMHTs had a manager (Onyett, 1997). Now the norm is for team leaders (ward managers in in-patient settings) to have overall managerial and budgetary responsibility for all staff within the team, with a degree of professional accountability and supervisory responsibility being held by service-wide professional heads. Currently, it is often only the doctors within teams who remain separately accountable, through a line from the consultant to the clinical director/associate medical director and ultimately the medical director.

Accountability and responsibility

Mental health services in England have, in recent years, moved rapidly towards prescriptively structured teams that are highly accountable to local management and responsible for delivering nationally determined targets, for example the implementation of guidelines from the National Institute for Health and Care Excellence (NICE), and allocating the case-load to 'care clusters'. There are clear tensions within this framework that affect professional staff, who have traditionally valued their autonomy. The organisational literature strongly suggests that staff work best when they experience a degree of control over their workload and working environment.

Failures in health and social care tend to result in calls for improvement in the external monitoring of team performance. The Francis report (2013) is an example of this, since the majority of its recommendations relate to the regulation of service providers and individual practitioners. There has been a countervailing argument that excessive monitoring of staff in the pursuit of increased effectiveness was demotivating, due to the implied lack of confidence and trust in staff (Handy, 1981). This argument is, in the contemporary era of clinical governance and health informatics, now lost.

Transparency and accountability are the current watchwords. In responding to the Francis report, the Royal College of Psychiatrists (2013) acknowledged five key principles underpinning care:

1 Always put patients first, engaging openly and transparently with patients and carers about care and treatment – respecting their wishes wherever possible.
2 Prioritise patient safety and well-being.
3 Provide high-quality clinical leadership within teams of professionals and in organisations.
4 Respect regulation, inspection and accountability as supporting care.
5 Value the importance of outcomes and accurate data in improving patient care.

Presumably, the authors of the report assumed that the psychiatrist would have adequate technical skills.

There are knotty issues surrounding the responsibility and accountability of members of multi-professional mental health teams. The consultant psychiatrist is not the undisputed leader of the team (Department of Health, 2010). Responsibilities can be divided into *employee responsibilities* (as set out in contracts and job descriptions), *professional responsibilities* (as set out in codes of conduct and defined standards of professional practice, with the doctor's professional regulator being the General Medical Council) and *legal responsibilities* (as defined by statute and common law, e.g. the duty of care and specific responsibilities set out in the Mental Health Act and Mental Capacity Act).

There is particular controversy over the degree of responsibility held by individuals (notably the team leader/manager and the consultant pychiatrist/responsible clinician), the extent to which responsibility can be distributed among team members who undertake specifically agreed tasks and whether responsibility can be held collectively by the team (an idea that would appear to be unlikely to survive legal challenge). One particularly onerous role within a mental health team is that of care coordinator (Department of Health, 2010: pp. 18–19). Employers, of course, have responsibilities, notably in spelling out the expectations on staff and ensuring appropriate structures are in place for these expectations to be met (in terms of, for example, staff selection, supervision and training, and the available resources, policies and procedures).

Power and multidisciplinary working

The organisational literature emphasises the roles of power, influence and authority in making any complex organisation work (Onyett, 2003). For Handy (1981: pp. 111–144), power can: be *physical* (e.g. bullying); lie in the control of *resources*; be related to a particular *position* within the organisation; be inherent in some form of *expertise*; or be purely *personal*, flowing from individual charisma. The final source of power that Handy identifies is *negative* power – the capacity to ensure that any initiative does not succeed. In professionally dominated organisations, such as the NHS, professionals, particularly doctors, wield considerable negative power.

Handy goes on to describe how these forms of power can be used to influence the actions of others – which is the key issue for an organisation – by means of *coercion*, the application of *rules or procedures*, *bargaining* (as in a *quid pro quo*), *persuasion* (appealing to the other's rationality and professional values) or *altering the work environment*. Hunter (1999) suggests that when managing in the public sector, it is more effective to take on the role of 'servant leader', supporting and guiding staff rather than exerting status and power. This may not sit well with some consultant psychiatrists, but may provide an indication of how to lead more effectively.

Influencing the culture of the team

Teams work best when the members agree on the common cause, rather than merely functioning according to power relationships. The key issue for members of a well-functioning team, once its task is clarified, is how to achieve their common objectives. Here, *persuasion* is the most effective form of power. Other forms of power become relevant when there is no agreement about team objectives or methods. Consultant psychiatrists may then have to resort to *bargaining* and appealing to relevant *rules or procedures* to ensure that the work is done. It is also valuable for their credibility within the team if consultants can influence the allocation of resources, even in a small way: this will depend crucially on their skills at working within the larger organisation. The consultant will be anxious to foster a team culture that is healthily focused on appropriate tasks and outcomes, although this is by no means easy.

The consultant psychiatrist and the team leader/ manager

Although there are some who advocate that the consultant psychiatrist should automatically be the leader of any multidisciplinary team, this is not commonly the case in practice. Because of the multiple, time-consuming aspects of the team leader role, it would be a poor use of scarce senior clinical time. This is, of course, not to say that psychiatrists should not be providing clinical leadership to teams within which they work (Royal College of Psychiatrists, 2010b; Jenkinson *et al*, 2013).

Where the team leader is not a psychiatrist, there is a potential tension between the role of the team leader, who has clear managerial accountability for service delivery and wide-ranging responsibilities for the work of staff within the multidisciplinary team, and that of the consultant, who has authority over non-consultant doctors. In the community setting, team leaders have a key role in allocating work to individual team members and managing the overall case-load. This can be a source of conflict. The consultant will generally have strong (and hopefully well-informed) opinions about the needs of patients in contact with the service, as well as a rather clear idea about the functioning of team members. Team leaders are responsible for meeting external targets that reflect organisational priorities about which the consultant may be ignorant or dismissive. The consultant may fall outside the management structure but will also feel responsible for the performance of the team: neither the psychiatrist nor the team leader has the authority to constrain the other's activity.

In its response to the Francis report, the Royal College of Psychiatrists (2013: p. 15) stated:

> 'Psychiatrists, whether or not in formal medical management roles, must: advocate and implement excellent care within their teams; promote a patient-safety-first culture, and embed this in daily practice support and enable colleagues to deliver high-quality care; [and] promote a culture where colleagues feel safe and supported in raising concerns.'

This is an excellent starting point for defining the consultant role within a team.

Managing demand in mental health teams

One particular difficulty for many teams is the management of demand, which for health and social services continually threatens to overwhelm available resources. Doctors have traditionally taken a leading role in this, using mechanisms that have been far from transparent to the public (or the Department of Health). Writing in the context of the covert rationing of healthcare, New (1996) identified some well-worn strategies employed to control workload (see Table 13.1). Developments in health policy have sought to block off some of the ways community mental health services have managed demand, by, for example, bearing down hard on waiting lists,

Table 13.1 Strategies for managing excessive demand

Strategy	Manifestations and outcomes
Deterrence	Service charges, gate-keeping by primary care, unfriendly staff, inconvenient appointment times, poor-quality care environments
Deflection	Passing referrals to other agencies – shifting between health and social care, primary and secondary care, mental health and intellectual disability services
Dilution	Thinly spreading service provision, adopting minimal standards of care, reducing skill mix in a nursing team
Delay	Waiting lists (which for psychological treatments can become infinitely long)
Denial	Not providing a treatment or service at all – using eligibility criteria

Adapted from New (1996).

removing the health/social care divide and demanding written protocols defining the responsibilities of services. However, as resources shrink, these measures are now again being increasingly used.

The contemporary emphasis is on services using strategies that ensure the rapid flow of patients through the metaphorical 'care pathway', retaining in secondary care a deserving few who will be in receipt of clearly defined and regularly reviewed 'packages of care' offered within 'care clusters' (Jacobs, 2014). Doctors in all disciplines no longer have the same degree of control over their workload and that of the teams within which they work, this role now being shared in psychiatry with the bed manager and the team leader.

The current economic climate has led to significant financial pressures on mental health service providers in the UK, probably to a greater degree than in the acute sector, despite the lip service paid to 'parity of esteem'. These pressures result in organisational 'turbulence', which can appear to some to be chaos. For example, the past decade has seen the development of assertive outreach teams across England, only to see their widespread destruction in response to developments in the evidence base and, more pertinently, the need to make savings. Currently, teams are continually being formed and reformed, as service structures are altered in an attempt to deliver efficiency savings (i.e. cost reductions) and, in some cases, align the overall service to a set of care clusters. There will be a limit on how far efficiency savings can be driven before the effectiveness of mental health services is significantly challenged.

The psychiatrist as a clinical leader

Psychiatrists commonly take on leadership roles and much of this book is devoted to describing these roles. Psychiatrists in training should be familiar with contemporary thinking on the competencies expected of their role in medical leadership, which are now included in specialist training curricula (Academy of Medical Royal Colleges & NHS Institute for Innovation and Improvement, 2010; Jenkinson et al, 2013).

A variety of leadership styles have been identified, including the *laissez-faire* style (which might be described as hands-off), *transactional* leadership (getting the job done) and *transformational* leadership, where the overall vision counts most (Harrison & Gray, 2003). The contemporary NHS is much taken by transformational leadership and this is obviously most required when there is a need for change, when, for example, a team or service is underperforming. Important though the transformational style may be, there are often prosaic tasks that have to be undertaken to ensure that teams can function (Reynolds & Thornicroft, 1999). These tasks are outlined in Table 13.2. Few consultants would wish to undertake all of them for the teams within which they work, but all should be willing and able to contribute their expertise to ensure that the tasks are carried out effectively.

179

Table 13.2   Key leadership tasks in mental health teams

Leadership tasks	Effects for the mental health team
Managing change	Motivation of staff; managing anxiety and opposition to change; breaking down change into achievable steps
Managing staff	Recruitment; producing job descriptions; managing staff performance; supervision; assessing and meeting training needs; dealing with conflict
Managing budgets	Producing budgets; interpreting budget statements; implementing financial controls; managing underspends and overspends
Managing the team	Maintaining service quality; enhancing communication within the team; producing and interpreting information; delegation of responsibilities
Working with stakeholders	Managing team boundaries; working within the larger organisation to achieve local and shared goals; accessing resources; user and carer involvement; working with primary care and commissioners
Anticipating the future	Awareness of key organisational drivers (e.g. targets, star ratings); awareness of policy and practice trends

Adapted from Reynolds & Thornicroft (1999).

The NHS Leadership Academy (2013) has published a revised Healthcare Leadership Model, which builds on the NHS Leadership Framework and the Medical Leadership Competency Framework (Academy of Medical Royal Colleges & NHS Institute for Innovation and Improvement, 2010). The model has nine components, each of which has a description and a set of competencies (Box 13.3). Levels of competency range from the 'essential' to the 'exemplary'. One of the nine competencies is 'Engaging the team', which is defined as:

> 'Involving individuals and demonstrating that their contributions are valued and important for delivering outcomes and continuous improvements to the service.'

To quote the model:

> 'Leaders promote teamwork and a feeling of pride by valuing individuals' contributions and ideas; this creates an atmosphere of staff engagement where desirable behaviour, such as mutual respect, compassionate care and attention to detail, are reinforced by all team members.'

Essential to this competency is *involving the team* (listening to what team members have to say). Proficiency is described as 'fostering creative participation' (seeking feedback and involving the team in identifying potential problems and solutions). Those who aspire to being strong need to 'cooperate to raise the game' (a rather banal expectation to encourage team members to work together and be available to support other teams).

Box 13.3 The NHS Leadership Model: leadership dimensions

1 Inspiring shared purpose
2 Leading with care
3 Evaluating information
4 Connecting our service
5 Sharing the vision
6 Engaging the team
7 Holding to account
8 Developing capability
9 Influencing for results

Source: NHS Leadership Academy (2013)

To be exemplary, the healthcare leader must be 'stretching the team for excellence and innovation'.

Conclusion: how to succeed and how to fail in team-working

Psychiatrists need to cultivate an interest in how teams work and an understanding of the complexities surrounding leadership roles within

---

Box 13.4 How psychiatrists succeed with a multidisciplinary team

- High degree of technical competence
- Specialist expertise
- Effective response to crisis
- Respect from patients and carers
- Meeting (time) commitments
- Getting through the required work
- Respect for other members of staff
- Genuine interest in other professional roles (ask questions!)
- Listening to others' opinions
- Making (good) decisions
- Clear communication
- Availability
- Politeness
- Consistency
- Taking responsibility
- Acknowledging error
- Learning from mistakes
- Praise – specific rather than generalised
- Supporting team with management
- Evidence of strategic vision

Box 13.5　How psychiatrists fail with multidisciplinary teams

- Rudeness to patients, staff and carers
- High-handedness
- Inconsistency
- Favouritism within the team
- Not listening to staff, patients and carers
- Bullying team members
- Unwillingness to take responsibility
- Blaming others when things go wrong
- Refusal to make decisions
- Unavailability generally and in crises
- Poor timekeeping
- Poor technical competence
- Undermining the team leader
- Disliked/ignored by management and consultant peers
- Failure to learn from mistakes
- 'Pigeon-holing' other professions – holding outdated/inaccurate views about their role

---

a team (Jenkinson *et al*, 2013). There are some obvious ways for the psychiatrist to be an effective member of a multidisciplinary team (Box 13.4). Equally, although rarely acknowledged, there are ways for the consultant to fail (Box 13.5). Broadly speaking, a consultant's success within a team depends on both a modicum of technical competence and a range of interpersonal skills and abilities. Outright failure with a team is generally due to a lack of interpersonal skills.

Rightly the consultant will feel responsible for how well the team is working. In reality, teams ebb and flow. There will be, even in the best of services, times of excellent functioning and times when the team is going through a difficult period. Difficulties can be due to external or contingent factors, such as seemingly unreasonable demands from management, changing political circumstances, funding problems, staff turnover or some demoralising adverse event. They can also be due to factors internal to the team, of which the most obvious are lack of agreement about what the team is supposed to do, poor leadership and personal or professional conflicts between team members.

The effective consultant psychiatrist will support the team leader in ensuring that the key management tasks required to maintain good team working are undertaken, and will also be aware of when the predominant task becomes one of transformation.

References

Academy of Medical Royal Colleges & NHS Institute for Innovation and Improvement (2010) *Medical Leadership Competency Framework. Enhancing Engagement in Medical Leadership* (3rd edition). NHS Institute for Innovation and Improvement.

Baker DP, Day R, Salas E (2006) Teamwork as an essential component of high-reliability organisations. *Health Services Research*, **41**: 1576–98.

Borrill CS, Carletta A, Carter A, *et al* (2000) *The Effectiveness of Health Care Teams in the National Health Service*. Aston Centre for Health Service Organisation Research.

Department of Health (2008) *Refocusing the Care Programme Approach*. Department of Health.

Department of Health (2010) *Responsibility and Accountability. Moving on for New Ways of Working to a Creative, Capable Workforce*. Department of Health.

Department of Health (2012) *Transforming Care: A National Response to Winterbourne View Hospital. Department of Health Review: Final Report*. Department of Health.

Francis R (2013) *Report of the Mid Staffordshire NHS Foundation Trust Public Inquiry. Executive Summary*. TSO.

Handy CB (1981) *Understanding Organizations*. Penguin.

Harrison T, Gray AJ (2003) Leadership, complexity and the mental health professional. A report on some approaches to leadership training. *Journal of Mental Health*, **12**: 153–9.

Hunter D (1999) *Managing for Health. Implementing the New Health Agenda*. Institute for Public Policy Research.

Jacobs R (2014) Payment by results for mental health services: economic considerations of case-mix funding. *Advances in Psychiatric Treatment*, **20**: 155–64.

Jenkinson J, Oakley C, Mason F (2013) Teamwork: the art of being a leader and a team player. *Advances in Psychiatric Treatment*, **19**: 221–8.

Johnson S, Osborn DP, Araya R, *et al* (2012) Morale in the English mental health workforce: questionnaire survey. *British Journal of Psychiatry*, **201**: 239–46.

Martin JP (1984) *Hospitals in Trouble*. Basil Blackwell.

Nancarrow SA, Booth A, Ariss S, *et al* (2013) Ten principles of good interdisciplinary teamwork. *Human Resources for Health*, **11**: 19.

New B (1996) The rationing agenda in the NHS. *BMJ*, **312**: 1593–601.

NHS Leadership Academy (2013) *The Healthcare Leadership Model, version 1.0*. NHS Leadership Academy.

Onyett S (1997) The challenge of managing community mental health teams. *Health and Social Care in the Community*, **5**: 40–7.

Onyett S (2003) *Teamworking in Mental Health*. Palgrave.

Øvretveit J (2001) The multidisciplinary team. In *Textbook of Community Psychiatry* (eds G Thornicroft, G Szmukler): pp 207–14. Oxford University Press.

Reynolds A, Thornicroft G (1999) *Managing Mental Health Services*. Open University Press.

Royal College of Psychiatrists (2010*a*) *Psychiatrists' Support Service. Information Guide: On Dealing with Difficult Colleagues*. RCPsych support service website, http://www.rcpsych.ac.uk/workinpsychiatry/psychiatristssupportservice/informationguides/difficultcolleagues.aspx (accessed April 2016).

Royal College of Psychiatrists (2010*b*) *Role of the Consultant Psychiatrist. Leadership and Excellence in Mental Health Services* (Occasional Paper OP74). Royal College of Psychiatrists.

Royal College of Psychiatrists (2013) *Driving Quality Implementation in the Context of the Francis Report* (Occasional Paper OP92). Royal College of Psychiatrists

Salas E, Dickinson TL, Converse SJ (1992) Toward an understanding of team performance and training. In *Teams: Their Training and Performance* (eds R Swezey, E Salas): pp 3–29 Ablex.

Tuke S (1813) *Description of the Retreat: An Institution Near York for Insane Persons*. W Alexander. .

Tyrer P (2000) The future of the community mental health team. *International Review of Psychiatry*, **12**: 219–26.

West MA, Borrill CS, Unsworth KL (1998) Team effectiveness in organizations In *International Review of Industrial and Organizational Psychology, Vol. 13* (eds CL Cooper, JT Robertson): pp 1–48. Wiley.

West M, Alimo-Metcalf B, Dawson J, *et al* (2012) *Effectiveness of Multi-Professional Team Working (MPTW) in Mental Health Care. Final Report.* NIHR Service Delivery and Organization Programme.

Xyrichis A, Ream E (2008) Teamwork: a concept analysis. *Journal of Advanced Nursing,* **61**: 232–41.

CHAPTER 14

Managing multicultural and multinational teams in healthcare

Oyedeji Ayonrinde

This chapter highlights considerations for leaders and managers of multi-national healthcare teams. A number of theoretical frameworks are applied to understanding these multinational teams. For the manager, additional competencies may be required to ensure effective work towards shared goals as high levels of cultural heterogeneity influence team functioning and healthcare delivery. As multinational teams will all have their own unique characteristics, the manager should recognise and adapt to this.

While the National Health Service (NHS) is the primary health provider in the UK, health services more generally have a diverse and global workforce. The multinational and multidisciplinary workforce interacts daily with patients and carers of cultural, ethnic and social diversity. Clinical teams, on the other hand, experience an interplay of variables such as professional status, age, gender, years of experience and complexity of roles carried out. Interspersed with this are individual staff cultures, language competencies, countries of origin, values and beliefs.

The workforce

Table 14.1 gives a breakdown of NHS staff (2015 figures) by professional category. About 11% of this healthcare workforce, 14% of the professionally qualified clinical staff and 26% of doctors were born outside the UK.

Doctors

As of April 2016, doctors from 152 different countries are registered with the UK medical regulatory body, the General Medical Council (GMC), with the largest numbers from India, Pakistan and South Africa (GMC, 2016) (Fig. 14.1). Medical workforce demography and migration trends are continuously changing (full details available on GMC website). The number of graduates from the European Union (EU) joining the UK medical register is greater than the number of international medical graduates (IMGs), exceeding the numbers from South Asia. European graduates were

Table 14.1   NHS workforce, 2015

Category	Number employed
Professionally qualified clinical staff	658661
All doctors	115303
Total non-medical staff	1127480
Qualified nursing, midwifery & health visiting staff	363610
Total qualified scientific, therapeutic & technical staff	160799
Qualified ambulance staff	18949
Support to clinical staff	369054
NHS infrastructure support	215068
Total	1242783

Source: Data from http://www.hscic.gov.uk/catalogue/PUB17807 (accessed April 2016).

about a tenth of all doctors in 2013, whereas IMGs represented a quarter. The number of UK graduates leaving to work abroad is also increasing. Regarding ethnicity, 47.7% of doctors on the register describe themselves as White, 18.7% Asian and 2.6% Black, 3.6% as belonging to other ethnic groups and 1.4% as being of mixed origin.

In psychiatry, 59% of doctors on the specialist register are UK graduates, 32% IMGs and 13% European graduates. More than a third of psychiatrists in training are non-UK graduates.

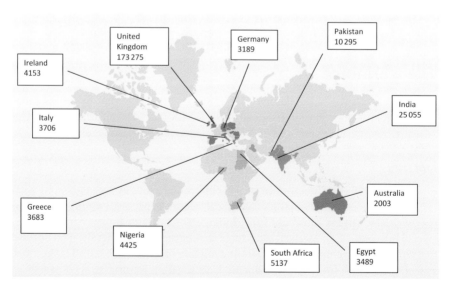

Fig. 14.1   World map indicating countries of primary medical qualification for doctors working in the UK (data from GMC, 2016).

While it has been contended that a diverse workforce benefits the culturally and ethnically diverse patient population in the UK, there is little empirical evidence to support this. Undoubtedly, though, better understanding of the workforce is necessary for effective management and leadership.

With globalisation, country of medical qualification may not correspond with the clinician's culture or ethnicity. A study commissioned by the GMC found that a number of overseas-trained doctors experienced challenges associated with legal, ethical, cultural and professional standards. In addition, organisational knowledge was inadequate among some doctors when they entered the workforce (Slowther *et al*, 2009). Communication and cultural awareness were problematic for some doctors, for instance 'subtleties of language, dialects and misunderstandings of the nuances of non-verbal communication, social behaviour and norms' (Slowther *et al*, 2009). Though medically knowledgeable, some struggled with 'cultural literacy' and consequently a higher proportion of complaints, suspensions and exclusions than UK graduates. Some 60% of complaints to the GMC from employers and 34% from the public were about IMGs or European graduates. Psychiatry is the second highest specialty complained about to the GMC. Male doctors joining the register aged 40–50 have a higher chance of facing sanctions.

Nurses

The UK nursing and midwifery workforce is also diverse, with 69% of initial nursing registration from England, 17% from the rest of the UK, 4% originally registered in the EU and 10% from outside the EU (Migration Advisory Committee, 2016: p. 19). The international nursing population are from nearly 200 different countries, with the largest non-EU numbers from the Philippines (22 773) and India (16 759) in 2015, according to the Nursing and Midwifery Council (2015).

Organisational culture concepts

The team

Although the terms 'group' and 'team' are occasionally used interchangeably, they refer to two different concepts. A 'group' is a collection of individuals 'which has been consciously created to accomplish a defined part of an organization's collective purpose' (Huczynski & Buchanan, 2007: p. 291). The evolution of a group into a team involves a five-stage process (Tuckman & Jensen, 1977):

1 forming (orientation phase)
2 storming (conflict)
3 norming (cohesion)
4 performing (effective team working)
5 adjourning (team disbanding).

Effective teams transition through these maturation processes. The individual and cultural characteristics of team members may influence the transitional processes and ensuing outcomes.

The psychiatric team

Psychiatric teams consist of clinical and non-clinical staff, who bring a breadth and depth of experience to patient care. The membership will typically include:

- manager
- consultant
- middle-grade/junior doctor
- nurse
- nursing assistant/support worker
- psychologist
- occupational therapist
- social worker
- administrator/clerk
- housekeeper.

In conjunction with clinical roles, the characteristics of team members may either be surface or deep level (Fig. 14.2). Surface-level characteristics are predominantly explicit and associated with visible demographic features such as age, gender, race and ethnicity. Deep-level characteristics are psychological or cognitive attributes such as values, personality, attitudes and beliefs, which require interpersonal interaction (perhaps some probing) to discern.

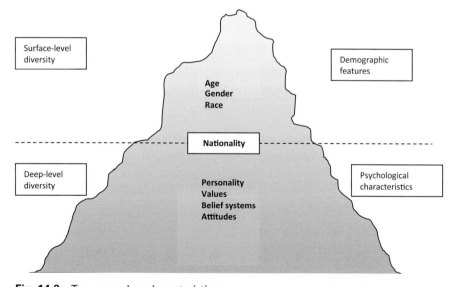

Fig. 14.2 Team member characteristics.

The visible nature of surface-level features may trigger spontaneous or stereotyped responses within teams, while deep-level attributes are likely to be recognised (or even appreciated) with familiarity over time. Research into cultural diversity frequently explores themes such as the interaction between ethnicity or nationality and social, overt and surface-level features (Ely & Thomas 2001; Mannix & Neale, 2005).

Cultural differences affect teams in different ways to other types of diversity, with both positive (McLeod *et al*, 1996; Thomas *et al*, 1996; Earley & Mosakowski, 2000) and negative (Watson *et al*, 1993; Kirkman *et al*, 2004; Jehn & Mannix, 2001) associations proposed.

Earley & Mosakowski (2000) hypothesise that 'transnational teams do not begin with shared meaning systems and that successful heterogeneous teams create hybrid team cultures over time'. 'Hybrid' team culture refers to emergent sets of rules, norms, expectations and roles that team members share and 'enact'. This offers a shared, group-specific identity and so provides a basis for team member self-valuation, while enabling team interaction and performance.

The members of homogeneous teams (e.g. with respect to culture) share salient characteristics, or have perceived commonalities, such as expectations of how each should behave within the professional role in a multidisciplinary clinical team (doctors, nurses, social worker, occupational therapist and psychologist). In teams with moderate heterogeneity (different cultures), subgroup identities dominate (Lau & Murnighan, 1998). As the team faces difficulties, members retreat toward pre-existing, pre-group or subgroup identities such as their nationality, culture or professional group, creating a potential for interpersonal conflict. The highly heterogeneous team (e.g. culturally and professionally) has few shared characteristics for subgroup formation. In such situations, unique categories and identities emerge and prevail. The team creates a new shared understanding of roles and status, and evolves its own communication methods. This emergent 'hybrid' culture is dependent on group understanding and interaction. In stressful times, a highly heterogeneous team cannot easily fall back on pre-existing group or subgroup identities, unlike homogeneous or moderately heterogeneous teams, as they have few characteristics in common. Lau & Murnighan (1998) suggest that when a highly heterogeneous team is challenged, it must form a hybrid team culture to progress. This may require time and determination.

Diversity and the team

In multinational teams the following three theoretical processes may occur (Mannix & Neale, 2005).

- *Similarity attraction*. Individuals find shared values, beliefs and attitudes appealing and are therefore more likely to work together well when these are present.

- *Social identity and social categorisation.* Individuals have a tendency to categorise themselves into specific groups (e.g. doctors, nurses, psychologists and social workers) with a sense of belonging (in-group) or not belonging (out-group).
- *Information processing.* Diverse teams have a greater capacity to access and process a broader range of information through networks and hence an increased capacity for innovation and problem-solving compared with less diverse groups.

Cultural diversity and team productivity

Stahl & Voigt (2008) suggested that diversity (a team input) affects a variety of team processes and affective reactions, which in turn influence team performance (output). Merging two models, they developed a concept to explore the interplay between team diversity and performance and productivity:

- *Divergence and convergence* (Earley & Gibson, 2002). Divergent processes present different thoughts, ideas and values while convergence restricts these.
- *Process losses and process gains* (Steiner, 1972). Process gains are the positive contributions to group performance; process losses are the negative consequences.

The interplay between these models is summarised in Table 14.2.

- *Divergent – process gain* – enriches teams as broad experiences and ideas are incorporated into team creativity and may manifest in effective problem-solving and brainstorming.
- *Divergent – process loss* – team or group members pull in different directions, and disagreement and conflict may occur, adversely affecting team performance.
- *Convergent – process gain* – having shared goals and objectives enhances team performance and productivity through cohesion and effective communication.

Table 14.2 The interplay between divergence and convergence, and process loss and process gains

	Process gain	Process loss
Convergence	Cohesion Communication Social integration Satisfaction	Group-think
Divergence	Creativity	Conflict

Source: Based on Stahl & Voigt (2008).

- *Convergent – process loss* – reduced flexibility within the team, with marginalisation or disregard for new ideas, which may lead to 'group-think' (unquestioning agreement with a leader or an assumption that team members with specific expertise are consistently more knowledgeable).

Nationality

Multinational teams, cross-national teams, hybrid national teams

Nationality involves belonging to a particular nation. This cannot be verified by demographic features alone and may be confounded by variables such as the country of birth, country of parental heritage, the independence of nations, the merging of countries into a union (e.g. the EU) and the naturalisation of individuals. Migration following conflict or disaster or for economic reasons influences the geographical spread of health professionals, some of whom may hold multiple nationalities; the global dispersal of families has led to multiple nationalities within the same family.

An important consideration for health services is that individuals with shared nationalities are more likely to have similar backgrounds and a closer degree of likeness in values, language and communication, which may influence team cohesion.

Homogeneous, intra-national teams

Assuming individuals from the same country or geographical region share high degrees of homogeneity, there should be cohesion. However, other differences surface upon closer inspection; for instance, within Indian teams, caste, religion, language, ethnic and geographical differences may emerge. West African teams may experience differences in colonial history, educational structures, social class and tribes. These may manifest as a polarisation on the grounds of Yoruba versus Igbo (ethnic), Nigerian versus Ghanaian (national), or Francophone versus Anglophone colonial identities. Within Europe, differences between German, French, Italian and British nationals can be striking. On closer scrutiny, British team members may also vary greatly if they are English, Welsh, Scottish and Northern Irish. The salience of these variables may depend on the situation, priorities and needs of the interaction. Multinational and single-nation team members may share strong bonds and identity based on faith, language and history. Deep-level diversity may go unrecognised within national organisations (Weber *et al*, 1996; Stahl & Voigt, 2008).

National culture: the Hofstede model

Hofstede (2001) proposed a compelling model of five cultural dimensions reflecting differences between national populations. In multicultural teams, the differences in some of these dimensions can influence team dynamics. Two are particularly salient:

- *Power distance.* This dimension captures hierarchy and authoritative relationships. The more hierarchical a culture is, the greater is the power distance. In clinical settings, this may manifest in both cultural and professional hierarchies (e.g. the trainee and consultant psychiatrist).
- *Individualism versus collectivism.* The stronger the ties are people have with their social group, such as family, company or nation, the more their culture is oriented towards collectivism or internalised 'we-ness'. Conversely, individualism promotes a greater sense of 'I-ness' and individual pursuit. Clinicians with collectivist backgrounds may experience additional pressures, such as supporting extended family needs or mediating family conflicts.

Other team variables

Task complexity

This is the degree to which tasks are ambiguous, require intricate decision-making, are mutually dependent or are lacking in routine and require structure (McGrath, 1984). Greater task complexity has been associated with poorer performance by diverse groups (De Dreu & Weingart, 2003).

In healthcare teams, roles and hierarchy often reflect task complexity. For instance, in a surgical team there are differences in roles, responsibilities and task complexity between the neurosurgeon, anaesthetist, theatre nurse, the porter and the cleaner. That notwithstanding, there are high levels of interdependence required to complete a team task effectively.

Team size

The larger a clinical team is, the greater is the potential for differences between members. In large multidisciplinary teams, the interfaces between professional role, experience, gender, age and culture enrich the team as well as increasing the likelihood of conflict, with less effective communication.

Team duration and stability

The length of time for which a team is together, including the stability of the team's membership over that period, has an influence on team cohesion and can benefit processes and output. A more stable multinational team will develop a common or shared hybrid identity, which can improve team performance (Earley & Mosakowski, 2000). Harrison *et al* (1998) observed that the early challenges of cultural diversity decreased over time. Conversely, these benefits would diminish in teams with frequent structural changes and high staff turnover. On balance, established multinational teams experience less conflict and better communication than new ones.

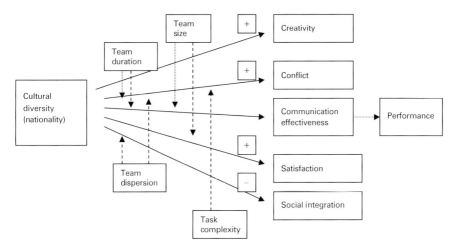

Fig. 14.3 Impact of cultural diversity on team outcomes (+ positive, – negative). Adapted from Stahl & Voigt (2008).

Summary

Multinational teams are characterised by high degrees of divergence, but more diverse teams have a greater potential for creativity, albeit with an increased potential for conflict, especially when taking on complex tasks. Communication may be less effective in large teams, where demographic or surface-level factors (e.g. ethnicity, gender, age) are salient, and improved when underpinned by deep-level or psychological factors (e.g. values). Smaller diverse teams had higher levels of satisfaction. Stahl *et al* (2010) found no direct relationship between cultural diversity and team performance. Fig. 14.3 summarises the impact of cultural diversity on team outcomes.

Cultural intelligence

Culture transcends all structures of society. Rockstuhl *et al* (2011) observed that different types of intelligence influenced leadership effectiveness in different situations:

- general intelligence predicted both national and international leadership
- emotional intelligence was a stronger predictor of national leadership
- cultural intelligence was a stronger predictor of international leadership effectiveness.

In health services, general intelligence may determine academic success and professional qualifications yet emotional intelligence facilitates the empathy required to be a caring clinician. Cultural intelligence is a critical leadership competency required by leaders and managers of multinational teams.

Components of cultural intelligence have been described by Earley & Mosakowski (2004) as:

- *head (cognitive)* – the ability of an individual to learn about the beliefs, values, norms and taboos of a culture
- *body (physical)* – the ability to adopt mannerisms, gestures and behaviours characteristic of a culture
- *heart (emotional/motivational)* – the desire to acquire, improve or master another culture.

Communication and multicultural situational awareness

Situational awareness is the ability to accurately evaluate a situation and related information for relevance (Wright & Endsley, 2008: pp. 101–103). In healthcare, this is important in teamwork across different disciplines to ensure that goals and outcomes are shared. Health professional training is geared towards shared awareness. However, the different mental models (cultural, national or linguistic) within teams can have a significant effect on perception and decision-making. Team members sharing erroneous views may dangerously impair situational awareness. The more diverse the team is, the greater will be the options, and multinational, cultural and linguistic heterogeneity may increase this further.

Effective multinational team situational awareness and communication should lead to shared perceptions (clarity of information), comprehension (information interpreted as intended) and actions (carried out as intended or expected) (Fig. 14.4). Ineffective communication can lead to a series of disconnects and errors.

Interplay of multinational and multidisciplinary situational awareness in a healthcare team

The manager focusing on inter-professional situational awareness should be sensitive to the national and cultural differences in the team as the

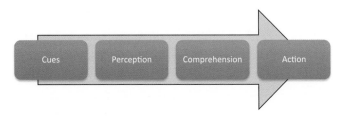

Fig. 14.4 Situational awareness and communication

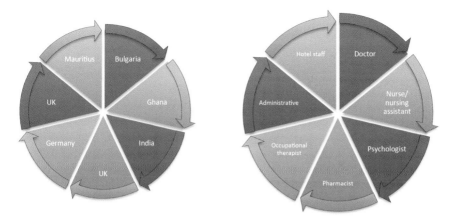

Fig. 14.5 Interactions within multinational and multidisciplinary teams

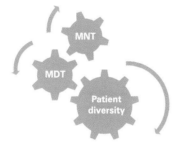

Fig. 14.6 Interactions between a multinational team (MNT) and a multidisciplinary team (MDT) and patients

interplay can produce a kaleidoscope of situations within services (Fig. 14.5). A common daily interface would be clinical hand-overs within teams.

In psychiatric practice, a multinational clinical team is likely to interact with a diverse and often multinational client group, and this presents both challenges and opportunities (Fig. 14.6).

Analysis of the multinational team

The manager is encouraged to reflect on the multinational composition of the team. This may become more visual when mapped. An example of such mapping is presented in Fig. 14.7; in this team, 21 different countries and four continents were represented. In this example team, the non-UK staff form a majority group.

Illustrated with a frequency plot (Fig. 14.8), the spread and prevalence of different nationalities is visible and may provide important insight into team dynamics.

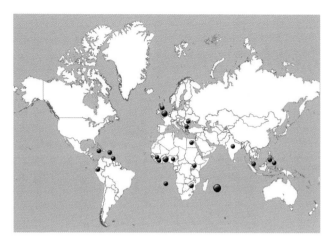

Fig. 14.7 Map showing countries of origin of a healthcare team

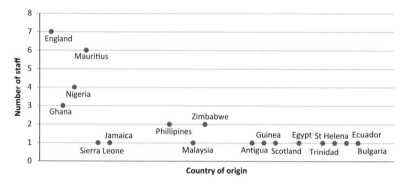

Fig. 14.8 Frequency plot of the countries of origin of a healthcare team

Staff membership of a 'minority' group outside the workplace may yet present membership of a 'majority' group at work. However, this does not guarantee status or influence in the workplace.

Generalisation of staff identity based on geographical region of origin such as 'European', 'Asian' and 'African' is fraught with limitations. While 'African' staff share continental origins, they may identify with regional groupings, for instance Southern African and West African (Fig. 14.9). West African staff may further differentiate colleagues by nationality, such as Nigerian, Ghanaian or Sierra Leonean. Nigerian staff may, however, associate with national ethnic identities, for example Yoruba or Ibo. It is not uncommon for some individuals to fall back on values and beliefs about other regional or national ethnic groups based on pre-migration beliefs or stereotypes, such as perceptions of aggression, attitudes towards relationships, educational achievement and entrepreneurship.

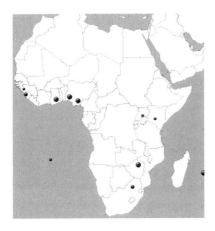

Fig. 14.9   Different regions of origin of African staff in a healthcare team

Important considerations for the manager

Communication difficulties

Communication difficulties are a common challenge faced within multinational teams, manifesting as the manner and speed of speech, accent and comprehension.

Accents

Some multicultural team members may speak with a 'strong accent' – an accent with pronunciation that is non-standard (i.e. not similar to that of a native speaker and therefore more difficult to understand). It is not uncommon to have multiple accents within teams, in which case even more attention to communication is required.

Large variation in accents within teams requires sensitivity with communicating clinical information, as some individuals risk being misunderstood. Tolerance of different accents may vary across teams. As surface-level and overt characteristics, accents do not reflect an individual's knowledge or ability.

Language and vocabulary

Variation in syntax, fluency and vocabulary can have an impact on staff confidence in team situations such as hand-over, ward rounds, tribunals and meetings with patients or carers. Some individuals adjust communication style to accommodate their multilingual colleagues. As telephone communication is solely verbal, some individuals may, notwithstanding the best of intentions, come across as abrupt, not listening and requiring repeated clarification due to style of speech or accent.

Idiomatic and colloquial use of phrases or slang poses challenges (e.g. 'spending a penny' or 'I was gutted'). Furthermore, familiar words may have a different interpretation, connotation or nuance.

Some individuals experience greater difficulty with comprehension in stressful or emergency situations. Misinterpretation, misrepresentation or inconsistent accounts of critical events can have unforeseen consequences.

Tone of voice

Culture, country of origin and the main language spoken may influence an individual's tone of voice. There may also be urban–rural or regional differences within countries. Anecdotally, New Yorkers are described as louder in tone than their neighbours in Boston.

It is not uncommon for loud communication to be perceived as aggressive and threatening, while soft and quiet speech is often felt to indicate a lack of confidence or assertiveness.

Written communication

As with the spoken word, differences in the quality and consistency of written communication can be a concern as they can lead to error, misunderstanding and conflict. Note that there may be some inconsistency between spoken and written communication, such as a clinician with a strong accent or limited eloquence but exceptional written English.

Non-verbal communication

Cross-national differences in non-verbal communication are common, and include reduced eye contact and gaze avoidance when communicating with authority figures. There are different cultural norms of non-verbal communication, such as expressive gesticulation, which may come across as argumentative or aggressive when trying to stress a point. Cultural codes regarding handshakes differ; for instance, the 'firm' handshake would not be the norm for many African and Asian staff. Eye contact and handshakes seen as non-verbal communication of sincerity and forthrightness in one culture may be perceived as disrespectful in another.

Staff speaking in their vernacular or native tongue

Conversations between staff in an unfamiliar foreign language can be offensive and disrespectful to team members. When such conversations are loud or indiscreet this negative effect is accentuated, but when they are quiet and discreet they may arouse suspicion. Some professionals are oblivious of the negative feelings evoked in patients and colleagues until these are brought to their attention. Conversely, additional language skills may benefit services when dealing with non-English-speaking patients and carers.

Unintended risk

Risk situations can unwittingly occur as a consequence of multinational communication confusion or errors in verbal, non-verbal and written communication. These errors can have very serious and harmful consequences on the care and well-being of patients. While health professionals have language codes for their specialty, they have no control over the language patients use. This is illustrated with the following examples:

- A worker said a patient 'was stinking of piss' (Australian slang for beer) and an alcohol problem was misinterpreted as urinary incontinence in a hand-over.
- A patient was thought to have said she had left a candle in her 'bowel' – leading to exploration in an emergency room. She had actually said 'bowl'.
- A British nurse said to a West African relative of a patient, 'I will deal with you soon'. This was perceived as a threat as this phrase is often used by African police before delivering harsh treatment.

Stereotypes

Stereotypes are often based on the overt or visible features of an individual, such as skin colour, accent, tone of voice and style of non-verbal communication. At times, generalisations are made on the basis of nationality or culture. Some team members are discerning about individual differences while others stereotype or generalise behaviours as cultural or national.

With staff and colleagues, managers should reflect on the pitfalls of stereotyping, which may manifest in recruitment, disciplinary or other processes.

Etiquette

Differences in etiquette between countries of origin and the UK may be observed in multinational teams, such as expressions of politeness, deference or respect, especially concerning the use of clinical titles – 'Doctor' – or avoiding the use of first names. Not all multinational team members (or indeed managers) are familiar with generic British etiquette and failure to conform to this may unwittingly be perceived as rude or impolite. Conversely, some behaviour considered polite and respectful in one culture may be unfamiliar to the recipient of the 'respect' and come across as ingratiating in another. Some staff adapt cultural etiquette to different interactions.

Deference/power distance

Power distance (Hofstede, 2001) and respect for those in authority can manifest in team hierarchies. This may be more noticeable among same-culture staff from non-Western cultures than among their British counterparts (Fig. 14.10). Latent but powerful cultural hierarchies may

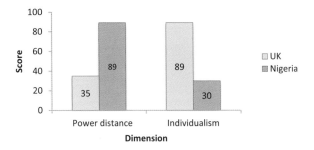

Fig. 14.10 Country comparison on Hofstede dimensions

influence tasks, communication and perceptions of group membership. Status such as age or faith group leadership or gender may even override team hierarchy.

Gender

Gender roles and perceptions of authority among individuals of the same country of origin may disadvantage some female staff. Younger female staff from large-power-distance cultures sometimes feel doubly disadvantaged when trying to assert themselves or to seek parity with men from their culture or region of origin. Unfortunately, some men have manifest or latent culture-rooted expectations of their female colleagues. This may take the form of bullying or harassment.

Attitudes towards faith

Faith is a personal value that transcends country of origin. Multinational staff may share or practise different faiths, expressed through different symbols or artefacts such as turbans, crosses or growth of facial hair. Expression of faith and participation on key religious days may affect staff rotas and resource allocation. Some individuals are more expressive of faith, yet in the UK open expression of faith in clinical practice is discouraged. Some staff may have their first direct interactions with other faiths in the UK.

Attitudes towards sexuality

Staff from countries that prohibit or criminalise homosexuality may struggle with internalised feelings, although some may feel liberated and able to express previously concealed sexual preferences. Faith-based views about sexual preferences can influence, and possibly impair, clinical judgement. The transgender health professional or patient finds him/herself particularly marginalised in diverse or polarised groups. The manager may be confronted with personal prejudice or 'homophobic' views within teams.

Ethnocentrism

Ethnocentrism is the processing of information through one's own cultural lens. At times, clinical opinions are influenced by the cultural or national background of the team member, for instance empathy, the perception of adversity, or norms of child-rearing practice; there may be polarised views regarding the assessment of psychopathology and treatment decisions.

Intra-national or cross-regional differences

Intra-national or cross-regional differences can be subtle and go unnoticed within teams. Tensions can arise in situations linked with historical or pre-migration issues among groups. Unfamiliar differences from countries of origin can include caste issues (higher-caste Indian staff versus the 'untouchables') or latent regional national hierarchies among Asian, African and Caribbean nations. Team members may come from regions that are in or have been in conflict.

Social and leisure activities

Multinational team members can have different concepts of leisure and social activities outside work. Some may socialise with alcohol in the pub, at the theatre or the opera, or go clubbing, while others mingle with their faith groups or largely socialise only through rites-of-passage activities (birthdays, weddings, etc.). Shared social activities among some team members may stratify the team further.

Identification with patients from the country of origin

While cultural insights at times enrich patient care, staff risk identifying with or even colluding with patients of a shared cultural heritage with heightened empathy or countertransference. It is not uncommon for patients to avoid clinicians of shared heritage due to confidentiality concerns.

Knowledge

Perception of knowledge within teams is linked to professional roles, qualifications, hierarchy and years of experience, social class and country of education. Command of English, eloquence or fluency can erroneously be perceived as indicating people are more knowledgeable than they actually are. Understandably, less fluent team members may feel their opinions are overlooked because they present less well than others.

Taboos

With the best of will and sensitivity, team members may breach a taboo or code in another culture through inappropriate jokes, faith opinions or oblivious use of gestures. The innocuous use of a left hand, offering a pork meal or wearing shoes may cause unintended distress. While some tolerate taboos, others might complain. The manager should be considerate with regard to taboos and ensure complaints are not rebuffed or deemed irrelevant to work.

Misidentification

Mislabelling individuals or ascribing another group identity (e.g. Indian-Pakistani, Ghanaian-Nigerian, Jamaican-Trinidadian, Irish-Scottish) may cause unintended upset.

Stereotyped assumptions about professional roles on the basis of appearance (gender or ethnicity) can also be disconcerting. Managers may be oblivious of additional skills members of staff possess (e.g. support workers with accountancy, law and business qualifications in roles pending professional conversion in the UK).

Subgroups and subcultures

Groups of staff with a shared culture or nationality can reduce their sense of isolation by congregating. However, this national, cultural and ethnic cohesion may cause difficulty and split teams. The presence of these cliques or subgroups within teams can be divisive, although their members will likely feel they provide support and safety in numbers.

Perceived prejudice and discrimination

Perceptions of an invisible ceiling that limits career achievements are not uncommon among international staff. Experiences of discrimination can be associated with a sense of disadvantage, of not belonging to specific groups, or of lacking key attributes of the host nation group. Managers need to ensure staff appointment, promotion and disciplinary processes are not perceived as discriminatory. Experiences of marginalisation or discrimination can cause significant dysphoria within team members and reduce organisational effectiveness, staff recruitment and retention.

Expectations of patients

Some professionals experience difficulty understanding or being understood by patients, some of whom may even be hostile or abusive towards them. Patient expectations at odds with the clinician's may heighten this. In some instances, team members may feel inadequate to meet some patients' cultural needs, such as unfamiliar eating disorders.

Subgroup behaviours

Managers should be vigilant regarding the development of cliques and subgroups, for instance a skewed preponderance of staff from a particular country during a shift through rota manipulation, or certain staff consistently showing a preference for working with colleagues from the same culture or nationality. Marginalisation could reduce the engagement of key team members, thereby reducing productivity (process loss).

Investigations/disciplinary issues

It is not uncommon for there to be a perception of 'scapegoating' or disproportionate outcomes for particular groups following a crisis. It is important to ensure there are no conscious or unwitting biases within the organisational culture which may disadvantage certain individuals. Governance structures to monitor, record and report this are important. In addition, investigations involving cultural themes should be carefully considered. This is a very sensitive area to explore within teams. Belonging to a national subgroup can at times be felt to be protective or supportive.

Acculturation

Organisations sometimes assume that most foreign-trained employees are familiar with British culture, while they may still be in the process of acculturation. Early acculturation in the new immigrant may inhibit confidence and reduce engagement in decision-making. The induction process, supervision and longitudinal review of performance can be important facilitators of acculturation.

Benefits of working in a multinational team

While there may be some challenges, team diversity can also increase effectiveness and productivity through the following.

Knowledge

Multinational clinical teams can enhance knowledge of other cultures through daily cross-cultural interaction beyond what might be experienced outside the workplace. Through this interaction, some staff have opportunities to alter preconceived views about other groups or nationalities, although stereotypes are reinforced in some situations.

Enhanced professional practice

The multinational team provides opportunities for its members to observe and learn from the different approaches and practice of colleagues. Furthermore, cross-national acquisition of clinical skills enriches clinical practice, particularly with diverse patient groups. Team members will be able to familiarise themselves with different and uncommon clinical presentations, such as culture-bound syndromes, faith-related issues and ranges of explanatory models. Diverse patient populations can be a considerable incentive for clinicians to broaden cross-cultural knowledge. Ultimately, the multicultural and multinational team has the potential to increase their breadth and depth of expertise (which represents value creation).

Benefit to patient care

Multinational teams can enhance the care given to patients of diverse faith, nationalities, languages and belief systems. The broader range of clinical expertise and understanding of patient distress enriches the range of therapeutic options, with teams better equipped to work with complex cases, a role at times burdened on interpreters.

Improved communication

The well-integrated hybrid multinational team develops improved communication between colleagues, with members adapting the way they communicate to fit the team's global culture. The manager should be vigilant to changes in the team's composition and the impact this may have on new members. Staff from homogeneous (same culture and nationality) teams would understandably need time to adjust.

Box 14.1 Recommendations for managers and teams on approaches to successful multinational teamwork

- Be aware of the team mix and manage rotas with awareness of subgroup dynamics
- Recognise power distance across different cultural and national groups
- Promote understanding of cultural differences within the team
- Provide training regarding individual cultures within the team
- Provide communication skills training (team–team and team–patients)
- Build a team based on similarities rather than differences
- Make the team's goals and vision clear to each team member and reinforce them within the team
- Encourage managers to respect multinational differences
- Get to know each team member as an individual and not an ambassador of a nation
- Recognise the individual skills and achievements of team members
- Encourage active listening within the team, no matter how people speak or come across
- Provide coaching on cross-cultural and cross-linguistic communication
- Provide mentorship across culture and nationality
- Develop specific expertise from the multinational skill mix
- Encourage a balance between general, emotional and cultural intelligence

---

Customs and values

Beyond the workplace, multinational team members exchange cultural values, knowledge, social practice, dietary customs and mannerisms through team social events. The unintended benefit is sometimes manifest during other cross-cultural interactions.

Conclusions

The mental health workforce is professionally, culturally and internationally diverse. Leadership and management of these multinational teams can be both rewarding and challenging. Challenges are often associated with the mode of communication rather than the content of the message itself. Difficulties may increase clinical risk and interpersonal conflict in teams. However, culturally diverse and international teams also have the potential to improve clinical practice, innovation and patient care. Managers are encouraged to develop their own cultural intelligence to harness the team's potential (Box 14.1).

References

Ayonrinde OA (2003) Importance of cultural sensitivity in therapeutic transactions: considerations for healthcare providers. *Disease Management and Health Outcomes*, **11**: 233–48.

De Dreu CKW, Weingart LR (2003) Task versus relationship conflict, team performance, and team member satisfaction: a meta-analysis. *Journal of Applied Psychology*, **88**: 741–9.

Earley PC, Gibson CB (2002) *Multinational Work Teams: A New Perspective*. Lawrence Erlbuam Associates.

Earley PC, Mosakowski EA (2000) Creating hybrid team cultures: an empirical test of transnational team functioning. *Academy of Management Journal*, **43**: 26–49.

Earley PC, Mosakowski EA (2004) Cultural intelligence. *Harvard Business Review*, **82**, October: 139–46.

Ely RJ, Thomas DA (2001) Cultural diversity at work: the effects of diversity perspectives on work group processes and outcomes. *Administrative Science Quarterly*, **46**: 229–73.

GMC (2016) List of registered medical practitioners – statistics. Available at http://www.gmc-uk.org/doctors/register/search_stats.asp (accessed May 2016).

Harrison DA, Price KH, Bell MP (1998) Beyond relational demography: time and the effects of surface- and deep-level diversity on work group cohesion. *Academy of Management Journal*, **41**: 96–107.

Hofstede G (2001) *Culture's Consequences* (2nd edition). Sage.

Huczynski AA, Buchanan DA (2007) Group formation. In *Organizational Behavior* (eds AA Huczynski, DA Buchanan) (6th edition). Pearson Education.

Jehn KA, Mannix EA (2001) The dynamic nature of conflict: a longitudinal study of intragroup conflict and group performance. *Academy of Management Journal*, **44**: 238–51.

Kirkman BL, Tesluk PE, Rosen B (2004) The impact of demographic heterogeneity and team leader-team member demographic fit on team empowerment and effectiveness. *Group and Organization Management*, **29**: 334–68.

Lau DC, Murnighan JK (1998) Demographic diversity and faultlines: the compositional dynamics of organizational groups. *Academy of Management Review*, **23**: 325–40.

Mannix E, Neale MA (2005) What differences make a difference? *Psychological Science in the Public Interest*, **6**: 31–55.

McGrath JE (1984) *Groups: Interaction and Performance*. Prentice Hall.

McLeod PL, Lobel SA, Cox TH (1996) Ethnic diversity and creativity in small groups. *Small Group Research*, **27**: 248–64.

Migration Advisory Committee (2016) *Partial Review of the Shortage Occupation List: Review of Nursing*. Available at https://www.gov.uk/government/uploads/system/uploads/attachment_data/file/510630/Partial_review_of_the_shortage_occupation_list_-_review_of_nursing.pdf (accessed May 2016).

Nursing and Midwifery Council (2015) Data from https://www.whatdotheyknow.com/request/269442/response/659545/attach/5/COM034%20Effective%20Practitioners%20by%20Country%20of%20Training%202%20June%202015.xls (accessed May 2016).

Rockstuhl T, Seiler S, Ang S, *et al* (2011) Beyond general intelligence (IQ) and emotional intelligence (EQ): the role of cultural intelligence (CQ) on cross-border leadership effectiveness in a globalized world. *Journal of Social Issues*, **67**: 825–40.

Slowther A, Lewando HG, Taylor R, *et al* (2009) *Non UK Qualified Doctors and Good Medical Practice: The Experience of Working Within a Different Professional Framework*. Report for the General Medical Council. University of Warwick.

Stahl GK, Voigt A (2008) Do cultural differences matter in mergers and acquisitions? A tentative model and meta-analytic examination. *Organization Science*, **19**: 160–76.

Stahl GK, Maznevski ML, Voigt A, *et al* (2010) Unraveling the effects of cultural diversity in teams: a meta-analysis of research on multicultural work groups. *Journal of International Business Studies*, **41**: 690–709.

Steiner ID (1972) *Group Process and Productivity*. Academic Press.

Thomas DC, Ravlin EC, Wallace AW (1996) Effect of cultural diversity in work groups. *Research in the Sociology of Organizations*, **14**: 1–33.

Tuckman B, Jensen N (1977) Stage of small group development revisited. *Group and Organizational Studies*, **2**: 419–27.

Watson WE, Kumar K, Michaelsen LK (1993) Cultural diversity's impact on interaction process and performance: comparing homogeneous and diverse task groups. *Academy of Management Journal*, **36**: 590–602.

Weber Y, Shenkar O, Raveh A (1996) National and corporate cultural fit in mergers and acquisitions: an exploratory study. *Management Science*, **42**: 1215–27.

Wright MC, Endsley MR (2008) Building shared situation awareness in healthcare settings. In *Improving Healthcare Team Communication: Building on Lessons from Aviation and Aerospace* (ed CP Nemeth): pp 97–116. Ashgate Publishing.

CHAPTER 15

Management of change

Zoë K. Reed

One of the most important tasks requiring management is securing the implementation of change. That is the focus of this chapter and the approach will be to provide some overall concepts which people have found help them to be effective in these turbulent times.

On one level, the management of change needs no introduction, since it is something we cope with throughout our lives. As we go through the different stages and different educational and economic opportunities, we manage each transition. On a micro-level, our bodies and our social relations are always undergoing minor, and sometimes major, changes and we manage the necessary adjustments. However easy or difficult we find these changes, we manage. The issue is whether we manage them well and whether having the right theories to help guide our thoughts, feelings and behaviours might move us from coping with, to thriving in, change.

'Skills and ability to manage change' is a phrase appearing in most organisations' job descriptions and person specifications these days. Psychiatrists as individuals will be skilled in supporting service users through their personal changes – the clinical change task. This chapter offers an approach which should enable psychiatrists to have a way of thinking which will give them confidence in approaching the managerial and organisational change task.

Why is the management of change necessary?

Society in the UK, as elsewhere in the world, is changing rapidly and will continue to do so. The effects of developments in information and communications technology are well known and support the prediction that constantly adjusting services and provider practices will be a feature of the modern world. This has an impact on all parts of the economy, including the delivery of mental healthcare. The context for that delivery is one where the right to choice is an expectation of service users and being subject to contestability is a fact for service providers. As the public becomes more educated about options and more prepared to voice their needs and wants, the requirement is for services and clinicians to offer flexible and responsive services which are experienced as personalised by each service user.

The other big organisational driver for change is an economic one. All industries have to be constantly aware of the competition, and to check out the relative quality and cost of their products. In the UK, the concepts of *contestability* and *choice* have been introduced into the National Health Service (NHS) as a way of bringing a focus on quality and cost into healthcare. The constant drive to increase the efficiency and cost-effectiveness of services is as important as increasing their clinical effectiveness. This is because the need for services will always outstrip available resources and the money for new services is usually locked within existing services.

The final driver for change which is offered here is that of medical advances. Research is continually being undertaken and generates evidence which points to more effective ways to secure the desired outcomes for service users. However, these ways can be at odds with clinical practice as taught during training to become a doctor. Providing evidence-based care therefore requires good change management skills – to secure changes in both personal practice and in the practice of others.

What change has to be managed?

At its most basic, the change which has to be managed is that of personal behaviour. Individuals have to start to do things differently. Ensuring that the change is sustained in each individual and applied consistently by all individuals is the change management task. To secure this, organisations frequently implement change programmes. These programmes often work on the idea that if you change people's thoughts and feelings, then the *behaviour* change (which is the desired outcome or goal of the programme) is more likely to be sustained and spread throughout the organisation.

An area where there has been much debate about the design of change programmes is that of ensuring equal access, experience and outcomes for all service users, regardless of their ethnicity. The design of change programmes has evolved over the years from ones with the aim of winning 'hearts and minds' (i.e. a focus on thoughts and feelings and emphasising the moral case) to ones which focus on changing behaviours (i.e. emphasising the legal framework and business case).

An effective change programme will therefore include design components which aim to secure spread and sustainability (Fraser *et al*, 2003). This is because, although it is relatively easy to find a few enthusiastic individuals within an organisation to experiment with new ways of working, what is more difficult to achieve is a change programme which is replicable across an organisation and which secures and maintains the desired changes. Key to the success of any design is, first, to be very clear about what the required outcomes are, then to understand the organisational context within which the change has to be achieved, and finally to apply the right concepts to the design of the programme.

What concepts help?

For organisations and individuals to secure the change that is required and to thrive in a context where frequent change is the norm, it is important to work within a theoretical framework which is likely to lead to successful outcomes. Put simply, some ways of thinking can actually be unhelpful and lead to the person asked to lead the change feeling overwhelmed by the task. This is clearly not productive and the key to success is to construct a way of thinking about things that makes the change task seem doable and even enjoyable. The concepts can be grouped into categories in which they are most helpfully applied:

- organisations and systems
- individuals in groups – the leadership task
- individuals.

Theories about organisations and systems

Complexity sciences (Battram, 1998) draw on biological and physical sciences and contain a number of principles and ideas which help designers to shape change programmes. Central to these are the idea that organisations are *complex evolving systems* (Mitleton-Kelly, 2003). This term gives recognition to the fact that organisations are organic and, to quote Mitleton-Kelly, are 'co-evolving within a social ecosystem'. Wheatley describes organisations as:

> 'A collection of individual agents who have the freedom to act in ways that are not entirely predictable and whose actions are interconnected such that one agent's action changes the context for other agents.' (Wheatley, 1999)

This definition can be applied at every level of *nested systems,* which, in the present context, would be each team member within the team, each team within the organisation, each organisation within the health services community, each health services community within the broader public sector.

Thinking about organisations and individuals within them in this way leads to profoundly different designs to change programmes than views of a more traditional nature. Conventional management theories view organisations as machines and staff within them as component parts. From this world-view, designers assume people can be told what to do and that they will do it in a consistent manner. They assume that learning from one area will be automatically replicable in another. They believe that a plan for change can be worked out in advance in detail and that it must be and can be executed as planned.

Complexity perspectives provide a more organic and holistic view. Biological metaphors are frequently used to deepen understanding of successful approaches. Two of these are *birds flocking* and *termites building*. Both describe the idea that central command and control is neither necessary nor helpful in orchestrating action. Birds and termites achieve amazing results through the individual agents following a few *simple rules*. Some modern change management programmes focus on seeking to identify the few simple rules – often characterised as values or guiding principles – which will enable all individuals to shape their behaviour for themselves in accordance with organisational goals.

The termite hill *emerges* from the *patterns of behaviour* of the termites following their simple rules. There is no grand plan: the hills simply emerge from the behaviour. The *intrinsic motivation* of the termites coupled with the simple rules ensures that the termites *self-organise* to achieve the desired result. Emergence, intrinsic motivation and self-organisation are key concepts in the complexity sciences. They are the underpinning theory to techniques such as whole-group brainstorming and 'Post-It' note exercises. When design is guided by more conventional thinking, there can be a fear of asking a large group of people to generate as many ideas as possible and then to come out with a way forward, because it could feel uncontrollable and potentially non-productive. However, from a complexity perspective there is confidence (and tools and techniques coherent with the theory) that everyone has an intrinsic motivation to be cooperative, that they will self-organise to achieve the objectives and that the solutions will emerge from the process. The aim of such exercises is to involve everybody and to create a *possibility space* (Battram, 1998) in which solutions will emerge. This contrasts with more conventional management methods, where top management create a plan and then seek to persuade staff to follow it through consultation exercises.

Birds are also used to illustrate the need for *attractors* within the system. As a way of getting people to understand that organisations are living entities, not machines, a rock is contrasted with a bird. If you want to get a rock into the corner of a room, with a bit of practice on your aim you will be able to achieve it by throwing. By contrast, if you want to get a bird into the corner of a room you certainly will not achieve it by throwing the bird; instead, your only chance is by placing the attractor (for birds) of bird seed in the corner.

Using words like 'systems' and drawing on biological metaphors has another important message for organisations. It is that life proceeds: things are never static, and flow and movement are an intrinsic part of organisations. This contrasts with more conventional approaches, where there is an assumption that once the change has occurred and the problem has been fixed, the organisation will remain static. Many small changes or adjustments, quickly executed, are a key feature of change programme designs, which work in harmony with living systems.

Theories about individuals in groups – the leadership task

Understanding that the management task is about enabling a living system rather than controlling a machine brings a different set of leadership tasks. A metaphor that is frequently used to describe the organisation is a garden, and this can help managers understand that their role is to create the most favourable conditions for emergence and self-organisation. They must tend their gardens with care and continually work on improving the conditions to maximise the chance of healthy development, but what they cannot do is *make* the plants grow! This helps managers and leaders let go of thinking that their role is to figure it all out and then create a plan and force the system to implement it. Instead, the need for a much more nurturing role becomes apparent. A key role for managers and leaders in this world-view is to manage the context and the relationships around their work area to enable the part of the system they are responsible for to thrive and grow. Leaders start something, see what happens and give feedback in a continuous cycle; they watch to see when the required patterns of behaviour emerge and then manage the conditions so that those patterns are reinforced and sustained. Core skills are in the design of the possibility space and close observation in the search for the *tipping point* (Gladwell, 2000), when the whole system starts to move in the required (or desired) direction.

Helpful guidance for managers comes from the idea of *learning organisations,* with the leaders' new work being to act as *designers, stewards* and *teachers* (Senge, 1993): in learning organisations, leaders design the processes and systems within which the vision can be generated and articulated; they are stewards of that vision, with a special sense of responsibility but without being possessive of it; as teachers, they help people achieve more accurate views of reality and hold the creative tension which is generated. This description of leadership contrasts with the more conventional theories of a leader as a hero, leading from the front, or a leader as the most knowledgeable expert on the subject area. It calls for knowledge, skills and attention to process to get the best out of everyone – leadership as guardian of the co-created vision and expert in process rather than expert on content.

Complexity sciences help managers and leaders look for order rather than control; they provide a conceptual framework for inviting participation – every voice is valid – rather than curtailing contribution (for fear that someone will speak out against the plan). They foster a real belief in the intrinsic motivation of people. Even in chaotic circumstances, individuals can make congruent decisions when there are a few simple principles that everyone is accountable for but where the condition within which everyone is operating is one of individual freedom.

In this mind-set, much management time is spent on developing and sustaining a *shared vision* that will guide and shape the behaviour of the individuals in the team. Creating the conditions for *team learning* becomes an essential leadership task, since the way in which the organisation will move forward and adapt to its shifting context is to do something and see what happens – if it is what is wanted then repeat; if not, modify the conditions, do something and see what happens.

Theories that help individuals thrive in this context

To be effective in complex adaptive systems, people need to have highly developed *emotional intelligence*, which Goleman (1996) describes as:

'The capacity for recognising our own feelings and those of others, for motivating ourselves, and for managing emotions well in ourselves and in our relationships.'

The research evidence is that competent leaders who also exhibit high levels of emotional intelligence lead teams which have the competitive edge. Crucially, if managers are to lead from the perspective that all individuals have intrinsic motivation, then it follows that a high level of emotional intelligence needs to be developed in all members of staff.

Personal mastery and *mental models* (Senge, 1993) are crucial skill areas for continuous development. They complement the development of emotional intelligence and enable individuals to understand what motivates them and to work at clarifying and articulating how they are thinking about people and issues. People's responses to a set of circumstances are based on their particular mental models. Individuals have their own mental models and so crucial to progress in learning organisations is the development of the ability for people to articulate their mental models and suspend them before the group so that others can understand and respond. Individuals in learning organisations need to become skilled in *dialogue* (Battram, 1998) rather than discussion. This approach starts with listening and encourages reflection. Suboptimal suggested solutions are acceptable, as the focus is on generating many ideas and synthesising the way forward.

Implications for psychiatrists managing change

People who choose to work in the field of mental health are well placed to work within conceptual frameworks which emphasise the humanness of us all. Understanding human strengths and uniqueness is essential to effective clinical practice in the field. This means that psychiatrists, for example, are particularly well placed to assist in the design and implementation of change programmes. This contrasts with doctors who have chosen to specialise in surgery, for example, where it can be argued that the ability to understand the human condition is perhaps less essential to the delivery of quality healthcare.

For psychiatrists to influence and implement change programmes effectively, they have to be active players in the organisational system within which they operate. Each individual's views are valid, within the theoretical framework for change management advocated in this chapter, and so it follows that it is really important for each clinician to be actively engaged in the life of the organisation. Finding opportunities to influence and shape throughout a psychiatrist's career is a good way of proceeding – not leaving it until a role is secured (e.g. as clinical director) which has a specific management component. This is not necessarily easy given the design of university medical training programmes, which favour identification with the medical school rather than with the mental health trust where the clinical practice is being carried out. Nevertheless, participation in the life of the mental health trust will ensure that psychiatrists are fully part of the culture of the organisation and understand and enact its values. This is something which service users emphasise as particularly important, since for many of them their psychiatrist is the most important member of the clinical team.

Conclusion

All individuals at work need to develop their emotional intelligence and other skill sets (Box 15.1) to enable them to engage effectively with colleagues, whatever their location in the hierarchy and structure. This is the underlying essential set of competencies required to manage change effectively.

Developing a working knowledge of the other theories highlighted in this chapter should equip all who are asked to lead or implement change with a way of thinking about the context and the task such that they are confident

---

Box 15.1   Tips for successful change leaders

- Develop your emotional intelligence and your humanness
- Undertake continuing professional development in management and change leadership
- Think about your organisation as an organic entity that naturally keeps evolving
- Spend time with the team, building a shared vision
- Believe in people and their capacities and abilities to embrace change
- Develop a way of communicating that allows space for others to have opinions and contribute
- Demonstrate through your behaviour that you positively welcome and value diversity
- Pay attention to *process* as well as *content*
- Make change the norm in the team – doing many little changes quickly
- Catch people doing things right and continue to provide the conditions that have supported that behaviour
- Design processes that involve everyone and enable everyone to participate
- Offer sub-optimal proposals and invite genuine participation in co-creating the best solution
- Go where the energy for change is and support those who wish to achieve improvement – once the tipping point is reached the rest will come through

---

enough to involve those around them in designing the way forward. Taking the first small steps is the key to success, and in a way which involves as many as possible of those who will be required to implement the change. Applying complexity principles to shape the thinking gives the confidence to take those first essential steps. The references and further reading listed below are by way of a sample reading list that will give you all the tools you need to design and implement successful change programmes. Enjoy the management of change!

Acknowledgements

Grateful thanks to Arthur Battram for our early discussions and help in formulating my thinking.

Postscript for the fourth edition

A lot has happened in the NHS since the publication of the third edition in 2007 and if I were writing this chapter now I would begin by saying 'The *single* most important task requiring management is securing the implementation of change', rather than just saying that it was *one* of the most important tasks. In the intervening years the NHS has had unprecedented challenges due to the demographic shifts and government austerity drives across the whole of the public sector. The reductions in public spending on housing, social care, voluntary sector services and welfare benefit changes have had as much of an impact on people when they are suffering with mental health conditions as the funding reductions affecting NHS mental health services.

So, if the need for change has become even greater, are we any closer to a shared understanding of the nature of the change that will help us all continue to provide high-quality, effective services with great experience and outcomes for everyone when they need them? One idea, which is gathering a fair degree of consensus, is that people need to become fully activated in their own life and care. One of the places where this was first promoted was in the report *Securing Our Future Health: Taking a Long-Term View* prepared by Sir Derek Wanless for HM Treasury (Wanless, 2002). Wanless estimated the costs of meeting the healthcare needs of the population in 2022 and the report described three scenarios for how the UK could meet the vision. Scenario 3 was called *fully engaged* – and was described as follows:

> 'levels of public engagement in relation to ... health are high. Life expectancy increases and goes beyond current forecasts, health status improves dramatically and people are confident in the health system and demand high quality care. The health service is responsive with high rates of technology uptake, particularly in relation to disease prevention. Use of resources is more efficient.'

The idea of citizens *fully engaged* in their own health and care is becoming the dominant discourse across all services responsible for the care and treatment of people with long-term conditions (LTCs). This is the most pressing area for attention because treating LTCs currently takes up the majority of spending on health and care and, given demographic changes, is projected to rapidly take up an increasing amount of resources. The majority of people with mental health needs seen in secondary care can be considered to have LTCs. Given the frequent comorbidity with a number of physical health conditions, such as diabetes, the majority of patients whom psychiatrists treat are also in the category of people with multiple LTCs. The proposition is that if mental health services can be redesigned so that *self-management* and *peer support* are at the core of the delivery system then more people will remain well – thus stemming the tide of need that is currently in danger of overwhelming the system.

A number of different pieces of work and publications (e.g. Coulter, 2013) have promoted the fact that people with multiple LTCs spend on average 8755 hours per year in self-care and 5 hours in professional care. That is, people with LTCs are living their lives in their local communities, with their neighbours, families and friends, with only a tiny proportion of that time spent with doctors and clinicians. A big part of the change programme required is thus to find ways to support patients to make improvements in their self-care time.

In mental health, a number of fundamental changes are required to the model of operation and mind-set of clinicians. The King's Fund *House of Care* report (Coulter, 2013) emphasises that traditional practices create dependency, discourage self-care, ignore preferences, undermine confidence, do not encourage healthy behaviours and lead to fragmented care. So what psychiatrists as key leaders in the mental health system have to promote are the change programmes which make it more likely that the 5 hours of clinical contact a year can lever even small changes in the 8755 hours a year, such that health and happiness for patients improves and dependency on the NHS decreases.

The first change area is to take a co-production approach to clinical consultations with patients. A national programme called 'People Powered Health' (see www.nesta.org.uk/project/people-powered-health) worked in six development sites, including one in Lambeth, London, UK, to build the business case for a full co-production approach. This includes clinicians working in an equal and reciprocal relationship with patients and their family and friends. It also includes encouraging *peer support,* which is good for the mental health of both the peer providing the support and the patient (peer) receiving the support. Another aspect of co-production is to take an asset-based approach to the consultation – building on the positive in people's lives.

A tool that will help psychiatrists to take a co-production approach with their patients is MyHealthLocker (see https://www.myhealthlockerlondon.nhs.uk/). This is a patient-focused website that enables patients to hold their own records and to bring together information from, for example, their general practitioner and their secondary care psychiatrist. Encouraging patients to take control of their care record and to feel fully involved in their care is a crucial part of the way forward. This change in the practice of clinicians and teams is greatly supported by clinical records being seen by the patient as belonging to them and not to the clinical team. Continuing on the theme of changes, which will encourage patients to take control, is the idea of secondary care clinicians ceasing to set the date for a follow-up appointment. Working in a way whereby it is clear to patients that there will be no follow-up appointment but should patients think they would benefit from seeing the psychiatrist then they can make contact and will be guaranteed an appointment in a short period of time fundamentally shifts the power dynamic by putting decisions on future healthcare needs in the hands of patients. Patients then have to take responsibility for monitoring how they feel and to decide for themselves if they need NHS support.

The system redesigns that are required centre on the integration agenda and the acceptance that the NHS is just one small part in the whole system, which helps us all to take responsibility for and maintain our health and well-being. If we are to focus on the positive in people's lives and support them to take active control of their health then it follows that the NHS needs to recognise the valuable contributions which, for example, the community and voluntary sector make in local neighbourhoods and to encourage their development. The move to capitated budgets for a segment of the population across a number of health, social care and voluntary and community sector providers is one of the enablers which is helping to facilitate such a way of thinking.

My postscript has drawn on some current thinking on the nature of the change that is required if we are to survive and thrive as a healthcare system and a society. What has not changed, however, are the theories and world-views which will help psychiatrists lead and facilitate that change. The complexity tools and methods and ways of thinking and being described above are as useful and valid today as they were when the third edition was published. So, while the urgency has increased and the direction is clearer, complexity approaches are still recommended as the most effective way to secure the sustainable change that is required in individuals, teams and systems.

References and further reading

Battram A (1998) *Navigating Complexity*. Industrial Society.

Blinker BB, Alban BT (1997) *Large Group Interventions – Engaging the Whole System for Rapid Change*. Jossey-Bass.

Clarkson P (1995) *Change in Organisations*. Whurr.

Coulter A (2013) *Building the House of Care*. King's Fund.

Fraser W, Conner M, Yarrow D (eds) (2003) *Thriving in Unpredictable Times*. Kingsham Press.

Gladwell M (2000) *The Tipping Point – How Little Things Can Make a Big Difference.* Little, Brown.

Goleman D (1996) *Emotional Intelligence.* Bloomsbury.

Mitleton-Kelly E (2003) *Complex Systems and Evolutionary Perspectives on Organisations.* Pergamon Elsevier Science.

Senge P (1993) *The Fifth Discipline – The Art and Practice of the Learning Organisation.* Century Business.

Senge P, Kleiner A, Roberts C, *et al* (1999) *The Dance of Change – The Challenge of Sustaining Momentum in Learning Organizations.* Nicholas Brealey.

Wanless D (2002) *Securing Our Future Health: Taking a Long Term View.* HM Treasury.

Wheatley M (1999) *Leadership and the New Science – Discovering Order in a Chaotic World.* Berrett-Koehler.

See also http://www.wheelofwellbeing.org, an interactive website enabling you to record and monitor your progress in taking actions to improve your own well-being, developed by South London and Maudsley NHS Foundation Trust.

CHAPTER 16

Managing the psychiatrist's performance

Michael Holland

On 3 December 2012 the General Medical Council (GMC), with the introduction of revalidation, was the first medical regulatory body in the world to implement large-scale changes to the regulation of doctors. Since the start of the millennium significant changes have been made to how both the regulator and organisations now manage the performance of doctors in the UK. In this chapter I will outline the processes for managing doctors' performance through the use of appraisal and revalidation, job planning and finally, if all else fails, via the more formal processes of investigation and case management. (Further details of revalidation are presented in Chapter 17.)

Most doctors work hard to improve the quality of their work year on year, and provide excellent care to their patients. However, given the numbers of doctors working in the UK it is inevitable that some fail either to maintain standards high enough to keep patients safe or to maintain the quality of their own work. If we fail to address the poor performance of doctors then we place patients at risk of harm or even death, undermine the morale of the teams and erode public confidence in the profession.

In 1994 Professor Liam Donaldson wrote about doctors' performance problems in hospitals (Donaldson, 1994). These included disruptive and irresponsible behaviour, lack of commitment to duties, badly exercised clinical skills, inadequate medical knowledge, dishonesty, sexual overtones in dealings with patients or staff, disorganised practice and poor communication with colleagues. He found that 6% of doctors could be of serious enough concern to warrant the consideration of disciplinary action. Donaldson commented that the management of poorly performing doctors was 'difficult, distasteful, time consuming and acrimonious work'. He recommended that managers should: always adhere to policies and procedures for handling disciplinary problems; avoid precipitate action; remain non-judgemental; beware of manipulation by those who have axes to grind; and never avoid dealing with problems, as this may harm patients.

In the time since Donaldson was writing, the procedures have changed significantly, with a new framework for dealing with doctors' performance and a statutory obligation for employing organisations to provide a system for the revalidation of their doctors. This framework attempts to put in place a system that identifies performance concerns early and supports doctors to continuously reflect on their practice and improve its quality.

It would be wrong to think that the inquiry established in 2000 into the murders committed by general practitioner Harold Shipman was what brought about the changes in the regulation and management of doctors' performance. In the late 1990s there was a series of scandals. One of these led to the Bristol heart inquiry (Smith, 1998), where a hospital's chief executive officer, a doctor, and two paediatric cardiac surgeons, were struck off the medical register for the deaths of 29 children out of the 53 who were operated on at the hospital. That inquiry changed the landscape of medical regulation forever. The Bristol case threw up issues that needed to be addressed urgently about the management and regulation of the profession:

- the need for clearly understood clinical standards
- how clinical competence and technical expertise are assessed and evaluated
- who carries responsibility for team-based care
- the training of doctors in advanced procedures
- how to approach the so-called learning curve of doctors undertaking established procedures
- the reliability and validity of data used to monitor doctors' personal performance
- the use of medical and clinical audit
- the appreciation of the importance of factors other than purely clinical ones that can affect clinical judgement, performance and outcome
- the responsibility of a consultant to take appropriate actions in response to concerns about his or her performance
- the factors which seem to discourage openness and frankness about doctors' personal performance
- how doctors explain risks to patients
- the ways in which people concerned about patient safety can make their concerns known
- the need for doctors to take prompt action at an early stage when a colleague is in difficulty, in order to offer the best chance of avoiding damage to patients and the colleague and of putting things right.

At around the same time there was also the case of Rodney Ledward (Department of Health, 2000), the gynaecologist in Kent who is thought to have harmed almost 100 women through negligent practice. Prior to this there had been the cases of Haslam and Kerr, psychiatrists working in York in the 1970s and 1980s, who were convicted of the indecent assault of patients; a total of 67 patients declared themselves to have been victims of Kerr and 10 patients to have been victims of Haslam (Kennedy, 2006). The Shipman inquiry criticised the first proposed revalidation framework for being too weak (Smith, 2004) and following this the GMC redesigned it; that redesign led to the current framework. Post-Shipman, the way in which a doctor's performance is accounted for and monitored has changed and continues to at a rapid pace. All doctors, including doctors in training, are included in the programme of revalidation.

Reinertsen (2003) sees medicine as a combination of both art and science: the application of research science to the art of healing. All doctors are aware of the limits of evidence-based medicine and yet doctors often show marked variation in practice, even within the evidence base. With time, patients have become more aware of this practice variation and the lack of defensible arguments for it. The new performance management systems are attempting to change the culture of doctors to being open to critique and self-reflection and therefore allow for improvement to happen, through continuous learning but also through demonstration of competence and most importantly through demonstrating how our practice benefits our patients. This echoes an article by Lucian Leape (1994), who discussed the culture of medicine as one of a model of 'perfectibility'; through training and education, perfection is sought and blame is used to encourage better performance. This model in the safety literature is thought in fact to make practice more *unsafe*, as pressure is put on individuals to constantly perform and to admit to error is to elicit blame. Therefore the ability to learn from one's mistakes is substantially reduced. The framework for appraisal and revalidation, which will be discussed next, attempts to set up a process to improve on this.

Appraisal and revalidation

On 3 December 2012 revalidation became a statutory obligation for employing organisations in the UK. The process involves doctors compiling a portfolio that describes their practice and performance across their whole scope of work. In this section I will describe the process that the doctor undergoes when preparing for and having an appraisal and how this links through to the management of performance of the individual doctor.

The purpose of revalidation is 'to assure patients and the public, employers and other health care professionals that licensed doctors are up to date and fit to practise' (Revalidation Support Team, 2013). The appraisal itself is a single meeting between two medical professionals, one of whom is a trained appraiser. There are four potential purposes of the medical appraisal (see Box 16.1). These four purposes allow doctors, over time, to reflect on their current performance and with the help of a skilled appraiser make plans to improve it. The purpose of revalidation is not about trying to find the next Shipman, as it is not designed to find the criminal among us, but to help doctors improve their practice and deliver an assurance process for doctors. It is meant to be a supportive and developmental process that, with time, allows doctors to demonstrate improvement in their practice.

Box 16.1   Four potential purposes of the medical appraisal

- To enable doctors to discuss their practice and performance with their appraiser in order to demonstrate that they continue to meet the principles and values set out in *Good Medical Practice* (GMC, 2013) and thus to inform the responsible officer's revalidation recommendation to the GMC.

- To enable doctors to enhance the quality of their own professional work by planning their professional development.

- To enable doctors to consider their own needs in planning their professional development.

- To enable doctors to ensure that they are working productively and in line with the priorities and requirements of the organisation they practise in.

Prior to the appraisal the doctor should prepare a portfolio; this information falls under four broad headings (GMC, 2012*a*) (see Box 16.2).

There are six types of supporting information that the doctor needs to provide and these are listed under the following headings (GMC, 2012*a*):

1   continuing professional development
2   quality improvement activities
3   significant events
4   feedback from colleagues
5   feedback from patients
6   review of complaints and compliments.

Within each section the doctor provides evidence and is obliged to reflect on what has happened over the last year and the data on performance therein. Doctors should where possible compare their data against those of

---

Box 16.2   The four broad headings for the doctor's portfolio

- *General information*. This provides the context, describing what the doctor does and where the doctor practises (for all aspects of work).

- *Keeping up to date*. This is where the doctor demonstrates that he or she has maintained knowledge and skills and improved the quality of professional work.

- *Review of the doctor's practice*. The doctor demonstrates that she or he has evaluated the quality of all professional work.

- *Feedback on the doctor's practice*. This provides information demonstrating how others perceive the quality of the doctor's professional work.

Table 16.1 Types of information to be included for appraisal purposes

Heading	Requirement	Frequency of update
Personal details	Self-declaration of no change, or an update identifying any changes in role or qualifications	Annually
Scope of work	Any significant changes in a doctor's professional practice should be highlighted as well as any exceptional circumstances. This should cover all clinical and non-clinical activities (e.g. teaching, management, medico-legal, medical research)	Annually
Record of annual appraisals	Evidence of previous year's appraisal outcome	Annually
Personal development plans (PDPs) and their review	Demonstration of progress against previous PDP. Any additions made by the doctor should be confirmed by the appraiser as being relevant and carried forward into the next PDP if required	Annually
Probity	Self-declaration confirming the absence of any probity issues	Annually
Health	Self-declaration confirming the absence of any medical condition that could pose a risk to patients and that a doctor complies with the health and safety obligations set out in *Good Medical Practice*	Annually
Continuing professional development (CPD)	A description of CPD undertaken demonstrating: its relevance to the doctor's individual professional work; its relevance to the doctor's PDP; reflection and confirmation of good practice or new learning/practice change where appropriate A certificate of good standing for CPD from the Royal College of Psychiatrists should meet the GMC and College requirements	Annually

their peers, either internally or against national reporting. It is the reflection on the information provided that leads to the doctor identifying areas for development and improvement. The Royal College of Psychiatrists has produced guidance on what type of information should be included and how often for appraisal purposes (Royal College of Psychiatrists & Academy of Medical Royal Colleges, 2013); this is summarised in Table 16.1.

Through the use of this supporting information doctors are therefore able to demonstrate that their practice meets the four domains of the *Good Medical Practice* framework (GMC, 2011). These four domains (which each have three attributes) are outlined in Box 16.3. The Royal College of Psychiatrists (2009) has published *Good Psychiatric Practice*, which is aligned to the GMC's *Good Medical Practice* and sets out standards of practice for all psychiatrists.

For doctors to have an appraisal that is useful to improve their performance and quality of practice, it requires adequate preparation on

Table 16.1 continued

Quality improvement

Clinical audit	One complete audit cycle. If audit is not possible then other ways of demonstrating quality improvement activity should be undertaken, such as review of clinical outcomes or case discussions	Once every 5 years
Review of clinical outcomes	Where clinical outcomes are used instead of, or alongside, clinical audit or case reviews there should be evidence of reflection and change in practice	Once every 5 years
Case review or discussion	If the doctor is unable to provide evidence from clinical audit or outcomes, documented case reviews should be presented Evidence of case-based discussions with action points included in PDP	10 case reviews per 5 years

Significant events

Clinical incidents, significant untoward incidents or other similar events	All serious incidents that the doctor is either directly involved in or clinically or managerially responsible for must be reported and reflected on. If self-employed without a reporting system, a personal record of any incidents needs to be maintained and presented	Annually

Feedback on practice

Colleague feedback	At least one colleague multi-source feedback exercise should be undertaken	Once every 5 years (early in the revalidation cycle)
Feedback from patients and/or carers	At least one patient feedback exercise	Once every 5 years (early in the revalidation cycle)
Feedback from clinical supervision, teaching and training	Clinical supervisors and educational supervisors should provide evidence that they have met minimum training requirements set by the GMC	Once every 5 years
Formal complaints	Details and summary of any complaints received by the doctor or the team that doctor works in, with personal reflection on the complaint	Annually
Compliments	A summary of any unsolicited compliments received and reflection on these	Annually

the part of both the doctor and the appraiser. Appraisers should be trained to use their professional judgement during the appraisal to assess the quality of the evidence provided and the progress the doctor is making towards revalidation. This is seen as similar to the clinical judgements

---

Box 16.3 Four domains of *Good Medical Practice*

1 Knowledge, skills and performance
   • Maintain your professional performance
   • Apply knowledge and experience to practice
   • Keep clear, accurate and legible records
2 Safety and quality
   • Put into effect systems to protect patients and improve care.
   • Respond to risks to safety
   • Protect patients and colleagues from any risk posed by your health
3 Communication, partnership and teamwork
   • Communicate effectively
   • Work constructively with colleagues and delegate effectively
   • Establish and maintain partnerships with patients
4 Maintaining trust
   • Show respect for patients
   • Treat patients and colleagues fairly and without discrimination.
   • Act with honesty and integrity

---

that the appraiser is used to making as a clinician (Revalidation Support Team, 2012). Appraisers should not be afraid to challenge doctors in their view of their performance and, overall, should try to make the appraisal a positive experience for the doctor. Appraisers will need to balance their discussions according to the doctor's supporting information and progress towards revalidation; they should help the doctor address the different areas and therefore improve the overall quality of care given. The appraiser may suspend an appraisal if patient safety concerns are raised, in order to deal with them within the organisation. The appraiser should always have little reluctance to seek advice from senior medical managers and senior appraisers within the organisation where difficulties occur during the appraisal. There should be adequate support structures within the organisation for the appraisers so that they can seek timely and informed advice. This could be through appraiser forums, whereby appraisal issues are shared and discussed with other appraisers and appraisal skills can be honed and improved, or more directly through advice from the appraisal/revalidation lead or the responsible officer.

The appraisal links to revalidation by demonstrating to the responsible officer that the doctor is fit to practise, and has made progress on their personal development plan (PDP) and has made a further plan for the coming year. This thereby shows to the responsible officer that the doctor is continuing to try to improve the care delivered. The responsible officer will triangulate this information regarding the doctor's appraisal with information from the organisation's clinical governance systems and any relevant clinical governance information from other organisations that the doctor works in, to make a decision regarding the doctor's revalidation status.

The appraisal, when done well, is a very good mechanism for the majority of doctors, as it allows them to reflect on their current performance and make plans on how to improve it in the coming years through their PDPs. When the appraisal is performed badly, however, it serves little purpose for either doctor involved and may over time lead to the doctor becoming more defensive and less able to reflect on and improve performance. This is why the appraisers need adequate training and comprehensive support mechanisms to help them perform appraisals to the best of their ability. It is not, however, the best mechanism for the management of those with performance concerns or for the delivery of performance objectives related to organisational performance. These should be managed either through job planning, which I will now discuss, or through a more formal investigation process, with a remediation or rehabilitation plan, which I will discuss later in the chapter.

Job planning

Job planning has been in place since 1991 but became an integral part of an NHS consultant contract in 2003. It is defined as 'a prospective, professional agreement that sets out the duties, responsibilities, accountabilities and objectives of the consultant and the support and resources provided by the employer for the coming year' (British Medical Association & NHS Employers, 2011). The job planning process should be distinct from the appraisal process as they serve very different purposes. The appraisal is there as an assurance process that the doctor has maintained fitness to practise and made personal developmental objectives for the coming year. The purpose of the job planning process is to improve organisational performance and the quality of practice of the doctor as it aligns to the organisation.

In the job planning meeting, the clinical manager and doctor should meet to review the doctor's previous objectives and progress against these as well as planning the objectives for the coming year. These objectives should set out the relationship between the personal objectives of the consultant and those of the local service. These objectives could relate to any of the following areas:

- quality
- activity and efficiency
- clinical outcomes
- clinical standards
- local service objectives
- management of resources
- service development
- multidisciplinary team working.

Although the objectives that are set are personal to the individual doctor, if she or he works in a team setting with other doctors it may be more appropriate to consider objectives jointly with the whole team. This allows for the manager to share responsibilities across the team in an open way that gains the agreement of all the doctors involved. This could also be used where a single activity, such as investigations into serious incidents, which need to be carried for the hospital, are divided between a consultant workforce within a specific directorate. Often, job planning is used for little more than just setting an agreed timetable of activity for the consultant and few, if any, objectives are set.

Although job planning is on an annual cycle, it is the responsibility of both the doctor and the clinical manager to identify any potential problems if they arise that may limit the doctor's ability to meet the objectives set. It is advisable that if doctors feel that they are not going to be able to meet their objectives they discuss this early with their manager and possibly make changes to their job plan. It is through this flexibility that objectives can be altered to fit with other changes in the local context as and when they happen. Job planning should therefore not be a hurried process but one that should be helpful to both the organisation and the individual doctor. Organisations often spend little time on this, which can leave both doctors and the organisation resentful as neither feels that the other is delivering what they should. Job planning should match the objectives that the doctor can realistically achieve over the year with the resources required to complete these, in terms of both time available (i.e. through the agreed timetable) and equipment or staff. Time should be taken for the clinical manager and doctor to work collaboratively to set the right objectives that improve or develop the service that the doctor works in. Job planning, like appraisal, is therefore a useful process in particular for those doctors for whom serious performance concerns are not an issue.

Managing poorly performing doctors

Poor performance has not always been managed well and in recent years, with the rise in consumer power, increasing numbers of complaints are going to the GMC for investigation. The traditional approaches to dealing with difficult or poorly performing doctors were keeping quiet or conversations in corridors or corrosive emails being sent by third parties. There was often little in the way of a paper trail recording any direct discussions and a lack of objectively corroborated allegation; judgements were often made without investigation. There has, though, been a drive to improve this with the establishment of the National Clinical Assessment Service (NCAS) in 2001 and the development of clinical governance systems within organisations. The onset of revalidation has made organisations tighten up their governance systems for doctors, with regular reporting to the GMC of progress and outcomes of investigations. The regulatory environment has also changed dramatically since 1997 with the introduction of the health regulators – the Care Quality Commission (CQC) and Monitor – and this has led to greater board accountability for hospital performance and therefore for the quality of the staff that they employ. The recent dreadful events at Mid Staffordshire NHS Foundation Trust (Francis, 2013) highlighted the need for us all to pay attention to the quality of care that is delivered to our patients and to speak up early if we have concerns.

In line with the increase in governance and consumer expectations, service complaints about doctors have increased greatly in recent years. In 2009 there were 5773 enquiries made to the GMC about doctors' practice; by 2012 this figure had increased by 79%, to 10 347 (GMC annual statistics). In 2012 the greatest increase in referrals was from public organisations such as employers or police, with an increase of 35% from 2011; however, most of the enquiries (60%) currently come from members of the public. There has also been an associated increase in the likelihood that the GMC will investigate the doctor, from 1 in 68 cases to 1 in 64; however, 56% of all enquiries are closed without investigation. Psychiatrists are one of the more common groups of doctors for whom complaints are made to the GMC, making up 7.2% of the enquiries (GMC, 2012b).

Concerns may arise from any aspect of a doctor's performance or conduct which poses a threat or potential threat to patient safety, exposes the service to financial or other substantial risk, undermines the reputation or efficiency of services in some significant way, or is outside acceptable practices, guidelines and standards (NCAS, 2010). Concerns may be raised through a number of means, not least by the doctor herself or himself. They may come to light from colleague or patient complaints or through governance systems, incidents, audit or outcomes monitoring. They may also arise through criminal proceedings, appraisal or whistle blowing. Each of these triggers needs to be taken seriously and investigated thoroughly and objectively.

The concerns raised may be about the conduct of the doctor, or the doctor's ability or health. It is the responsible officer's responsibility to determine with others the type of concern it is and how serious it is. Many organisations have set up decision-making groups which consist of senior medical managers who will review these concerns to determine type and severity. There needs to be a clear and consistent approach across an organisation in this process. The first issue before investigating the concern is to determine whether there are any urgent safety issues for patient, staff or doctor. The responsible officer must determine whether the doctor's practice can continue, or whether there is a need for immediate restriction of practice or exclusion/suspension or, in rare circumstances, dismissal. In determining the type of concern, the responsible officer has a choice of three categories:

- *conduct* – the doctor chooses to do something he or she knows or should know is wrong (e.g. a refusal to comply with reasonable require-ments of the employer; or wilful, careless, inappropriate or unethical behaviour likely to compromise standards of care or patient safety)
- *capability* – the doctor is unable to do the right thing (e.g. outdated clinical practice; inappropriate clinical practice arising from a lack of knowledge or skills that puts patients at risk; ineffective team-working skills)
- *health*.

Establishing the type and the level of concern will help to provide an appropriate response from the organisation. In thinking through the level of concern, the NCAS (2013) provides the guidance set out in Box 16.4.

In addressing concerns that are raised about doctors, one must not underestimate the complexity that may be involved, as doctors often come into contact with multiple people across multiple organisations. There may well be a mix of concerns about conduct, capability and poor relationships and a further confusion with multiple conflicting expert reports. However, this should never prevent an objective evaluation of the evidence taking place.

When a concern has been raised, always try to get this in writing. If it is of a serious nature it must be put in written form. Unless there is a clear safety concern, the organisation should always try to keep the doctor at work; it can be very difficult to manage a remediation programme for a doctor if he or she has been removed from clinical activities. This could be done through close supervision, chaperones or limiting the doctor's scope of

---

Box 16.4 National Clinical Assessment Service guidance on levels of concern

Low level

- Unintended or unexpected
- Low possibility of recurrence
- Minimal impact
- No harm to patients, staff or individual

Medium level

- Potential for recurrence
- Potential for moderate impact or harm
- Staff member has raised concern
- Organisation or professional reputation may be at stake

High level

- Significant incident
- Interruption to delivery of care
- Likely or high potential of recurrence
- Critical or high potential for harm

In order to help with the decision regarding what level of response to make, the following questions may be of use:

- Is there any risk to patient safety?
- How much harm occurred?
- How likely is it to recur?
- How significant would a recurrence be?
- What is the reputational risk?
- Does the concern affect more than one area of practice?
- How much intervention is likely to be required?
- What is the mitigation?

work; in ideal circumstances the doctor will voluntarily agree to the actions taken. The process for the management of concern must demonstrate that it does not discriminate in any way against any employee. When a concern is raised, the process may be extremely stressful for the doctor involved and the organisation must support and communicate openly with any doctor where a concern has been raised. In managing a concern always refer to your local hospital policy and communicate quickly with the human resource professionals and the NCAS for advice on dealing with the matter.

A good system for managing and supporting doctors around their performance is one where there is a low threshold for concerns to be reported and acted on. The organisation should have a well-developed and supportive process for individuals to receive regular and full feedback, whether via appraisal, multi-source feedback or regular team meetings. The organisation should have a culture where staff members are supported and able to challenge practice and convention and where there are open discussions on performance, ideally a culture that places importance on helping doctors to learn about their own practice and continuously improve. A healthy staff group is equally important and efforts to improve the health of the staff should be made by the organisation; it should have clear systems to support those staff with ill health and disability.

Doctors are not always good at either recognising or acting on their own ill health (McKevitt *et al*, 1996). At times, doctors continue to work while suffering ill health, which puts patient safety at risk (Wallace *et al*, 2009). Doctors appear to be more likely to suffer mental health conditions than the general population and up to 7% will have a substance misuse problem during their lifetime. Suicide rates are particularly high for female doctors, anaesthetists, general practitioners and psychiatrists (Harvey *et al*, 2009). It is therefore extremely important for organisations to recognise and support those doctors who suffer from any illness.

Ill health should be managed in the same way as any other performance concern, with early attention and support offered to the doctor. In managing ill health within the workplace, patient safety should always remain central in the decision regarding return to work.

The future

There have been significant changes in the way doctors are regulated and performance is managed. Reports by the King's Fund (Nath *et al*, 2014) and research from Plymouth University (Archer *et al*, 2014) show that we are still in the early stages of accepting revalidation as a profession but that it is increasingly being seen as a process that has the potential to improve the quality of care that we provide and that supports doctors in improving practice. Several areas clearly need further work, such as consistency in the performance of appraisals and ensuring that appraisal does not become just another 'tick box' exercise.

With increased sophistication in data collection and management, the potential for psychiatrists to understand their own performance, in similar ways to cardiothoracic surgeons, can only lead to better understanding of our own variations in performance; if used for learning, that in turn will lead to improved outcomes for our patients.

References

Archer J, Regan de Bere S, Nunn S, *et al* (2014) *Revalidation in Practice: Shaping the Future Development of Revalidation*. Health Foundation.

British Medical Association, NHS Employers (2011) *A Guide to Consultant Job Planning*. BMA.

Department of Health (2000) *The Report of the Inquiry into Quality and Practice Within the National Health Service Arising from the Actions of Rodney Ledward* (Ritchie report). TSO.

Donaldson LJ (1994) Doctors with problems in an NHS workforce. *BMJ*, **308**: 1277.

Francis R (2013) *Report of the Mid Staffordshire NHS Foundation Trust Public Inquiry. Final Report* (Francis report). Mid Staffordshire NHS Foundation Trust Public Inquiry.

GMC (2011) *Good Medical Practice Framework for Appraisal and Revalidation*. General Medical Council.

GMC (2012*a*) *Supporting Information for Appraisal and Revalidation*. General Medical Council.

GMC (2012*b*) *Fitness to Practice Worksheet*. General Medical Council.

GMC (2013) *Good Medical Practice*. General Medical Council.

Harvey SB, Laird B, Henderson M, *et al* (2009) *The Mental Health of Health Care Professionals*. Department of Health.

Kennedy P (2006) Kerr/Haslam inquiry into sexual abuse of patients by psychiatrists. *Psychiatric Bulletin*, **30**: 204–6.

Leape LL (1994) Error in medicine. *JAMA*, **272**: 1851–7.

McKevitt C, Morgan M, Holland WW (1996) *Protecting and Promoting Doctors' Health: The Work Environment and Counselling Services in Three Sites*. Nuffield Trust.

Nath V, Seale B, Kaur M (2014) *Medical Revalidation: From Compliance to Commitment*. King's Fund.

NCAS (2010) *How to Conduct a Local Performance Investigation*. National Clinical Assessment Service.

NCAS (2013) *Case Manager Training*. National Clinical Assessment Service.

Reinertsen JL (2003) Zen and the art of physician autonomy maintenance. *Annals of Internal Medicine*, **138**: 992–5.

Revalidation Support Team (2013) *Medical Appraisal Guide: A Guide to Medical Appraisal for Revalidation in England*. NHS England.

Royal College of Psychiatrists (2009) *Good Psychiatric Practice* (3rd edition). RCPsych.

Royal College of Psychiatrists, Academy of Medical Royal Colleges (2013) *Supporting Information for Appraisal and Revalidation: Guidance for Psychiatry*. RCPsych & AoMRC.

Smith J (2004) *Fifth Report – Safeguarding Patients: Lessons from the Past – Proposals for the Future*. Shipman Inquiry.

Smith R (1998) Regulation of doctors and the Bristol inquiry. *BMJ*, **317**: 1539.

Wallace JE, Lemaire JB, Ghali WA (2009) Physician wellness: a missing quality indicator. *Lancet*, **374**: 1714–21.

CHAPTER 17

Revalidation for psychiatrists

Ellen Wilkinson

Since 1858, the General Medical Council (GMC), which is a registered charity, has held a statutory function to maintain a list of medical practitioners registered in the UK. There has always been an expectation and duty that doctors maintain their professional competence throughout their careers but until now this assumption has not been monitored, nor enforced, except through processes relating to their fitness to practise. In 2009, all registered medical practitioners were routinely granted a licence to practise. However, since December 2012, when revalidation commenced, this licence has been subject to review every 5 years. Revalidation is important but questions have been raised about its validity. Some of the issues are covered in the previous chapter.

According to the GMC's website:

'Revalidation is the process by which licensed doctors are required to demonstrate on a regular basis that they are up to date and fit to practise.... Revalidation aims to give extra confidence to patients that their doctor is being regularly checked by their employer and the GMC.' (http://www.gmc-uk.org/doctors/revalidation/9627.asp)

The change in legislation and guidance has created new relationships between doctors, employers, regulators, patients and the public. The full impact, costs and benefits remain to be seen.

History of revalidation

The Merrison report in 1975 introduced the concept of specialist training and certification and altered the composition of the GMC. It also suggested periodic tests of competence, but ruled these to be outside its terms of reference (Merrison, 1975). This task was passed to the Alment Committee, whose terms of reference were: 'To review the present methods of ensuring the maintenance of standards of continuing competence to practise and of the clinical care of patients, and to make recommendations' (Alment, 1976). The report, *Competence to Practise*, published in 1976, concluded that compulsory re-licensure was not indicated as it was too difficult but that professional development should be encouraged for all doctors on a voluntary basis.

Revalidation for the medical profession has therefore been under discussion for decades. Progress has been slow, through a series of government reports, the introduction of clinical governance, clinical audit and annual appraisal, and a series of scandals relating to doctors. In 2004, in *Safeguarding Patients – Lessons from the Past, Proposals for the Future*, the fifth report of the Shipman Inquiry, Dame Janet Smith asserted that 'any system of revalidation of registration must have wider aims than merely the detection of the activities of a mass murderer practising as a GP' (Smith, 2004). She expressed a view that appraisal alone, as proposed by the GMC to be implemented in 2005, did not provide adequate protection for patients. She described in detail activity within the GMC, including consultation papers, testing and cost–benefit analysis. This estimated significant cost to the GMC and medical time diverted from patient care. The proposed design in 2001 was a system of appraisal with periodic review by a local revalidation group and random quality assurance by the GMC. In 2002, the Medical Act 1983 was amended to allow for the 'licence to practise'. By 2003, the process appeared to have been diluted to only involve five consecutive appraisals, with the doctor deciding how to demonstrate compliance with the GMC's *Good Medical Practice* (discussed below). An independent route was proposed for doctors not working in a managed environment. The GMC was subsequently identified by the House of Commons Health Select Committee as having 'prime responsibility for planning and executing effective and timely revalidation'.[1]

Early pilots were conducted in 2008 and 2009. Pathfinder pilots in 2010 involved 3022 strengthened medical appraisals (SMAs); there were ten pilot sites across healthcare sectors. These pilot studies were reported to have been only partially successful in answering the questions posed, leading to a requirement for additional testing and piloting. The Medical Appraisal Guide (MAG) emerged – from a simplified strengthened medical appraisal.

Revalidation finally commenced on 3 December 2012 and the GMC stated its intention to revalidate the majority of licensed doctors in the UK for the first time by March 2016.

Introduction and implementation

Regulations for medical revalidation came into force on 1 January 2011. They are the Medical Profession (Responsible Officers) Regulations 2010.[2]

---

1 See http://www.publications.parliament.uk/pa/cm201012/cmselect/cmhealth/1429/142904.htm.
2 See http://www.legislation.gov.uk/uksi/2010/2841/contents/made; see also the Medical Profession (Responsible Officers) (Amendment) Regulations 2013 at http://www.legislation.gov.uk/uksi/2013/391/contents/made.

In 2010, the Medical Director of the NHS in England, the Chief Medical Officers of England, Northern Ireland and Wales and the Deputy Chief Medical Officer for Scotland issued a 'statement of intent' – a commitment to proceed with medical revalidation subject to an assessment of readiness in summer 2012. At the UK Revalidation Programme Board meeting on 20 September 2012, the four Revalidation Delivery Boards (from each part of the UK) and the GMC reported that they were ready to start revalidation in December 2012. The General Medical Council (Licence to Practise and Revalidation) Regulations Order of Council 2012 ('the Regulations') was submitted to the Privy Council for approval.

In England, the NHS Revalidation Support Team (RST), part of Guy's and St Thomas' NHS Foundation Trust, was funded by the Department of Health to support the implementation of revalidation. The RST worked in partnership with NHS England, the Department of Health (England), the GMC and designated bodies to deliver an effective system of revalidation for doctors in England. From 1 April 2014, this function was absorbed into NHS England. Scotland, Wales and Northern Ireland each have their own revalidation delivery boards which feed into the UK Revalidation Implementation Advisory Board (which commenced in March 2013). The Revalidation Implementation Plan for Northern Ireland was approved by the Confidence in Care Programme Board. In Scotland there is the Revalidation Delivery Board Scotland. Appraisal training has been provided through NHS Education for Scotland (NES) and there is a National Appraisal Leads Group. In NHS Scotland, the executive medical directors of NHS boards, special NHS boards and the Central Service Agency (CSA) are the responsible officers. In Wales, there is a Wales Revalidation Delivery Board.

Organisational readiness for revalidation

The Organisational Readiness Self-Assessment (ORSA) process was adapted from the Assuring the Quality of Medical Appraisal for Revalidation (AQMAR) tool. The ORSA exercise was an annual process designed to help designated bodies in England develop their systems and processes for the implementation of revalidation. Responsible officers submitted a self-assessment, using a tool based on the legislation, regulations and associated guidance and criteria suggested by the GMC. Regionally submitted data were pooled to give a national picture of organisations' readiness for the introduction of revalidation. In 2014, this process was replaced by the Framework for Quality Assurance.

The first ORSA exercise was completed in 2011. This covered 507 organisations out of 562 known designated bodies, believed to cover 85–90% of doctors in England. Overall, 73.7% of doctors had completed an appraisal, but with a difference between primary and secondary care: 85.2% in primary care trusts but only 55.7% in hospital trusts. For hospitals, there was a significant difference between appraisal rates for consultants (65%) and specialty and associate specialist (SAS) doctors (31.4%).

In 2012, the ORSA exercise was repeated. Of 691 organisations, 651 responded, including all such organisations within the NHS. Engagement from locum agencies was well below 50%. The general practitioner (GP) appraisal rate was improved, at 90.1%, and 73.1% of hospital consultants and 53.1% of SAS doctors reported appraisal completion.

In 2013, appraisal rates were reported as: GPs 90.3%; acute hospital consultants 75.1%; acute hospital SAS doctors 60.7%; mental health consultants 84.3%; and mental health SAS doctors 80.7%. By 2015, the total annual appraisal rate across all licensed doctors had increased to 86.2%.

New designated bodies were created to include locum agencies in the Procurement Services Framework, introduced on 1 July 2013. By January 2014, there were 832 designated bodies in the UK, including 760 in England.

In England, the chosen option for implementation was a 3-year roll-out, with 20%, 40% and 40% of doctors planned for revalidation in consecutive years, commencing in April 2013. The selection was coordinated and overseen by responsible officers. In Northern Ireland, revalidation dates were selected at random, based on GMC number.

Cost estimates

The cost–benefit analysis completed by the Department of Health in November 2012 estimated the cost to implement revalidation would be £97 million per year for the first 10 years (Department of Health Professional Standards Team, 2012). Costs to doctors, employing organisations and the regulator were included. This report included only the costs associated with appraisal for the 27% of doctors not currently engaging (using data from the ORSA) and estimated that 5% of doctors would be identified for remedial activity, with the majority requiring low-level interventions.

This cost–benefit analysis predicted greater benefit for the private sector, where appraisal was thought to be less well embedded. This view was based on the reported non-appraisal rate for private sector doctors as 56.4% in the 2011/12 ORSA return, when 7800 doctors reportedly worked solely in the private sector. It was estimated that 5% of remediation costs and 5% of patient safety and litigation benefits were incurred in the private sector.

The costs of revalidation were predicted to save money by reducing compensatory payments to NHS Litigation Authority (NHSLA) claimants and minimising the duration of exclusion for doctors (Department of Health Professional Standards Team, 2012).

Good Medical Practice

A revised version of *Good Medical Practice* came into effect on 22 April 2013. Although it was shorter than the previous version, a suite of explanatory guidance was made available through the GMC website. A supporting document for patients entitled 'What to expect from your doctor: a guide for patients' was issued to accompany the guide for doctors.

The status of *Good Medical Practice* is unambiguously stated in the introduction:

'Good medical practice describes what is expected of all doctors registered with the General Medical Council (GMC). It is your responsibility to be familiar with Good medical practice and the explanatory guidance which supports it, and to follow the guidance they contain.

'To maintain your licence to practise, you must demonstrate, through the revalidation process, that you work in line with the principles and values set out in this guidance. Serious or persistent failure to follow this guidance will put your registration at risk.' (GMC, 2013*a*)

Table 17.1 summarises its provisions.

Appraisal

In the Revalidation Support Team (2013) document *Quality Assurance of Medical Appraisers*, medical appraisal is defined as 'a process of facilitated self-review supported by information gathered from the full scope of a doctor's work'. Its uses are summarised in Box 17.1.

The cornerstone of revalidation is a quality-assured 'strengthened' appraisal process. This is achieved through increased rigour in the selection, training, support, feedback and review of appraisers. The appraiser for each

Table 17.1 Summary of *Good Medical Practice*, 2013

Domain	Attributes		
1. Knowledge, skills and performance	1.1 Maintain your professional performance	1.2 Apply knowledge and experience to practice	1.3 Ensure that all documentation (including clinical records) formally recording your work is clear, accurate and legible
2. Safety and quality	2.1 Contribute to and comply with systems to protect patients	2.2 Respond to risks to safety	2.3 Protect patients and colleagues from any risk posed by your health
3. Communication, partnership and teamwork	3.1 Communicate effectively	3.2 Work constructively with colleagues and delegate effectively	3.3 Establish and maintain partnerships with patients
4. Maintaining trust	4.1 Show respect for patients	4.2 Treat patients and colleagues fairly and without discrimination	4.3 Act with honesty and integrity

---

Box 17.1   Uses of medical appraisal

- To enable doctors to discuss their practice and performance with their appraiser in order to demonstrate that they continue to meet the principles and values set out in *Good Medical Practice* (GMC, 2013a) and thus to inform the responsible officer's revalidation recommendation to the GMC
- To enable doctors to enhance the quality of their professional work by planning their professional development
- To enable doctors to consider their own needs in planning their professional development
- To enable doctors to ensure that they are working productively and in line with the priorities and requirements of the organisation they practise in

---

doctor is selected as part of a managed process in accordance with the policy of the designated body. Appraisers require a role description, person specification, competency framework, feedback mechanism and assessment process. The outputs of appraisals also require quality assurance.

Appraisal was introduced into the NHS in 2001. It has been a contractual requirement for consultants in secondary care in the NHS since the consultant contract in 2003 and for medical practitioners in primary care since 2004. Appraisal was also included as a contractual obligation for SAS doctors in the 2008 contract.

In 2013, the GMC published a Good Medical Practice Framework, linked to the new edition of *Good Medical Practice*, which guides the structure of appraisals. The documentation for appraisal is usually determined by the designated body and commercial systems are available. The default document for medical appraisal in England is the *Medical Appraisal Guide*. In Wales, this is the Medical Appraisal and Revalidation System (MARS) for all doctors and in Scotland the Scottish Online Appraisal Resource (SOAR). In Northern Ireland, the Department of Health, Social Services and Public Safety provides appraisal forms for each grade of doctor, which are downloadable from its website.

There are three stages in the medical appraisal process:

1   inputs to appraisal, including a record of the doctor's scope and nature of work and relevant supporting information
2   the confidential appraisal discussion
3   outputs of appraisal, including the doctor's personal development plan (PDP) and a summary of the appraisal discussion and the appraiser's statements.

The PDP identified during appraisal uses the material reflected upon to direct and plan learning for the year ahead. It may include standard tasks, such as role-based mandatory training, completion of the College continuing professional development (CPD) certification process and

---

Box 17.2 Information required for appraisal

- Scope of current practice, encompassing organisations and locations worked in, including in a voluntary capacity if this activity requires a licence to practise (it is important for the appraiser to understand the scope and nature of each role)
- Statements of probity – relates directly to *Good Medical Practice*
- Statement of health – registration with a GP, appropriate immunisation, any serious condition which might pose a risk to patients
- Evidence of participation in annual appraisal
- Statements of good standing from the regulator (for work overseas)
- Evidence of achievement of a particular assessment or evaluation (if relevant)
- Personal development plans

Six further elements of supporting information are required:

- continuing professional development
- quality improvement activity
- significant events
- feedback from colleagues
- feedback from patients
- review of complaints and compliments

---

completion of appropriate clinical audit projects, quality improvement programmes and patient feedback. PDPs should also include bespoke actions in response to issues and concerns arising during discussion about the supporting information used in the appraisal meeting. The plans should be SMART (Specific, Measurable, Achievable, Relevant and Time-bound) and follow-up of progress during the year is desirable.

Supporting information

Over the 5-year revalidation cycle, supporting information should evidence practice relating to all 12 *Good Medical Practice* attributes. Collecting this information into a portfolio as evidence is necessary, but each item also requires reflection and consideration of how this information can inform the development and modification of practice. The definitive list of supporting information is contained in GMC guidance. An outline is presented in Box 17.2.

Continuing professional development (CPD)

Participation in a College CPD scheme to gain a certificate of good standing provides one possible (College-endorsed) way to demonstrate that a doctor has updated clinical knowledge and skills but even this should be checked at appraisal to ensure that it reflects the whole scope of practice. For career-grade psychiatrists (consultants and SAS doctors), peer group attendance is the recommended way to plan, approve and sign off that a

---

Box 17.3   The GMC's guidance on CPD

The purpose of continuing professional development (CPD) is to help improve the safety and quality of care provided for patients and the public.

- *Responsibility for personal learning.* You are responsible for identifying your CPD needs, planning how those needs should be addressed and undertaking CPD that will support your professional development and practice.

- *Reflection. Good Medical Practice* requires you to reflect regularly on your standards of medical practice.

- *Scope of practice.* You must remain competent and up to date in all areas of your practice.

- *Individual and team learning.* Your CPD activities should aim to maintain and improve the standards of your own practice and also those of any teams in which you work.

- *Identification of needs.* Your CPD activities should be shaped by assessments of both your professional needs and the needs of the service and the people who use it.

- *Outcomes.* You must reflect on what you have learnt through your CPD and record any impact (or expected future impact) on your performance and practice.

Passages quoted from GMC (2012).

---

course, conference or experience is reasonable, meeting identified learning gaps and satisfactorily completed. The GMC's guidance on CPD does not specify an annual number of hours but the GMC (2012) has issued guidance to doctors to clarify expectations for revalidation, reproduced in Box 17.3.

Quality improvement activity

Evidence of participation in quality improvement activity is the broadest component of supporting information. In surgical specialties, robust outcomes are published and there is a process to identify, check and remedy outliers. In comparison, for psychiatry, fewer hard outcomes are reliable and readily available, although nationally endorsed outcome measures are improving. The Royal College of Psychiatrists' College Centre for Quality Improvement supports accreditation programmes which can support best practice and allow benchmarking. It is recognised that organisations need to improve clinical governance information to identify concerns, to support the key role of the responsible officer and to allow psychiatrists to benchmark and achieve the best clinical outcomes for their patients.

Review of clinical outcomes is highly dependent on organisational information systems and the availability of national comparators, such as information from the national Mental Health Services Data Set, now called MHSDS.

Clinical audit

'Clinical audit is a quality improvement cycle that involves measurement of the effectiveness of healthcare against agreed and proven standards for high quality, and taking action to bring practice in line with these standards so as to improve the quality of care and health outcomes.' (Healthcare Quality Improvement Partnership, 2011)

For revalidation, participation in clinical audit demonstrates a willingness to evaluate one's own compliance with standards, but to obtain optimal value it requires reflection on practice and a contribution to action to make improvements based on the results. National clinical audits, such as the National Audit of Schizophrenia, run by the College Centre for Quality Improvement, allow comparisons across all participating health providers (see also Chapter 22, 'Clinical audit'). Similarly, the Prescribing Observatory for Mental Health enables comparison at organisational level and at team and/or clinician level, so that improvements can be introduced and evaluation against standards retested.

Case review or discussion

In psychiatry, the formalised assessment and discussion of a clinical case, based on the case-based discussion assessment used by trainees, has been piloted and mandated as a useful clinical quality improvement tool. The peer group has emerged as a specialty-specific vehicle to monitor and evaluate CPD as well as to assess and improve the management of live clinical cases.

Non-clinical evidence

For doctors with minimal clinical roles, it is still possible to engage in quality improvement, for example by monitoring the effectiveness of a teaching programme or evaluating the impact of a policy or management project. Like all supporting information, quality improvement evidence needs to be relevant, evaluated and reflective, with action taken and re-evaluated.

Significant events

The GMC defines a significant event as any unintended or unexpected event, which could or did lead to harm of one or more patients. This includes incidents which did not cause harm but could have done, or where the event should have been prevented. These events should be collected routinely by the employer, where the doctor is directly employed by an organisation, and organisations should have formal processes in place for logging and responding to all events. Self-employed doctors should make note of any such events or incidents and undertake a review.

NHS England (2015) has defined 'serious incidents' as follows:

'serious incidents are events in health care where the potential for learning is so great, or the consequences to patients, families and carers, staff or organisations are so significant, that they warrant using additional resources to mount a comprehensive response. Serious incidents can extend beyond incidents which affect patients directly and include incidents which may indirectly impact patient safety or an organisation's ability to deliver ongoing healthcare.

The occurrence of a serious incident demonstrates weaknesses in a system or process that need to be addressed to prevent future incidents leading to avoidable death or serious harm to patients or staff, future incidents of abuse to patients or staff, or future significant reputational damage to the organisations involved. Serious incidents therefore require investigation in order to identify the factors that contributed towards the incident occurring and the fundamental issues (or root causes) that underpinned these. Serious incidents can be isolated, single events or multiple linked or unlinked events signalling systemic failures within a commissioning or health system.'

A 'serious incident requiring investigation' may also be termed a 'serious untoward incident' (SUI) or 'serious incident' (SI). Organisations usually undertake an investigation into this level of incident, often using a root cause analysis technique. In primary care, this type of investigation is more usually referred to as a 'significant event audit'.

Doctors would be expected to report any such incidents but may also report less serious events from which personal learning is identified. Supporting information for appraisal would be expected to include as a minimum: participation in the incident and investigation; lessons learnt; and action taken to prevent recurrence.

Feedback from colleagues

Multi-source feedback or 360° feedback is a requirement within the 5-year revalidation cycle. The feedback is intended to help doctors to reflect on their practice and support their professional development by providing them with information about their practice through the eyes of those they work with. This is important because in the GMC National Training Survey 2013, an anonymous survey of around 50 000 trainees, 13.2% of respondents said that they had been victims of bullying and harassment in their posts (a slight increase from 13.1% in 2012) and 26.5% experienced undermining behaviour from a senior colleague (26.6% in 2012) (GMC, 2013b). Some doctors may be unaware of their behaviour and its potential impact on the experience of the trainee. Furthermore, in a report by the National Clinical Assessment Service (NCAS) based on 1198 cases in 2007–2008, behaviour was a concern in 56% of reported cases, with aggression in 1 in 13 practitioners, disruptive behaviour under pressure in 1 in 15 and bullying, harassment and/or discrimination in 1 in 30 (NCAS, 2009). In a team-based service model of mental health delivery, behaviour which disrupts team functioning is likely to have an adverse impact on the safety, effectiveness and experience of patient care. The GMC acknowledges that the selection of colleagues will depend on the nature of the doctor's practice and recommends asking as wide a range of colleagues as possible, including colleagues from other specialties, junior doctors, nurses, allied healthcare professionals, and management and clerical staff. Standards for colleague feedback and a feedback tool are available from the GMC website. For psychiatrists, the College Centre for Quality Improvement markets a 360° feedback system called ACP360 which has been validated for psychiatry.

Feedback from patients

The requirement for structured feedback from patients reflects an increased emphasis on customer feedback across the health sector and beyond. In February 2012, the NHS Patient Experience Framework was published; it was based on the Picker Institute's Principles of Patient-Centred Care, an evidence-based definition of a good patient experience. Organisations providing healthcare frequently request feedback from patients for internal service monitoring and improvement. The Friends and Family Test, introduced in 2013 to test whether patients or carers would recommend a service to family or friends, aims to generate openly available feedback data for health providers, emulating other widely available feedback systems in the retail and hospitality industries. The National Institute for Health and Care Excellence (NICE) has produced quality standards for generic adult NHS services and Quality Standard 14 (QS14) is entitled *Service User Experience in Adult Mental Health* (NICE, 2011). In this wider context of enhanced and structured patient feedback, the GMC recommends that the exercise should reflect the whole scope of practice and the type of patients providing feedback should reflect the range of patients seen. Again, importance is placed on reflection on this feedback and identification of opportunities for personal development. Moreover, a sufficient number of questionnaires should be distributed for the findings to be valid and useful. Patient representative and advocacy groups remain dissatisfied with patient feedback for revalidation on the grounds that it is too infrequent, and doctors remain concerned about the complexity and reliability of the exercise.

Review of complaints and compliments

Like significant events and outcome data, complaints are another element of supporting information that the employing organisation, or individual doctor if self-employed, is expected to collect systematically and regularly. These represent another format for patient feedback, although it can sometimes be difficult to tease out the component of care relating directly to a psychiatrist or doctor working with a multidisciplinary team. The revalidation portfolio requires evidence of complaints, participation in their investigation, actions taken to resolve and address them and any opportunities for professional learning, especially if there is a theme apparent across complaints or where there is triangulation with other elements of supporting information.

Box 17.4 The four stages of remediation

Stage 1: *Establishing the facts*. Standards or guidance from a College may provide helpful advice to the responsible officer. Several Colleges provide an 'invited review' service to untangle complex performance issues.

Stage 2: *Establishing the reasons for a performance problem*. Problems may arise as a result of issues relating to conduct, capability and health, often with a considerable overlap between these categories, and concerns may arise from any combination or all three of these. The assessment process is usually completed by a specialist agency such as the National Clinical Assessment Service.

Stage 3: *Planning and implementing remediation*. Colleges may assist others in specialist programmes of education or training or by providing a specialty curriculum or coaching.

Stage 4: *Evaluation of remediation*.

Remediation

The Academy of Medical Royal Colleges (2013) has produced useful guidance about remediation, and considers where the Royal Colleges and Faculties might align with this process. The primary responsibility for remediation rests, as previously, with the employer. If a concern is significant, the GMC may be involved through direct referral or through discussion with the GMC employer liaison advisor. The NCAS may offer assessment and remediation planning in some situations. Professional support units are planned to bring specialist resources together to support a remediation programme.

Remediation was defined by the Department of Health in *Tackling Concerns Locally* as:

'the overall process agreed with a practitioner to redress identified aspects of underperformance'. It also notes that 'Remediation is a broad concept varying from informal agreements to carry out some reskilling to more formal supervised programmes of remediation or rehabilitation.' (Department of Health, 2009)

The document describes a four-stage process (see Box 17.4).

Roles and responsibilities of the responsible officer

The roles and responsibilities of the newly created post of responsible officer are set out in legislation and regulations, the first of which were placed before Parliament on 24 November 2010 and came into force on 1 January 2011. New bodies, posts and functions and accountabilities were created.

The designated body must be based in the UK for the legislation to apply. The GMC website presents an updated list of all designated bodies recognised by the GMC. Each designated body must appoint a responsible officer and appoint or designate a second responsible officer if there is a conflict of interest. The responsible officer must have been a registered medical practitioner for at least 5 years, with capacity to carry out this responsibility. The designated body is responsible for providing resources to fulfil this role. The responsible officer must ensure that appraisals are regularly carried out, and include all relevant information across every area of practice. The responsible officer must establish and implement procedures to investigate concerns raised by patients or staff of the designated body or arising from any other source about a medical practitioner's fitness to practise. Where appropriate, the responsible officer must refer concerns about the medical practitioner to the GMC and monitor compliance with conditions or undertakings where these exist. The responsible officer must make recommendations to the GMC about medical practitioners' fitness to practise and maintain accurate records of these processes.

The responsible officer also has specific responsibilities in relation to the employment of doctors by the designated body. These include ensuring fitness for purpose – medical practitioners must have qualifications and experience appropriate to the work to be performed, appropriate references must be obtained and checked, and any necessary steps must be taken to verify the identity of medical practitioners. Where the designated body is an area team, the responsible officer also manages admission to the 'performers list', in accordance with the NHS (Performers Lists) Regulations 2004, and maintains accurate records of each of these processes.

When monitoring medical practitioners' conduct and performance, the responsible officer must: review regularly the general performance and clinical governance information held by the designated body, including clinical indicators relating to outcomes for patients; identify any issues arising from that information relating to medical practitioners, such as variations in individual performance; and ensure that the designated body takes steps to address any such issues.

The responsible officer must ensure that appropriate action is taken in response to concerns about medical practitioners' conduct or performance. This includes: initiating investigations with appropriately qualified investigators; ensuring that procedures are in place to address concerns raised; and ensuring that any investigation into the conduct or performance of a medical practitioner takes into account any other relevant matters within the designated body. The responsible officer must also consider the need for further monitoring of the practitioner's conduct and performance and ensure that this takes place where appropriate; ensure that the medical practitioner is kept informed about the progress of the investigation; and ensure that procedures include provision for the medical practitioner's comments to be sought and taken into account where appropriate. Further, the responsible officer must: take any steps necessary to protect patients; recommend to the medical practitioner's employer that the practitioner be suspended or have conditions or restrictions placed on practice; and identify concerns and ensure that appropriate measures are taken to address these. Such measures can include: requiring the medical practitioner to undergo training or retraining; offering rehabilitation services; providing opportunities to increase the medical practitioner's work experience; and addressing any systemic issues within the designated body which may have contributed to the concerns identified. The responsible officer must maintain accurate records of all steps taken.

Responsible officers must have regard to relevant guidance under the Health and Social Care Act, from the NCAS and in *Good Medical Practice*.

In 2013, further regulations came into force which made adjustments for new NHS architecture in England and recognised additional designated bodies. This placed an additional duty on responsible officers to ensure that medical practitioners for whom they are responsible have sufficient knowledge of the English language for the work to be performed in a safe and competent manner. This has subsequently been addressed through language testing and now forms a requirement for licensing.

Concurrent with the introduction of revalidation, the GMC introduced a new role – employer liaison advisors. These advisors offer support and advice to responsible officers, and provide a regular and proactive interface with the GMC. This enables a closer dialogue between the GMC and employers, allowing earlier discussion of potential problems.

Responsible officers have also been specifically trained for their role and meet in local peer networks, which provide for some continuing education, moderation and benchmarking.

There are some individuals who have been appointed as a 'suitable person'; they carry out the same functions as a responsible officer.

Responsible officers have a number of choices to make in relation to the revalidation of a doctor. They are responsible for making recommendations to the GMC on the revalidation of doctors. Responsible officers can only make recommendations about doctors with a prescribed connection to their designated body. There are only three options for action:

- a positive recommendation that the doctor is up to date and fit to practise
- a request to defer the date of the recommendation
- a notification of the doctor's non-engagement in revalidation.

The GMC responds to the recommendation by deciding whether to revalidate the doctor.

Roles and responsibilities of appraisers

A medical appraiser will normally be a licensed doctor with knowledge of the context in which the doctor works. An appraiser is linked with a doctor to be appraised according to the policy of the designated body. He or she should be the most appropriate appraiser for the doctor, taking into account the full scope of work, should be aware of the professional obligations placed on doctors by the GMC and the importance of appraisal for the doctor's professional status, and should have suitable skills and training for the context in which the appraisal is taking place.

Appraisers need to achieve a level of competence through initial training but this also needs to be maintained through support and continuing development. Quality assurance and performance review in the appraiser role is a responsibility of the designated body. This may involve direct observation of appraisals or evaluation of appraisal outputs.

There are a number of important but uncommon situations that every medical appraiser needs to know how to manage, should they arise. These include issues such as significant patient safety concerns, important health or behavioural problems, fraud or probity issues. Such topics should form the basis of regular continuing professional development activities.

Roles and responsibilities of the doctor

Every doctor planning to revalidate has a responsibility to keep up to date and informed. The best source of information is the GMC, which has issued and updated regular primary guidance. Additional secondary guidance can be obtained from Royal Colleges and the Academy of Royal Colleges. Maintaining a portfolio of supporting information, as described in the GMC guidance, is essential, as is processing what is available by reflection and critical review and recording this reflection in a format which can be discussed in appraisal.

The doctor must 'engage' with the revalidation process – indeed, the responsible officer has the option to report a doctor for non-engagement even if revalidation is not imminent.

For doctors without a designated body or suitable person, robust evidence needs to be provided directly to the GMC. Regular appraisal by a trained and experienced person who is a licensed doctor with a connection to a designated body or suitable person is required. A submission of evidence is required every 5 years, which the GMC states must be verifiable. An independent assessment of knowledge and skills is required: a computer-marked written examination and an objective structured clinical examination. This will attract a fee.

Evaluation of the first 12 months

Since early 2012, there has been a steady increase in doctors relinquishing their licence to practise. In 2012, 11 378 doctors left the medical register or gave up their licence to practise. Of these, 7288 told the GMC why they were leaving: 49% said they were planning to go overseas; 40% stated that they were retiring; and only 3% indicated that they did not want to take part in revalidation.

The expectations of revalidation were set out as: improved governance of professional development and standards; improved patient safety; improved quality of care; improved effectiveness and efficiency of systems and working practices, leading to improved public trust and confidence in the medical profession.

In 2014, several publications evaluated the impact of the first year of revalidation. The Revalidation Support Team (2014) issued a report entitled *The Early Benefits and Impact of Medical Revalidation*. This summarises research carried out in 2013–14 based on an analysis of 3500 responses to surveys from doctors, appraisers, responsible officers and designated bodies on the impact of medical revalidation in England. Appraisal rates are increasing, according to the ORSA returns, with an overall rate of 63.3% in 2010–11, 72.7% in 2011–12 and 76.1% in 2012–13, and the acceptability and perceived value of appraisal is increasing. There is some indication that concerns are being identified earlier, at a 'less serious' level. Support for the process is greater from responsible officers than appraisers, but the support among appraisers is higher in turn than among doctors. However, concerns remain for some that the time taken to complete the process is longer than expected and that this detracts from patient care. Patient groups remain dissatisfied by limited patient participation in revalidation and the general public has generally assumed that a licence review process already existed, so revalidation has failed to capture the public imagination. The majority of doctors found their appraisals supportive, and believed that they led to improvements in care and were a good use of their time. Continuing professional development was not thought to have changed much for doctors but has possibly become more visible for appraisers and responsible officers. Earlier identification of concerns was probably more a result of improved clinical governance processes than a direct result of appraisal.

The Revalidation Support Team identified a strong theme from its research into patient and public participation: patient feedback needs to be a more effective part of the appraisal and revalidation process; the public's voice needs to be represented more strongly in revalidation; and lay involvement is essential to the processes supporting revalidation. It reported that lay participants need to be engaged on a more formal basis. Patient feedback will be perceived as an effective component of revalidation only if doctors alter their practice as a result, with changes and improvements to patient care. The challenge is to seek regular and high-quality input from patients, to support doctors in responding to feedback and for healthcare organisations to inform patients about changes that have resulted from their feedback.

Conclusion

Despite delays in its planning and implementation, revalidation was finally introduced in December 2012. Those with the most complex new roles (responsible officers) appear to be most positive, perhaps as a result of more intensive preparation, support and training. There is significant resistance and reluctance from a minority of doctors, although the majority are engaged with the process. Patients do not feel adequately involved and the public are largely indifferent, possibly as a result of belief that a process was already in place. The potential for improving the quality of patient care or saving public money remains a tantalising but as yet unproven possibility. The extent to which revalidation is adopted by the NHS and other organisations as a whole-organisation responsibility and the extent to which its introduction changes culture may determine its ultimate value in improving the whole healthcare system. The relationships between doctors, employers, regulators and the public continue to change in its wake.

References

Academy of Medical Royal Colleges (2013) *Investigation, Remediation and Resolution of Concerns About a Doctor's Practice – Where Do the Colleges Fit?* AoMRC.

Alment EAJ (1976) *Competence to Practise: The Report of a Committee of Enquiry Set Up for the Medical Profession in the United Kingdom*. Committee of Enquiry into Competence to Practise.

Archer J, Regan de Bere S, Nunn S, *et al* (2014) *Revalidation in Practice: Shaping the Future Development of Revalidation*. Health Foundation.

Department of Health (2009) *Tackling Concerns Locally: Report of the Working Group*. Available at http://webarchive.nationalarchives.gov.uk/20130107105354/http:/www.dh.gov.uk/en/Publicationsandstatistics/Publications/PublicationsPolicyAndGuidance/DH_096492 (accessed May 2016).

Department of Health Professional Standards Team (2012) *Medical Revalidation – Costs and Benefits. Analysis of the Costs and Benefits of Medical Revalidation in England*. Department of Health.

GMC (2012) *Continuing Professional Development: Guidance For All Doctors*. General Medical Council.

GMC (2013a) *Good Medical Practice*. General Medical Council.

GMC (2013b) *National Training Survey*. General Medical Council.

Healthcare Quality Improvement Partnership (2011) *New Principles of Best Practice in Clinical Audit*. HQIP.

Merrison AW (1975) *Report of the Committee of Inquiry into the Regulation of the Medical Profession* (Merrison report). HMSO.

NICE (2011) *Service User Experience in Adult Mental Health* (QS14). National Institute for Health and Care Excellence.

NCAS (2009) *Professionalism – Dilemmas and Lapses*. National Clinical Assessment Service, National Patient Safety Agency.

NHS England (2015) *Serious Incident Framework: Supporting Learning to Prevent Recurrence*. Available at https://www.england.nhs.uk/wp-content/uploads/2015/04/serious-incidnt-framwrk-upd.pdf (accessed May 2016).

Revalidation Support Team (2012) *Ready for Revalidation: Supporting Information for Appraisal and Revalidation*. General Medical Council.

Revalidation Support Team (2013) *Quality Assurance of Medical Appraisers*. General Medical Council.

Revalidation Support Team (2014) *The Early Benefits and Impact of Medical Revalidation: Report on Research Findings in Year One*. General Medical Council.

Smith J (2004) *Fifth Report – Safeguarding Patients: Lessons from the Past – Proposals for the Future*. Shipman Inquiry.

CHAPTER 18

Quality improvement tools

Oyedeji Ayonrinde

We as professionals aspire to deliver high-quality services and our patients desire and deserve high-quality services. We all know and recognise quality but often it is difficult to define and deliver high-quality services as there are variations in resources across healthcare systems. This chapter begins by defining quality and goes on to discuss quality improvement criteria and principles; tools for measuring improvements in the quality of services are then presented.

Definitions

What is quality?

Quality in healthcare is difficult to define and may have a number of different interpretations. A simple definition is the 'degree of excellence' in healthcare. The Institute of Medicine defines quality in healthcare as a direct correlation between the level of improved health services and the desired health outcomes of individuals and populations.[1] An understanding of the meaning of quality is key to the process of quality improvement. Healthcare excellence is multidimensional and has the following characteristics:[2]

- safe – avoiding harm from care intended to help patients
- effective – beneficial, evidence-based service provision
- person-centred – empathic and responsive care based on individual needs and values
- timely – short waiting times and no detrimental delays
- efficient – avoidance of waste
- equitable – little individual variation in access to or quality of care.

---

1 See http://www.nationalacademies.org/hmd/Global/News%20Announcements/Crossing-the-Quality-Chasm-The-IOM-Health-Care-Quality-Initiative.aspx (accessed May 2016).
2 See http://www.nationalacademies.org/hmd/Reports/2001/Crossing-the-Quality-Chasm-A-New-Health-System-for-the-21st-Century.aspx (accessed May 2016).

While these dimensions often complement each other, it is inevitable that different situations will determine the prioritisation of one area over another.

What is quality improvement?

Again, this is a term which is often bandied about without clear definition. We propose that it is both aspirational and descriptive. Quality improvement consists of systematic and continual actions that lead to measurable improvement in healthcare services and the health status of targeted patient groups.

> 'The combined and unceasing efforts of everyone – healthcare professionals, patients and their families, researchers, payers, planners and educators – to make the changes that will lead to better patient outcomes (health), better system performance (care) and better professional development (learning).'
> (Batalden & Davidoff, 2007)

What processes lead to quality improvement?

A number of processes have been linked with broad and enduring improvement to health services. The Health Foundation lists the following on its website (http://www.health.org.uk/about-us/what-is-quality):

- sustained focus on continuous improvement
- recognition of internal motivators – professionalism, skills development, organisational development and leadership, and encouraging individuals to deliver the improvement
- recognition of external motivators – regulation, economic incentives and performance management – which may be difficult to control
- aligning quality at every level and across systems of the organisation as far as is practical
- redefining the relationship between service users and providers – involving patients, their families and carers in service planning and service development
- building knowledge, skills and new practices, with learning from other successful sectors.

Principles of quality improvement

The basic principles of quality improvement relate to a number of factors which involve the organisation and national policies and then local clinical teams and individual clinicians, even though the aims of quality improvement may vary across various stakeholders. The aims are illustrated in Fig. 18.1.

An organisation's current system is the process by which things are done, whereas its performance is the organisation's efficiency, outcomes of care and degree of patient satisfaction.

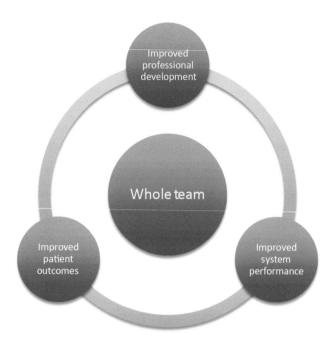

Fig. 18.1 Relationships between aims of improvement (adapted from Batalden & Davidoff, 2007)

Quality, on the other hand, is associated with the organisation's models of service delivery and healthcare systems. Change is often required to improve performance, improve results and raise quality.

Quality improvement programmes involve the following four key principles:

1 systems and processes
2 focus on patients (discussed in its own right under 'The service user/patient', below)
3 focus on being part of the team
4 focus on use of the data.

Systems and processes

Fundamental to improvement, organisations need a good understanding of their service delivery systems and the main processes. Quality improvement concepts recognise that both resources (inputs) and activities carried out (processes) have roles in the quality improvement of care (outputs/outcomes) (Fig. 18.2). While there are several quality improvement concepts, they are most effective when tailored to meet the needs of a specific organisation's health service delivery system.

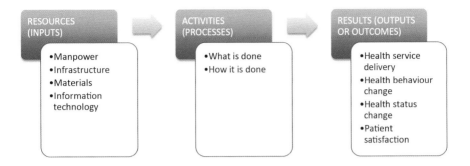

Fig. 18.2   Components of a healthcare system (adapted from Donabedian, 1980)

Another perspective is that health services consist of two key components:

*   What is done (care provision)
*   How it is done (where, when, and by whom).

A recurring theme in this chapter is that while each component can contribute to improvement, the best results come when these approaches are merged.

Quality improvement as a team process

First and foremost, teams have to own the concept of quality improvement and also work together to deliver that. In addition, within the team there may be specific individuals who can create a subgroup which can look after and help develop quality improvement.

With effective organisational culture, infrastructure and leadership, teams utilise the knowledge, experience and perspectives of their members in the quality improvement process. Institutions have to give teams the freedom to develop quality improvement targets and allow them to deliver these appropriately.

To achieve substantial and enduring improvements, team approaches operate best in the following conditions:

*   complex processes
*   innovation
*   multidisciplinary processes
*   multiple dimensions to issues
*   buy-in.

The role of data in quality improvement

Data are the key to the quality improvement process, through the measurement of current function, change and performance. The benefits include:

- the provision of objective rather than subjective measures
- the provision of baseline measures
- the evaluation of interventions
- the determination of whether intervention affords improvement
- the monitoring of improvements
- comparison of performance.

Quantitative and qualitative data have different roles and benefits. While quantitative methods provide numerical, measurable and analysable data, qualitative methods collect observable descriptive and contextual data as well as the relationship between structures.

Many health organisations have vast collections of data on a range of healthcare processes, treatments and outcomes, such as clinic activity records, incident reports, patient satisfaction surveys and public health indices; however, these data are not always 'mined' or processed with sufficient rigour to evaluate a service, monitor performance or identify opportunities for improvement. Standardisation of data collected with evidence-based measures helps focus quality improvement. Tools play an important role in this standardisation process.

Quality improvement tools

A combination of situation-specific and adaptable theories and techniques are referred to as quality improvement tools (Table 18.1). The choice of tool is influenced by the stage of the project, the task involved, the approach needed and the position in the patient pathway.

Table 18.1 Tools and methods in quality improvement

Area of interest	Tools or methods
Healthcare processes within system	Diagrams that illustrate relationships, flow, cause–effect, descriptive and qualitative data, case examples
Variation and measurement	Longitudinal data analysed on run charts and control charts
Service user/patient knowledge	Measures of illness burden, quality of life, patient feedback
Leadership and change	Knowledge development, leadership and team development, reflective practice
Collaboration	Managing conflict, team building, communication skills, 'situation–background–assessment–recommendation'
Social context and accountability	Recording undesirable variation, dissemination of information
Developing new and locally applicable knowledge	Making small tests of change ('plan–do–study–act' cycles)

Adapted from Batalden & Davidoff, 2007).

Conventional model of process mapping

Healthcare delivery involves numerous pathways (referral, assessment, treatment and discharge) which constitute the patient journey. Pathways involve individuals in both visible and less conspicuous organisational roles.

Mapping complete processes and journeys not only gives insight into current inefficiencies but also highlights opportunities for improvement. By observing naturalistic processes, variation and task or role duplication are recognised. Interestingly, process mapping is fertile ground for high-impact and often simple service improvement and innovation.

As mapping explores the complete process (Box 18.1), all staff and service users have the potential to contribute, since no one can be fully conversant with the details of all stages. Processes felt to be simple for patients may actually be quite complicated when broken down. Problematic bottlenecks may be identified.

Mapping output is dependent on the diversity of participants within the process and their familiarity with individual stages and transitions. A common mistake is the exclusion of non-clinical staff such as administrators and porters, who may have informative insights. Ideally, stakeholders should be identified and involved early in the process.

Box 18.1   The process map

- How many steps are there?
- How many processes are there?
- Are they necessary?
- Appropriate number of people carrying out tasks?
- Any role or task duplication?
- Are there any bottlenecks?
- How much error correction/rework is being carried out?
- Approximate time between each step?
- Which tasks help to achieve the purpose?
- Which tasks hinder or add no value?
- Can tasks that add no value be removed?
- Are processes achieving the set objectives?
- Are things being done in the right sequence?
- Is the most appropriate person doing the task?
- How relevant/useful is the information provided at each stage?
- Are some tasks performed in other processes better performed at this point?

Adapted from http://www.institute.nhs.uk/quality_and_service_improvement_tools/quality_
and_service_improvement_tools/process_mapping_-_a_conventional_model.html

---

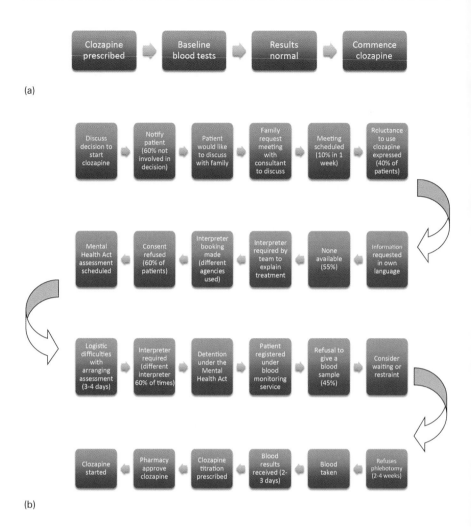

(a)

(b)

Fig. 18.3 Examples of process maps for the initiation of clozapine for a hypothetical patient: (a) high-level map (four stages) and (b) detailed map (24 stages).

The mapping process should focus on the service to be improved rather than branching into others, which may significantly protract the process. That notwithstanding, the process map should transcend functional borders and not be restricted to the team and department, as bottlenecks may lie in effluent or affluent processes.

Process mapping can enhance team engagement, as members share the processes and individual challenges are objectively highlighted. The team also collaborates in the design of new processes.

Other than the time commitment required, this tool is relatively low cost and can be rapidly implemented. Examples of process maps are shown in Fig. 18.3, for a hypothetical case involving the initiation of clozapine. The detailed process map (Fig. 18.3b) would require the input of the ward medical staff, on-call doctor, ward nursing staff, patients, carers, pharmacist, interpreters, phlebotomists, ward administrator, consultant secretary, porter, laboratory staff, emergency team, Mental Health Act office staff, approved mental health professional, independent section 12 approved doctor – at least 14 different inputs. Within groups, subgroup processes may differ (e.g. consultant processes versus the ward junior doctor or on-call doctor). While the high-level process map (Fig. 18.3a) gives an overview of the stages, the detailed process map (Fig. 18.3b) presents potential areas for service improvement and innovation in this hypothetical unit (presented in parentheses).

Readers may want to reflect on interventions they would carry out in these situations which may require redesign or removal of some elements while ensuring the patient is at the centre of the improvements. Consideration should also be given to the consequences of redesign on the larger organisation, such as impact on length of stay, financial or staff resources.

Spaghetti diagram

Imagine the journeys patients or staff may make to access different parts of a service, for instance the ward round, laboratory, pharmacy or dining area or the movement of patients in a unit at medication times. The spaghetti diagram is used to examine diagrammatically the optimum layout of a unit, department or ward. By schematically drawing people flows, it highlights problematic or inefficient layouts and identifies avoidable pathways and distances. This tool is a useful complement to process mapping.

The spaghetti diagram shown in Fig. 18.4 was used to investigate high rates of violence around room E. It was identified that at a particular time of day there was exceptionally high volume of traffic around the room, and the overcrowding increased the risk of conflict.

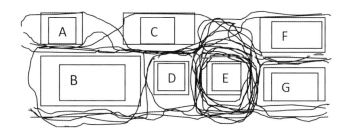

Fig. 18.4 Example of a spaghetti diagram, showing flow of people around rooms A–G

The service user/patient

Patient flow

In the process map considered in the previous section (Fig. 18.3), the 'patient flow' or smooth movement through the service was constricted by multiple 'bottlenecks'. Bottlenecks regulate the pace at which healthcare is delivered and the speed at which processes work. A simple yet common area of bottleneck is related to patient information. Accurate and appropriate written information is important for both patients and carers. Misinformation or miscommunication can impede appointments or protract interventions through lack of preparation, or delayed or even withdrawn consent. Reliable and consistent administrative input may be a more effective intervention here than additional medical staff.

The flow of tasks can either enhance or hinder pathways. For instance, the accumulation of referrals to a service, intermittent decision-making and batching of work may delay patient journeys and health outcomes. Higher mortality rates in hospitals over weekends may be linked to variation in interventions by senior clinicians. A review of systems can reduce variation in referral, waiting and treatment times.

Patient needs, expectations and satisfaction

The management and measure of patient needs, expectations and satisfaction form an important quality pillar which involves the following:

- Access to a health service may be influenced by its location, awareness of the service, cost of parking, and the availability of facilities for people with various disabilities.
- Evidence-based care can be enhanced by teaching, training and professional development programmes for clinicians.
- Patient safety systems include medication management, ligature audits and the management of slips, falls and infections.
- Patient engagement may manifest in service users' participation in health programmes and health awareness or stigma reduction activities.
- Integration with primary care and a range of physical health services, for example cardiology and endocrine clinics, is key to ensuring the parity of services and holistic mental healthcare.
- Multicultural healthcare presents challenges and opportunities to health providers, as some groups may be unwittingly marginalised or disadvantaged by specific structures and resources of the health system.
- Health literacy, awareness and communication are important in all patient interfaces. This may include signage, translated health information and plain use of English.

While the bulk of healthcare adds to patient well-being, the right referral, right diagnostic tests, right diagnosis, right information and communication, right advice, right treatment, right aftercare and right hand-over are all required. Eliminating waste can add value to patient care.

Readers are referred to the NHS Improving Quality website (http://www.nhsiq.nhs.uk) for more detail on tools and detailed illustrations.

Patient perspectives

With the best will and intention, services may not meet patient expectation or give satisfaction. A number of tools explore patient opinions on service improvement and ultimately satisfaction. Application of these tools depends on the specific patient group, scope and objectives. As patients are directly involved in most stages of healthcare they bring unique perspectives and observations often unnoticed by staff.

Four methods commonly used are:

- questionnaires
- semi-structured interviews
- focus groups
- patient shadowing.

Questionnaires

Questionnaires are an uncomplicated means of obtaining information from a large number of people. Often easy to administer, they can capture attitudes, satisfaction, experiences and perceptions of patients, carers and indeed staff. Questionnaires can provide baseline measures as well as sequential measures of change. However, it must be remembered that some groups of patients, such as children and those with dementia, may not be able to deal with questionnaires and their families or carers may be involved instead.

Important considerations for questionnaire design
- Have clear objectives for the use of the results.
- Involve service users in devising carefully structured questions.
- Consider the merits of multiple choice questions (MCQs), binary responses (yes/no), Likert scales and free text responses.
- Keep the instrument concise (approximately 10 minutes to complete it is ideal).
- Pilot the questionnaire and refine where necessary.
- Consider the merits and demerits of anonymising responses.
- Consider channels of access to and return of the questionnaire (e.g. reception, post, electronic).
- Consider technology (e.g. text, email, online survey such as Survey Monkey, which collates and analyses numerical responses).

Semi-structured interviews

Semi-structured interviews are useful in the collection of qualitative data from the respondent's perspective rather than group generalisations. The probing of responses provides more information, prioritisation, personalisation and idea generation than questionnaires. Beneficially, respondents can elaborate on comments. However, semi-structured interviews demand more time to implement and analyse.

Tips
- Use open-ended questions.
- Seek clarification to avoid misunderstandings.
- Attempt a conversational style.
- Empathically apply wording.
- Consider having an independent interviewer.

Focus groups

Focus groups are an informal collection of people with shared characteristics convened to explore an issue. The facilitator encourages free expression of opinion (agreement and difference). Groups usually convene on just one occasion.

Tips
- A group membership of 6–12 works best.
- The group should be convened for 1–2 hours.
- Clarify its purpose and objectives.
- Explain the process, expectations and potential outcomes.
- Ensure the facilitator has strategies to shift gridlocks.
- Give feedback to the group.

Patient shadowing

This process involves an observer accompanying a patient through the different stages of the healthcare journey. Unbiased observations are best made when the 'shadower' is inquisitive and unfamiliar with the process, thereby being able to question or seek clarification. Observations need to be objectified and contextualised by also getting the perspectives of the service staff. The comprehensive real-world picture of movement is best provided when a qualitative narrative is given in conjunction with a flow diagram. Findings can help evaluate and monitor services, and can inform training.

Tips
- Establish goals, objectives and process.
- Determine the relevance and the characteristics of the pathway.
- Develop a process template to record phases.
- Ensure the shadower does not influence care.
- Observe how the patient is treated by staff and the ease or difficulty of navigating the hospital environment and check for task duplication.

Tracer study

Unlike patient flows, the tracer study looks at administrative flows and the trails they leave (akin to emails with recipient details, times and when read) and is used to identify delays around paperwork tasks by using 'tags' attached to documents. With electronic communication, this method is declining.

Other aspects of the patient journey

A process of verifying the ongoing needs of people on out-patient or in-patient appointment lists is particularly useful in the management of waiting list capacity and demand. Where there is a significant range of clinical presentations, a systematic process can improve waiting-list management. One good method is for patients to be seen in accordance with their clinical need, urgency and priority (Clinically Prioritise and Treat – CPaT). This is similar to the triage process in emergency rooms.

Waiting lists and backlogs are not uncommon in clinical services, and identifying the problem and any bottlenecks can significantly improve flow. Demand management involves using planning and forecasting expertise to understand demand while ensuring patients receive the right care, in the right place, at the right time. For instance, managing staffing levels during the winter and over the summer holidays and bank holidays ensures the appropriate mobilisation of resources.

Missed appointments have significant resource implications and deny other patients an opportunity to be seen. An analysis of what can be done to reduce the level of 'did not attends' (DNAs) may identify short notice given of appointments, wrong contact addresses, and stigma or poor service reputation affecting attendance. Interventions such as telephone reminders, text reminders, checking patient availability before sending appointments and 'choose and book' initiatives can all increase attendance rates and thereby reduce waiting lists.

Comprehending and reducing the length of hospital stay will help achieve a smoother pathway by freeing bed capacity and increasing throughput. Predetermination of a discharge date with the team collectively working towards this has been found to reduce length of stay compared with open-ended admissions. Preparation for discharge and taking account of the patient's requirements or limitations (for example in relation to accommodation) should not be left until the end of the treatment episode; this will help ensure patients are prepared to leave hospital.

Stakeholder analysis

A stakeholder analysis helps identify and group different parties and individuals associated with an organisation or situation. An awareness of the different players and their impact or support can help in the planning of roles and involvement in a change project. Stakeholders may have different levels of commitment and influence in different situations (e.g. patient groups unhappy with a service change).

In mental healthcare, stakeholders may include local police, general practitioners, schools, the council, traffic managers and small businesses. On the surface, some of these do not appear to have direct health links; however, if the focus is on patient access and road safety or raising awareness of a service the relevance of these stakeholders becomes clearer.

Managers and leaders

Communication and leadership skills can play important roles and act as tools in quality improvement, particularly given the buy-in and team engagement required to implement initiatives. A number of leadership skills such as listening, building trust, engagement, empowerment and the recognition of stress are integral parts of change management, as are some of the therapeutic skills some psychiatrists apply. It is also valuable to identify areas of resistance to change.

Communication

Communication is key to interaction within services; inadequate communication can lead to incidents, cause delays and wastefully consume resources. 'Situation–background–assessment–recommendation' (SBAR) is a simple and structured outline which enables staff to share situational awareness while ensuring unambiguous and reliable information regarding patients is provided. Imagine a clinical emergency (such as a collapsed patient) requiring urgent attendance: the SBAR allows organised communication of critical information.

Pareto analysis

The Pareto principle is that 20% of sources cause 80% of problems. This helps a team to focus on problems that have the greatest potential for improvement and to identify which changes may yield the most benefit. It is valuable when deciding between multiple options. The problem is identified (e.g. complaints) and the frequency of problem categories is derived in descending order, taking into account duration and variation (e.g. day of the week). In the situation illustrated in Fig. 18.5, communication of diagnosis was most problematic and more attention was given to patient education programmes and information leaflets.

Driver diagrams

These diagrams are simple structured logic algorithm charts that show how an improvement goal can be staged into focal drivers and projects (see Fig 18.6).

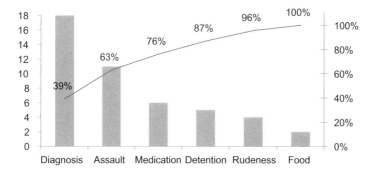

Fig. 18.5 Pareto analysis of complaints identifying communication of diagnosis as priority intervention required.

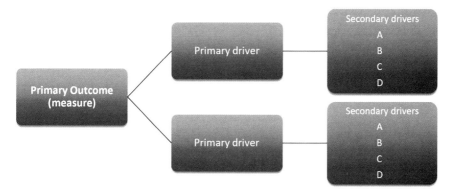

Fig. 18.6 A driver diagram showing the impact of secondary and primary drivers on outcomes.

The main levels are:

- goal, vision or primary outcome
- primary drivers – high-level factors that require influencing
- secondary drivers – specific activities, tasks or projects that are associated with or act on the primary driver.

Driver diagrams facilitate communication of improvement strategies and the development of a framework for monitoring and measurement of progress.

Activity

Consider the primary and secondary drivers for the following primary outcomes:

- medicines management
- mandatory training
- risk assessment documentation
- discharge summaries.

Team and staff performance measures

Clear roles and responsibilities are integral to efficient multidisciplinary team working. Role redesign helps restructure, amend and improve roles and clinical services, adjusting to staff shortages while ensuring job satisfaction. The sort of problems addressed could include administrative management of post and multiple consultant reviews of low patient numbers on the same day. This is also the principle of phlebotomy services and pathology lab pooling of investigations.

Responsibility charting involves visibly charting individual roles and responsibilities. Team members are made fully aware of their duties. The avoidance of duplication or uncertain roles is key to team efficiency. This tool is effective within and between teams as well as for project management and strategic management.

Alongside charts, action plans are an important component of effective and successful project management. They summarise how objectives are achieved, by whom and when. While relatively simple, action plans focus on tasks and provide clear roles and responsibilities.

Problem-solving

There are a number of helpful tools for the investigation and exploration of problems, including the actual root cause. Apart from system problems, these tools can be applied in the review of incidents or in carrying out investigations. This section provides an overview of some of them.

Brainstorming

This is a process of idea generation around problems, solutions and developing the next steps. This can be quite effective in teams and has the benefit of a 'fresh eyes' approach to challenging problems. Brainstorming can be effective with idea generation (ideation) and problem analysis, as seen below with the affinity diagram and fishbone diagram.

Affinity diagram

This is a method of creative thinking (brainstorming) for the organisation of considerable amounts of language data (opinions, issues, ideas) and puts information into understandable categories, with increased meaning. This grouping process is best applied in the clarification and comprehension of large and complex problems. It is also applied in the promotion of new ways of thinking. It is illustrated in Fig. 18.7.

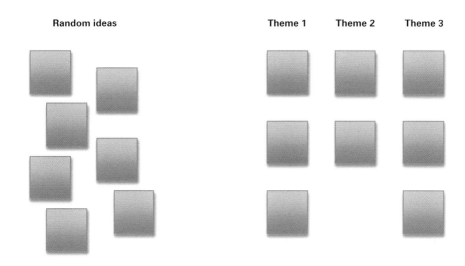

Fig. 18.7 Affinity diagram: ordering ideas into specific themes.

Tips
- Have five or six informed participants.
- Generate a list of ideas (e.g. on sticky labels).
- Display the ideas randomly on a wall or tabletop.
- Sort the ideas into themes by making connections between ideas or recurring themes.
- Create headers (phrases or sentences) on cards, reflecting clear concepts, for each group.
- Draw the completed diagram (with a problem statement above).

Cause and effect (fishbone) diagram

Cause and effect analysis helps individuals to think through the causes of a problem meticulously, and then arrange and cluster them appropriately, with a view to diagnosing the problem rather than focusing on the symptoms.

To construct a fishbone diagram (see Fig. 18.8 for an example), the following steps are required:

1 *Problem statement* – drafted with team agreement (this is the head of the fish, which is followed by a 'backbone'). In Fig. 18.8, the problem is the delayed discharge of patients in August (i.e. during the summer holidays).

2 *Categorisation.* This is a process of brainstorming in which the 'ribs' are attached to the backbone. These might include, for example, staff, management, process, budget and patient factors.

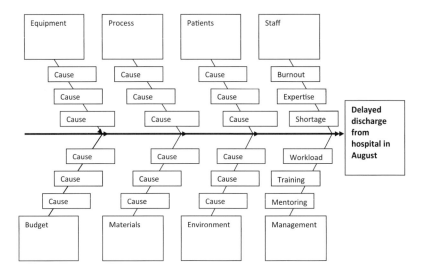

Fig. 18.8 Example of a fishbone diagram.

3 *Causes or contributory factors.* These are explored further and elaborated upon during brainstorm (e.g. staff burnout, shortage, expertise).

4 *Ask 'why'?* With each factor, ask why it occurs. For instance, why is there staff burnout? Why a recruitment problem? The 'five whys' approach can produce insights (see below).

5 *More ribs/more causes.* This helps the team probe deeper into causes and seek clearer understanding. Agree when to stop.

6 *Test for root causes.* A number of causes may recur within categories and can be tested for cause–effect correlation.

Root cause analysis using the 'five whys'

Application of this tool is through repeatedly asking the question 'why?' over several layers of an issue. While the number of layers may vary, five is a manageable standard. The stripping away of each layer can contextually lead you to the root cause of a problem.

Activity

Readers are encouraged to try this exercise in their services (or clinical practice) by probing further with each question below by asking five whys or preparing a fishbone chart.

- Why does ward X have the longest length of stay?
- Why are there so many complaints?
- Why are there delays in writing reports?
- Why don't staff attend meetings?

Creativity and innovation

Creativity tools

Recognition and measurement of problems can be significantly easier than the generation of ideas and solutions. Furthermore, new ideas relevant to a particular team or service may not be applicable or transferable to other situations or organisations. Creativity tools assist with the development of new perspectives, ideas and solutions.

As the team is ultimately going to be involved in the application of innovation, staff perceptions are important to generating ideas for service improvement as well as their buy-in with interventions.

Readers are referred to the NHS Improving Quality website (http://www.nhsiq.nhs.uk) for more information.

Quality improvement models

Following the evaluation or assessment of organisational structures or systems, data analysis may identify opportunities for improvement. The implementation of change is through the application of quality improvement models. These models focus on tested approaches as well as innovative methods.

An informed awareness of quality improvement models guarantees a more systematic and versatile approach to healthcare improvements. Presented here are three models that are widely applied in the development of healthcare interventions and in improving patient care: the lean model, FADE and Six Sigma.

The lean model

The lean model derives from Toyota's car plant methodology. The 'lean' concept is about getting the right things in the right quantities to the right place at the right time, while minimising waste and being open to change. In the medical context this model appreciates and defines value based on patients' needs and wants. The model maps how value can flow to the patient if a competent, cost-effective and time-efficient process is in place.

Lean waste is anything that does not add value to the patient experience and satisfaction, such as waste in terms of resources, services, time or work. Examples typically concern clinic scheduling, staffing, working additional hours, remote access to clinical records and medication flow management.

FADE

The FADE model consists of four key stages:

1   *Focus* – determine and define the process in need of improvement
2   *Analyse* – collection and analysis of data

3 *Develop* – development of action plans for improvement
4 *Execute* – implement, evaluate and monitor the system to consolidate gains.

Some aspects of the FADE model are similar to the plan–do–study–act (PDSA) cycle discussed below.

Six Sigma

Six Sigma is a measurement-based strategy for process improvement and problem reduction. Applied through the course of the quality improvement process, two Six Sigma techniques are recognised, namely:

- DMAIC – Define, Measure, Analyse, Improve, Control – intended for the scrutiny of existing processes
- DMADV – Define, Measure, Analyse, Design, Verify – used to develop new processes.

The 'lean Six Sigma'

The Six Sigma and lean models both require process analysis and mapping to accomplish improvement. An emergent model is the 'lean Six Sigma', an amalgamation of the two models. For example, a service facing difficulties (e.g. disruptive behaviour, violence and injuries to staff) may realise after initial interventions that increased staffing numbers do not reduce the violence but actually increase it. The core problems may be overcrowding, substance misuse and boredom, thereby requiring new structures to engage patients better in activities, security measures and testing for drug use.

Change

While all improvement requires a process of change, not all change guarantees improvement. Some change may actually worsen or damage situations and the manager must carefully monitor its implementation. Healthcare staff are key to the process of quality improvement through change. In healthcare there may be particularly high stakes or narrow margins of error.

Strategies to implement change include:

- experimentation through trial and error
- extensive research or analysis of problems
- adopting best practice from others
- top-down decisions from managers.

Each of these strategies has its strengths and weaknesses; however, a cautious approach is best applied in high-stakes situations.

Force field analysis

Force field analysis is a tool geared at understanding the pressures for and against change in systems (Fig. 18.9). At times, the challenges associated with change or the factors against change may be so overwhelming that the change is not appropriate at the time or additional negotiation is required. Force field analysis can be used with individuals, teams and organisations with planned changes or tasks.

By way of illustration, the forces against a change to consultants working a 7-day week might include cost, morale, staff shortages and lack of support staff.

The two-part Model for Improvement

The two-part Model for Improvement (Langley *et al*, 2009) is a strategic and systematic process for effective change management (see Fig. 18.10).

Part 1
- What is the goal?
- Is change an improvement?
- What improvement changes can be introduced?

Part 2
- Plan–do–study–act (PDSA) cycle.

Testing change can be iterative with testing, development, retesting and further development cycles of design prototypes. The design team learns from each test with continuous improvement and refinement (consider

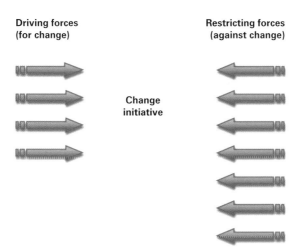

Fig. 18.9 Example of the application of force field analysis: introduction of 7-day weeks for consultants.

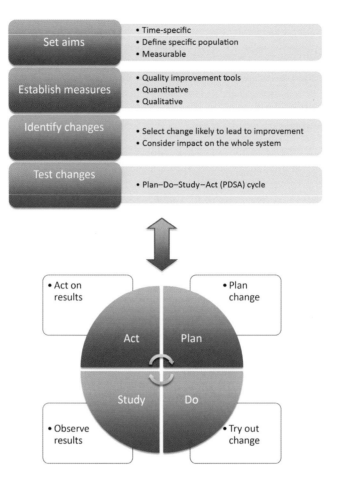

Fig. 18.10 The two-part Model for Improvement (adapted from the website of the Institute for Healthcare Improvement, http://www.ihi.org/resources/Pages/HowtoImprove/default.aspx, accessed May 2016).

the example of the unit experiencing violence, boredom and drug misuse above).

PDSA tips[3]

- Make small changes with in-built testing.
- Develop a motivated and engaged team.
- Review the outcome of each change.

---

3 Adapted from the webiste of the Health Resources and Services Administration, http://www.hrsa.gov/quality/toolbox/methodology/qualityimprovement/index.html (accessed May 2016).

- Discontinue (discard) the testing of faulty interventions.
- Involve non-team members if other experience is needed.
- Ensure the change is improvement.
- Avoid destabilising the larger complex system.

The metrics and the measure

NHS performance reporting is often focused on the attainment of targets and reporting mechanisms for audit and governance. Inappropriate selection of measures, interpretation out of context or inadequately focused interventions may have serious consequences. Bed occupancy, for instance, is an unreliable and potentially meaningless measure of effective bed utilisation, as illustrated by the following situations which may increase consumption of resources:

- delayed clinical reviews
- delayed discharges due to social factors such as loss of accommodation, homelessness, domestic disputes
- low frequency of ward rounds and batching discharge
- delay in carrying out investigations or obtaining results
- hospital-acquired infection or procedure complications.

In addition, the comparison of two data points (Fig. 18.11) employed in some management performance systems and clinical audit processes may not factor in complex longitudinal system changes. Improvement interventions based on such variation could have consequences for services.

Interestingly, none of the data point comparisons in Fig. 18.11 provides an accurate measure and the perception and implementation of quality improvement may be wrongly founded. If these data points were used to compare clinic performance, bed occupancy or length of stay, some parts of the service may be felt to have significantly better performance than others.

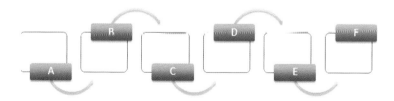

Fig. 18.11 Comparison and interpretation of data points: A–B, C–D or E–F suggests an increase; A–C, A–E or A–C–E suggests no change; B–C, D–E or B–E suggests a decline.

Table 18.2 Numbers of patients who did not attend clinics over a 5-week period.

Clinic	Week 1	Week 2	Week 3	Week 4	Week 5	Total
A	0	0	1	0	1	2
B	1	1	0	2	0	4
C	1	0	0	0	0	1
D	0	0	1	0	0	1
E	2	1	3	0	0	6
F	0	1	0	0	0	1
G	0	0	0	0	0	0
H	1	0	2	1	0	4
Total	5	3	7	3	1	19

Understanding variation

Table 18.2 shows 5 weeks of data on DNAs for a series of out-patient clinics. Assuming the clinics are approximately the same size, a series of questions can pertinently be asked:

- What patterns emerge in the data?
- Which clinics have a significantly better record than others?
- Which clinic should be copied or even awarded for best practice?

At first glance, the data in Table 18.2 may appear to have some patterns. Clinic G appears to have a very good record – what are they doing right? Clinic E is responsible for nearly one-third of all DNAs – is it in difficulty? Was week 3 a holiday week, in which patients would not attend?

However, there is actually no long-term statistical difference between the clinics as the numbers above were derived from a page of random numbers (with a skewed binomial distribution). Should managers fail to appreciate the random variation of performance statistics, service models may be encouraged to copy clinic G's practice, which may actually not produce an overall performance improvement. Clinic E may wrongly face the risk of being cited as underperforming.

Two types of variation are classified in the behaviour of systems:

- *Common cause variation* – variation following a wide variety of constant causes. Such variation is inevitable. Interventions are geared at reducing but not eliminating this variation.
- *Special cause variation* – variation can be associated with external factors that are unlikely to happen constantly (e.g. risk of ward closure due to winter norovirus infections). Other than making contingency plans

for such situations, a major structural or behavioural change is not warranted as recurrence of the event cannot be guaranteed.

Artificial variation may be caused by work patterns and organisational systems. This variation is particularly important to recognise so that appropriate interventions are put in place. A run-chart can be useful here.

Understanding and measuring the impact of change

Systems theory provides the theoretical framework for understanding the true impact of change, particularly in hospitals with multiple complex processes and where the root causes of problems may not be the causes initially identified. The failure to appreciate the relationships between individual parts of a single system can trigger flawed change interventions. In fact, 'trigger relief' or 'symptomatic relief' may worsen rather than improve situations. Furthermore, some improvements projected to bestow long-term solutions cannot be guaranteed as systems evolve over time. A perceived winter bed crisis may lead to a temporary increase in beds with unforeseen consequences for admission processes, ward rounds and additional discharge duties; these in turn may slow the discharge rate, increasing the length of stay and paradoxically worsening the bed crisis.

Statistical process control

Statistical process control (SPC) is the most practical and useful statistical tool in the measurement of problem-solving processes. This established way of assessing process variation can be used:

- to monitor a process
- to measure the quality of process output
- to understand the behaviour of a process
- to measure impact of process change on performance.

This shows how a system works over time and shows the sustainability of change, rather than relying on comparisons of behaviour from two samples taken at the same point in time. Assessment of management interventions does not determine whether a change in behaviour is caused by the change introduced.

The standard SPC chart

In healthcare, the most commonly found SPC chart is the XmR chart (Fig. 18.12), which takes single data points and estimates the likely spread of that data owing to variation. A minimum of 20 data points are required for a meaningful initial estimate and the measure of spread is used to generate control limits above and below the mean value.

The XmR chart is used because it does not need a lot of data to apply. Alternative sampling methods may be difficult to justify in healthcare processes that are too small or require more data.

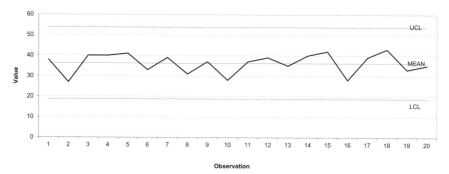

Fig. 18.12   The standard SPC chart. LCL, lower control limit; UCL, upper control limit.

Moving range computation from data values

The 'moving range', on the other hand, is used to estimate the degree of common cause variation and can be used to generate the process control limits. The moving range is computed by finding the difference between adjacent numbers in the sequence. The mean of the moving range figures provides an indication of the spread of the data.

Occasionally data may present outside of the limits that are not due to a special cause. When these new data points are plotted the behaviour of the systems being measured may be better interpreted.

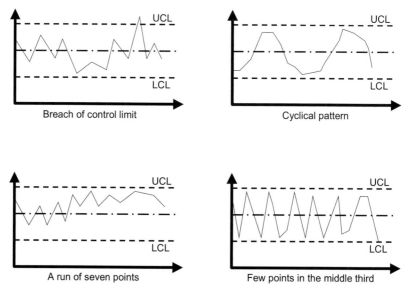

Fig. 18.13   The identification of unusual system behaviour. LCL, lower control limit; UCL, upper control limit.

There are four circumstances when data need to be checked to see if there is any unusual process behaviour change. Fig. 18.13 shows these.

There are rules of system behaviour data analysis:

1   *Data falls outside the control points.* Here the goal is to determine whether there has been a special cause event, or if the process performance has deviated without being noticed.

2   *Seven points above or below the mean or a seven-point trend.* Seven points consecutively above or below the mean is statistically very unlikely. Likewise, a seven-point increase or decrease requires investigation.

3   *Trends and patterns.* Cyclical behaviour of data would indicate some time-based factor that needs to be considered.

4   *Unusual distribution of points.* Where very few data points occupy the middle third of the range, this is a clue that some system behaviour has not been anticipated. Examples would be where we are inadvertently measuring two separate processes with their own different behaviours or where the process is affected by two people with different capabilities.

Use of SPC in mental healthcare improvement

Consider the example of an adult in-patient mental health service, with a total bed capacity of 88 across four wards. Service pressures require a reduction in bed numbers; however, there are very high rates of occupancy and leave beds are used to meet excess demand for emergency admissions. Length of stay has, though, been increasing. A run-chart analysis can illustrate this and confirm or refute the hypothesis that there is an excess of acute beds and that the pressures are secondary to flow issues.

The outcome may be addressing the 'inflow' by setting up a gate-keeping bed-management team working 24 hours per day and the impact can be monitored on a weekly admission chart. In addition, dedicated in-patient consultant roles may be developed with increased availability of senior medical input on admission ('front-loading') as well as eliminating batched weekly ward rounds in preference for discharge when patients recover.

Two years on, the daily bed availability run-chart would capture the impact of interventions such as:

•   the bed-management team reducing admissions through effective gate-keeping
•   having dedicated in-patient consultant sessions to ensure timely assessment of admissions and eliminating the batched discharge process.

Modelling and simulation

Forecasting and modelling tools can help decide which service improvement changes have the potential for maximum impact.

A financial tool: return on investment

The return on investment (ROI) calculates the quality of improvement initiatives by processing the financial benefits and costs data from the quality improvement interventions. This can be presented with the following formula:

benefits – costs = dividend

or, as a percentage figure,
[(benefits – costs) / costs] × 100 = percentage dividend

ROI can give very useful information on the efficiency of an improvement investment or can be used to compare the efficiency of different investments. By comparing the baseline and outcome measures ROI can validate a project, or can be the basis for the project to be reviewed, modified or even terminated. Alternatively, ROI can be used to monitor a project throughout its lifetime to ensure expected benefits are achieved.

Quality improvement in other health organisations

Royal College of Psychiatrists

The Royal College of Psychiatrists promotes quality improvement initiatives through the College Centre for Quality Improvement (CCQI), which 'aims to raise the standard of care that people with emotional or mental health needs receive by helping providers, users and commissioners of services assess and increase the quality of care they provide' (http://www.rcpsych. ac.uk/workinpsychiatry/qualityimprovement.aspx). The CCQI has engaged more than 90% of mental health services in the UK.

The CCQI:

- sets standards for the organisation and delivery of mental health services
- engages with front-line staff and supports them to measure their own service against these standards
- recognises local achievement, including by offering accreditation, and identifies areas for improvement
- works with local teams to develop and implement plans for service improvement
- works actively with other professional bodies, so that staff of all disciplines are engaged in the work
- works in partnership with service users and carers, and encourages local mental health services to do the same
- works with both NHS and independent sector services in the UK and has proved to be of interest to services in other countries

- encourages mental healthcare staff from different services to support each other and share good ideas through peer-review, newsletters, email discussion groups, and workshops.

National Institute for Health and Care Excellence

The quality standards produced by the National Institute for Health and Care Excellence (NICE) are concise sets of prioritised statements designed to drive measurable quality improvements within a particular area of health or care. They are independently derived from the best available evidence in collaboration with health and social care stakeholders. These standards are relevant to commissioners, public health and social care services, primary care services, local authorities, social care providers, public health services, hospitals, the community and service users and their carers.
NICE quality standards enable:

- health, public health and social care practitioners to make decisions about care based on the latest evidence and best practice
- people receiving health and social care services, their families and carers and the public to find information about the quality of services and care they should expect from their health and social care provider
- service providers to examine quickly and easily the performance of their organisation and assess improvement in standards of the care they provide
- commissioners to be confident that the services they are purchasing are high quality and cost-effective and focused on driving up quality.

(See http://www.nice.org.uk/standards-and-indicators#/standards)

Mental health trusts

Interested readers are encouraged to contact their organisation's quality improvement, clinical governance and audit departments to familiarise themselves with local projects and initiatives.

Conclusion

With a background in industry, quality improvement tools now play an important role in the improvement of healthcare processes. Their role in all spheres of clinical service development and the evaluation of change is visible in daily care at the clinic, ward, departmental and hospital levels. At a national level, quality improvement tools and methods are also incorporated into the development of guidance, accreditation and health innovations.

As healthcare systems consist of interdependent and complex processes, care should be taken to ensure change to one part of a process does not have a negative impact on the system as a whole. Sustained improvement requires regular re-evaluation of change with both quantitative and qualitative tools. This chapter is an introduction to a large body of quality improvement literature.

References

Batalden PB, Davidoff F (2007) What is 'quality improvement' and how can it transform healthcare? *Quality Safety Health Care*, **16**: 2–3.

Donabedian A (1980) *Explorations in Quality Assessment and Monitoring. Vol. I: The Definition of Quality and Approaches to Its Assessment*. Health Administration Press.

Langley GL, Moen R, Nolan KM, *et al* (2009) *The Improvement Guide: A Practical Approach to Enhancing Organizational Performance* (2nd edition). Jossey-Bass.

Further reading

Carey RG (2002) *Improving Healthcare with Control Charts*. ASQ Quality Press.

Walley P, Baugh S, Silvester K (2007) Quality improvement tools for healthcare. In *Management for Psychiatrists* (3rd edition) (eds D Bhugra, S Bell, A Burns): pp 313–23. Royal College of Psychiatrists.

Wheeler DJ (2003) *Making Sense of Data*, SPC Press.

Wheeler DJ (2003) *Understanding Variation: The Key to Managing Chaos*. SPC Press.

Womack J, Jones D (1996) *Lean Thinking: Banish Waste and Create Wealth in Your Organisation*. Simon and Schuster.

See also Royal College of Psychiatrists CCQI – publications, resources and projects (http://www.rcpsych.ac.uk/workinpsychiatry/qualityimprovement.aspx)

Internet

BMJ Quality and Safety, http://qualitysafety.bmj.com
Health Foundation, http://www.health.org.uk

Journals

BMJ Quality and Safety
Journal of Healthcare Quality
International Journal of Quality in Health Care
American Journal of Medical Quality

CHAPTER 19

Quality and quality governance

Sarah Cornick, Eleanor Cole and Rosalind Ramsay

'Quality improvement is everyday business and work.' (Juran, 1951)

Quality of care in mental health services is important. Not only does it impact directly on health outcomes, safety and patient experience, but it also impacts on the cost of care and the reputation of each local organisation and the NHS as a whole.

The *Oxford English Dictionary* defines quality as:

'the standard of something as measured against other things of a similar kind; the degree of excellence of something.'

Within healthcare, it has been less easy to define the concept of quality. The current definition of quality (see also Chapters 1 and 18) as applied in the NHS and enshrined in law through the Health and Social Care Act 2012 considers three dimensions:

* safety
* patient experience
* clinical effectiveness.

This definition fits with the US Institute of Medicine concept of quality which is often used in healthcare settings:

'[quality is] the degree to which health services for individuals and populations increase the likelihood of desired health outcomes and are consistent with current professional knowledge.' (Lohr, 1990)

The US Institute of Medicine also identified six dimensions of healthcare quality (Committee on Quality of Health Care in America & Institute of Medicine, 2001), stating that healthcare must be:

* safe – avoiding injuries to patients from the care that is intended to help them
* effective – providing services based on scientific knowledge to all who could benefit and refraining from providing services to those not likely to benefit (avoiding underuse and overuse)

- patient-centred – providing care that is respectful of and responsive to individual patient preferences, needs and values, and ensuring that patient values guide all clinical decisions
- timely – reducing waits and sometimes harmful delays for both those who receive and those who give care
- efficient – avoiding waste, in particular waste of equipment, supplies, ideas and energy
- equitable – providing care that does not vary in quality because of personal characteristics such as gender, ethnicity, geographical allocation and socioeconomic status.

History of quality initiatives in the National Health Service

Our current understanding of quality has, however, developed over many years of quality initiatives within the NHS and it is worth thinking about the development of the quality agenda over the longer term.

For the first 40 years of the NHS there was an implicit notion of quality, with the assumption that providing well-trained staff and good facilities and equipment was synonymous with high standards (Halligan & Donaldson, 2001; Palmer, 2002). The arrival of the Thatcher government in 1979 saw the start of the first major reforms to the NHS. These initially focused on funding, management and organisational reform (also see Chapter 1).

Quality management ideas that had been developed in the Japanese car industry and taken up by business in the USA crept into the American healthcare system in the 1970s before arriving in Europe. The new concepts included total quality management and continuous quality improvement, but these were not widely accepted. However, the rise of consumerism in the post-war generation started to challenge the traditional paternalistic role of healthcare professionals in general, and of doctors in particular. Patients wanted more information, choice and involvement in decisions regarding their healthcare.

There were also questions about variations in practice as clinicians adopted the principles of evidence-based practice, taking a more rigorous approach to their work. A series of high-profile service failures – an example being paediatric cardiac surgery in Bristol – raised concerns about professional self-regulation and doctors' accountability. These service failures prompted more urgent demands for change and attempts to address quality in a more systematic and explicit way.

Table 19.1 provides a summary of how the framework for quality monitoring developed up until Darzi's *Next Stage Review* (2008) (discussed below).

As the idea of quality became more formalised, the concept of clinical governance developed. Clinical governance was described as:

'the opportunity to understand and learn to develop the fundamental components required to facilitate the delivery of quality care – a no blame,

Table 19.1 Early development of the NHS quality agenda

Year	Development
1979	Conservative government: start of first major NHS reforms, initially focused on funding, management and organisation
1982	Managers become accountable for outcome measures, although these at first concentrate on financial and workload concerns
1990	National Health Service and Community Care Act: quality becomes a statutory duty; prior to this, quality was seen as inherent in the system, sustained by the ethos and skills of health professionals, and quality initiatives were generally not integrated across services
1992	Patient's Charter introduced and rise of the service user movement
1997	Labour government – development of duty around quality
1997	Department of Health white paper *The New NHS*. This clarifies that quality is the responsibility of everyone in and every part of the NHS. It introduced the concept that quality = clinical result and patient experience. It outlined structures to support quality: by setting standards; introducing national service frameworks and the national performance framework, as well as the National Survey of Patient and User Experience; by monitoring standards; and by establishing two bodies, the National Institute of Clinical Excellence (NICE; now the National Institute for Health and Care Excellence) and the Commission for Health Improvement (CHI)
1998	Department of Health consultation paper *A First Class Service: Quality in the New NHS*. This introduced the concept of clinical governance as a means to discharge duty in providing high-quality, safe and effective healthcare
1999	Department of Health consultation paper *Supporting Doctors, Protecting Patients*, with proposals for professional regulation
2000	Department of Health consultation paper *An Organisation with a Memory*, which concerned learning from incidents and which prompted the creation of the National Patient Service Agency (NPSA) in 2001
2003 onwards	Legal duty for NHS bodies to involve and consult the public. This led to establishment of patient advice and liaison services (PALS), patient and public involvement (PPI) forums and independent complaints advocacy services (ICAS)
2003	The Health and Social Care (Community Health and Standards) Act 2003 replaced the CHI with the Commission for Healthcare Audit and Inspection (presently known as the Healthcare Commission) in 2004, which had the overall function of encouraging improvement in healthcare and public health
2004	The Department of Health's NHS Improvement Plan increased the focus on the individual, patient choice and public health The Department of Health's document *National Standards, Local Action* provided a framework for quality and standards for better health (minimum 'core' standards and 'developmental' standards to promote improvement)

questioning, learning culture, excellent leadership, and an ethos where staff are valued and supported as they form partnerships with patients. These elements have perhaps previously been regarded as too intangible to take seriously or attempt to improve. Clinical governance demands re-examination of traditional roles and boundaries – between health professions, between

279

doctor and patient, and between managers and clinicians – and provides the means to show the public that the NHS will not tolerate less than best practice.' (Halligan & Donaldson, 2001)

A more succinct and more commonly used definition of clinical governance was:

'a framework through which NHS organisations are accountable for continuously improving the quality of their services and safeguarding high standards of care by creating an environment in which excellence in clinical care will flourish.' (Scally & Donaldson, 1998)

To review different areas, the inspections by the Commission for Health Improvement (CHI) used the seven pillars of clinical governance:

1 clinical audit
2 risk management
3 research and effectiveness
4 use of information
5 patient and public involvement
6 staffing and staff management
7 education and training.

NHS Next Stage Review

Lord Darzi's report *High Quality Care For All: NHS Next Stage Review* (Department of Health, 2008) further considered the definition of quality in healthcare services and how to make quality integral to the NHS with the focus of all NHS organisations being to improve patient care. Three dimensions of quality were considered essential for a high-quality service:

• patient safety (do no harm to patients)
• patient experience (patients' satisfaction with their own experiences, chiefly the quality of caring)
• clinical effectiveness (measured by both clinical and patient-related outcomes).

This definition of quality is now enshrined in law through the Health and Social Care Act 2012. Quality is achieved only if there is delivery against all three dimensions.

Darzi also suggested that making 'the achievement of high quality care an obsession within the NHS' would require seven steps to build on existing local clinical governance work:

1 bring clarity to quality
2 measure quality
3 publish quality performance
4 recognise and reward quality
5 raise standards
6 safeguard quality
7 stay ahead.

Recent high-profile service failures

Mid Staffordshire and the Francis report

Robert Francis QC chaired a public inquiry into the appalling standards of care which were uncovered between 2005 and 2008 at the Mid Staffordshire General Hospital NHS Trust. During this time, the trust board had led the trust to achieve foundation trust status (when it became the Mid Staffordshire NHS Foundation Trust), which meant that the trust had been scrutinised and assessed by various bodies involved in assurance and regulation. The trust had been largely compliant with the then applicable standards set by the Healthcare Commission and no systemic failures had been identified. The failures were eventually uncovered primarily following the persistent complaints made by a group of patients and their supporters, and in part due to attention paid to the trust's high mortality rates.

The final inquiry report (Francis, 2013) made it clear that there needed to be a culture throughout an organisation to promote quality of care, from board level to individual clinicians. Altogether there were 290 recommendations, with the additional recommendation that all trusts should consider and report on how they would implement these recommendations.

The initial government response in 2013 included the introduction of a new hospital inspection regime and legislation for a duty of candour (i.e. to be open with patients and relatives regarding mistakes). In November 2013, the government published a full response to the recommendations made by the Francis report. This focused on honesty and transparency, safe staffing levels and the introduction of criminal sanctions against wilful neglect. Progress against the recommendations in the Francis report will be reported to Parliament annually to ensure ongoing delivery of the required changes to practice to ensure an improvement in patient safety and the quality of care.

The government also commissioned Professor Don Berwick to carry out a review of patient safety following publication of the Mid Staffordshire report. His report, *A Promise to Learn* (Berwick, 2013), made ten key recommendations, directly quoted below:

'1. The NHS should continually and forever reduce patient harm by embracing wholeheartedly an ethic of learning.
2. All leaders concerned with NHS healthcare – political, regulatory, governance, executive, clinical and advocacy – should place quality of care in general, and patient safety in particular, at the top of their priorities for investment, inquiry, improvement, regular reporting, encouragement and support.
3. Patients and their carers should be present, powerful and involved at all levels of healthcare organisations from wards to the boards of Trusts.
4. Government, Health Education England and NHS England should assure that sufficient staff are available to meet the NHS's needs now and in the future. Healthcare organisations should ensure that staff are present in appropriate numbers to provide safe care at all times and are well-supported.

5. Mastery of quality and patient safety sciences and practices should be part of initial preparation and lifelong education of all health care professionals, including managers and executives.
6. The NHS should become a learning organisation. Its leaders should create and support the capability for learning, and therefore change, at scale within the NHS.
7. Transparency should be complete, timely and unequivocal. All data on quality and safety, whether assembled by government, organisations, or professional societies, should be shared in a timely fashion with all parties who want it, including, in accessible form, with the public.
8. All organisations should seek out the patient and carer voice as an essential asset in monitoring the safety and quality of care.
9. Supervisory and regulatory systems should be simple and clear. They should avoid diffusion of responsibility. They should be respectful of the goodwill and sound intention of the vast majority of staff. All incentives should point in the same direction.
10. We support responsive regulation of organisations, with a hierarchy of responses. Recourse to criminal sanctions should be extremely rare, and should function primarily as a deterrent to wilful or reckless neglect or mistreatment.'

There has been some criticism that although the first Francis report, in 2010, made sensible recommendations, the final Francis report (2013) was too long, with too many recommendations, which were too complex to implement, and which did not provide closure for those who had questioned the quality of services being delivered at Mid Staffordshire. Multiple responses to the final Francis report have been published (including the Berwick report commissioned by the government) and there are some schools of thought that these have not resulted in any significant change in different services.

Keogh mortality review

In February 2013, Professor Sir Bruce Keogh, NHS Medical Director for England, was asked to review the quality of care and treatment provided at 14 hospital trusts identified as being persistent outliers on mortality indicators. Consistent with the definition of quality found in the Darzi report, the following key themes were identified as being core elements of high-quality care (Keogh, 2013):

- patient experience
- safety
- clinical and operational effectiveness
- governance and leadership
- workforce.

In terms of 'governance and leadership', only limited evidence was found to suggest that trust boards and clinical leaders were effective in driving quality improvement. Otherwise, the following concerns were identified:

- poor articulation of any quality improvement strategy
- lack of a consistent approach to learning from issues arising from quality and safety reviews
- a disconnect between what leadership said were key risks and issues and the reality of what was happening within the hospitals
- weaknesses in the assurances presented to the boards
- significant issues highlighted during the review not being on the boards' agenda in any form.

The findings of the Keogh review will be used to develop understanding of the roles and responsibilities of the various NHS bodies to inform the approach to assuring quality in the new NHS architecture.

Quality governance – development of a new concept

An imbalance between the need for quality and a focus on meeting performance targets which were closely linked with the financial well-being of organisations was apparent. The *Next Stage Review* and more recent reports following the high-profile failures within the NHS led to a reformulation of the concept of clinical governance, which brought together the renewed emphasis on quality and the historical clinical governance work under a new single banner of 'quality governance'. Quality governance is:

'the combination of structures and processes at and below board level to deliver trust-wide quality services. If implemented effectively, assessment against the Framework should provide boards with assurance over the effective and sustainable management of quality throughout their organisation.' (Monitor, 2013)

The existing ideas about clinical governance have not been lost, but rather with the updated quality agenda there has been a shift in emphasis with regard to responsibilities, accountability and the assurance of quality. The roles of the regulators, organisations and individuals within an organisation have also been clarified, and there have been some changes in the regulatory bodies.

Regulation of quality in the NHS

The Francis inquiry commented that regulation in the NHS was complicated and uncoordinated and that this complexity contributed to failures in the quality of care being identified in a timely manner. The Health and Social Care Act 2012 clarified roles and responsibilities, with the intention of improving quality within the NHS. Following the reforms made by the Act, the main bodies with a role in quality are as follows:

- *NHS England*. This was previously the NHS Commissioning Board. It has responsibility for the allocation of funding to commissioning groups and direct commissioning of primary care and some specialised services and a duty to secure continuous improvements in quality of services provided. It has a role in convening and chairing quality surveillance groups, which enable all relevant parties to meet and share information to facilitate coordinated feedback to services, although they are not accountable bodies themselves in relation to implementation and delivery.

- *Monitor*. This is the sector regulator for health services in England, established in 2004 under the Health and Social Care (Community Health and Standards) Act 2003. Additional duties were given to Monitor in the Health and Social Care Act 2012. Monitor has powers granted by Parliament which include setting and enforcing a framework of rules for commissioners and providers.

- *Care Quality Commission* (CQC). This is the single integrated regulator for health and adult social care which in 2009 replaced the Healthcare Commission, the Commission for Social Care Inspection and the Mental Health Act Commission. It is responsible for safeguarding appropriate standards of quality and safety within health and social care. The CQC registers and monitors the compliance of providers of health and social care with their registration requirements.

- *NHS Trust Development Authority*. This oversees the performance of NHS trusts and drives improvements in their quality and efficiency.

- *Clinical commissioning groups* (CCGs). These are responsible for commissioning services which meet local needs and for promoting improvements in quality. They must ensure the quality of the services they commission.

- *Health Education England*. This is responsible for assurance of the quality of education delivered by the providers it contracts and for addressing any quality concerns in relation to education and training.

- *Healthwatch England*. This is the independent consumer champion for health and social care in England. It ensures that the opinions of service users become known to decision-makers.

- *National Institute for Health and Care Excellence* (NICE). This produces national guidance, standards and information to help professionals deliver the best possible care using the best available evidence. The guidance is also used to ensure the effectiveness of commissioning.

- *National Quality Board*. This champions quality and ensures consistency in quality throughout the NHS.

For the regulatory and assurance system to work effectively, it is essential that regulators, commissioners and other relevant bodies are able to share, openly and transparently, information and intelligence gathered about the quality of services within an organisation. There also needs to be coordinated feedback and action taken, where appropriate, if a quality failure is identified. Following the Keogh review, further work between the above bodies has been encouraged to develop a clear understanding of their roles and responsibilities. The 2013 Berwick report also emphasised the importance of the role of the government and regulators to simplify the complexity of the regulatory system and ensure cooperation among regulators.

Quality across the UK

With devolution have come some differences in the development of clinical governance and its supporting structures.

Scotland

The white paper *Designed to Care* (Scottish Executive Health Department, 1997) introduced the term 'clinical governance' to NHS Scotland. The white paper defined it as 'corporate accountability for clinical performance' and made trust chief executives responsible for the quality of care provided by their organisations. NHS Quality Improvement Scotland was set up in 2003 as the lead organisation to improve the quality of healthcare delivered by NHS Scotland. The Crerar review (Crerar, 2007) reviewed healthcare scrutiny and regulation in Scotland and concluded that the provisions were unnecessarily complex and too difficult for the relevant stakeholders to understand. Reorganisation resulted in the creation of Healthcare Improvement Scotland, which includes all component parts of NHS Quality Improvement Scotland, including the Healthcare Environment Inspectorate, Scottish Intercollegiate Guidelines Network (SIGN) and the Scottish Health Council. The key purpose of this organisation is to improve the quality and safety of healthcare and it has taken over responsibility for the regulation of independent healthcare. As well as developing evidence-based guidance and standards, it provides advice regarding local improvement cycles and leads work on assurance, scrutiny, measurement and reporting to demonstrate accountability.

Wales

Healthcare Inspectorate Wales is the independent inspectorate and regulator of all healthcare in Wales. It has a focus on: the safety and quality of services; patient, carer and staff experience; strengthening the voice of patients; and ensuring that timely and accessible information on the quality of services is available.

Northern Ireland

The Regulation and Quality Improvement Authority (RQIA) has a similar role in Northern Ireland with respect to health and social care services.

Implementing quality governance

Whereas historically clinical governance was felt to be the realm of individual clinicians and clinical managers, the move towards quality governance recognised that trust boards are ultimately responsible for quality within their organisations. A robust governance framework is essential in every organisation to ensure that essential standards of quality (and safety) are maintained and to provide assurance that quality governance processes are embedded throughout that organisation. They have a duty to ensure that data on their results are reported transparently.

Quality governance at the organisational level

To assist trust boards to fulfil their responsibility to ensure quality within their organisation, Monitor (2010) published the Quality Governance Framework, which is embedded into the assessment process for aspiring NHS foundation trusts and the compliance framework for existing trusts. This guidance is intended to raise the profile of the quality agenda at board level and help boards to deliver on their responsibilities. The Framework comprises four domains and ten questions for organisations to consider (Table 19.2).

In addition to the four domains, the guidance states that good quality governance should be based on the concepts of 'engage and cascade', that is, engaging with stakeholders and communication across the organisation, and 'assure and escalate', that is, ensuring that high-quality care is delivered and that the risks affecting quality are managed. The guidance is delivered under four themes, which highlight the challenges many trusts may come across when implementing an effective quality governance programme, and these fit with the above concepts:

- engagement on quality (*assurance*)
- gaining insight and foresight into quality (*engage*)
- accountability for quality (*cascade*)
- managing risks to quality (*escalation*).

Questions from the Framework are highlighted under each section of the guidance.

It is expected that quality will be a permanent item for consideration by an organisation's board. The guidance also supports trusts in making the corporate governance statement required under Monitor's licence conditions.

Further guidance for boards on their role and responsibilities has been provided by the NHS Leadership Academy's (2013) updated publication *The Healthy NHS Board 2013: Principles for Good Governance*. This guidance was first published in 2010 by the National Leadership Council, and since then has been updated following research and guidance published in the post-Francis era.

Table 19.2 The ten questions in four domains of Monitor's (2010) Quality Governance Framework

Strategy	Capabilities and culture	Processes and structure	Measurement
1A. Does quality drive the trust's strategy?	2A. Does the board have the necessary leadership, skills and knowledge to ensure delivery of the quality agenda?	3A. Are there clear roles and accountabilities in relation to quality governance?	4A. Is appropriate quality information being analysed and challenged?
1B. Is the board sufficiently aware of potential risks to strategy?	2B. Does the board promote a quality-focused culture throughout the trust?	3B. Are there clearly defined, well-understood processes for escalating and resolving issues and managing quality performance?	4B. Is the board assured of the robustness of the quality information?
		3C. Does the board actively engage patients, staff and other key stakeholders on quality?	4C. Is quality information used effectively?

Mapping the Gap: Highlighting the Disconnect Between Governance Best Practice and Reality in the NHS (ICSA, 2011) reported on a research project undertaken to examine the understanding of governance issues at NHS board level and the extent to which boards adhered to best practice governance guidance. It looked at four broad areas: strategy; decision-making; clinical and quality matters; and probity and transparency. In respect of clinical and quality matters, the project had the following findings:

- Only 5% of boards had clinical and quality matters clearly aligned to strategic objectives.
- Clinical and quality matters accounted for between 4% and 13% of the top five agenda items, depending on the type of trust, whereas the governance guidance recommends a minimum of 20%.
- The acquisition of information on clinical and quality matters from a range of sources, including site visits and patient feedback, did not appear robust.

However, it should be noted that this research used data gathered around the time that the new guidance from Monitor came into force and prior to publication of the Francis report and related commentary, and the more recent Keogh review, and it would be hoped that if the research was repeated now, the results would demonstrate that the quality agenda has been more fully incorporated into work undertaken by trust boards.

Guidance produced by the National Quality Board (2011) provided evidence to suggest that there is a correlation between governance initiatives and behaviour at board level and the overall performance of an organisation. The serious failings identified at the Mid Staffordshire NHS Foundation Trust are a good example of the link between board structures and processes to support the quality agenda and the overall performance of the organisation with respect to quality of care.

The Berwick report (2013) suggested that the leaders of NHS organisations and trust boards should:

- listen to and involve patients and carers in every organisational process, at every step in their care
- monitor the quality and safety of care constantly, including variation within the organisation
- respond directly, openly, faithfully and rapidly to safety alerts, to early-warning systems, and to complaints from patients and staff
- embrace complete transparency
- train and support all staff all of the time to improve the processes of care
- join multi-organisational collaboratives – networks – in which teams can learn from and teach each other
- use evidence-based tools to ensure adequate staffing levels.

Quality in the mental health sector

No Health Without Mental Health: A Cross-Government Mental Health Outcomes Strategy For People Of All Ages (Department of Health, 2011) is a mental health outcomes strategy, and following on from the Department of Health (2010) white paper *Healthy Lives, Healthy People* it continues the theme of establishing parity of esteem between services for people with mental health problems and those with physical health problems.

The strategy commented that there was top-down direction, with an emphasis on structures and processes rather than outcomes, and with fragmentation of some services and variability in the accessibility of care. It was recognised that commissioning of mental health services had often specified what providers should do rather than having a focus on improving the quality of commissioning.

Quality is a theme throughout the strategy, with the aim of improving outcomes within an efficient framework. 'Payment by results' is being developed for mental health services, to promote efficient allocation of resources and to provide a stronger incentive to maintain and raise the quality of care. The strategy also recognises the importance of NICE quality standards, 'quality accounts' and providing a more competitive market.

Closing the Gap: Priorities for Essential Change in Mental Health, a further policy document (Department of Health, 2014), set out 25 areas in which action will be visible in the shorter term, while keeping the longer-term aims of the overall mental health strategy of *No Health Without Mental Health* in mind. Again, quality was a theme throughout the document. Among other targets, the policy set out: plans to provide further guidance for those commissioning services; the development of a Mental Health Intelligence Network (MHIN); clear outcome targets for waiting times; and the development of a payments system that reflects quality and outcomes as well as volumes of activity. Identifying poor-quality services earlier was recognised as a key target. With this in mind, the CQC was developing a new model for monitoring, inspecting and regulating mental health providers to ensure that poor-quality services or gaps in provision would be identified sooner.

Value and the work of Porter

'Failure to improve value, means well, failure.' (Porter & Lee, 2013)

'Value' is defined as the health outcomes achieved that matter to patients relative to the cost of achieving those outcomes. Porter makes reference to the 'countless incremental fixes' adopted by clinicians and policy makers, that have had limited impact, when instead we should be aiming for 'high-value care' through a fundamentally new strategy in which value for patients is maximised and the best outcomes obtained at lowest cost. Our services need to be organised around what patients need.

The role of individual clinicians

Senior healthcare professionals working in clinical teams providing NHS services are in a crucial position, being at the front line, for ensuring quality of care to patients and are known to express strong support for the principles of quality patient care (National Quality Board, 2011). However, such beliefs may not translate into changes in everyday practice.

For individual professionals, care is delivered within a framework of professional regulation and responsibilities, which encourages personal accountability for the quality of care delivered. The General Medical Council (GMC) and Royal College of Psychiatrists provide frameworks and guidance that support the role of medically qualified professionals in delivery of quality healthcare. The GMC has 'safety and quality' as one of four domains in the core guidance for doctors (General Medical Council, 2013) and the College in its formal response to the Francis report (Royal College of Psychiatrists, 2013) set out a work programme to promote quality improvement following five key principles (Box 19.1).

Role of the consultant psychiatrist

Leadership skills are necessary to sustain and encourage engagement with quality improvement and are an integral part of the consultant psychiatrist's

---

Box 19.1   Frameworks to support the role of psychiatrists in delivering quality healthcare: the importance of outcomes and accurate data

General Medical Council (2013)
Duties of a doctor – safety and quality (domain 2):
'medical staff contribute to and comply with systems to protect patients.'

Royal College of Psychiatrists (2013)
• Always put patients first
• Prioritise patient safety and well-being
• Provide high-quality clinical leadership
• Respect regulation, inspection and accountability as supporting care

---

role. It is beneficial to have a leadership style which emphasises the importance of integrated and collaborative working between the professional disciplines, where there are shared visions, purposes and objectives. The consultant psychiatrist is a key link between the multidisciplinary team and the wider organisation (the trust). However, this needs to marry with nurses being the larger workforce and their and other professionals' contribution to delivery of services. Delivery of quality care cannot be done alone.

As part of their leadership role, consultant psychiatrists need to consider beyond the needs of individual patients and to think more in terms of the needs of the population being served.

Evidence has been limited for a specific effective leadership style in quality improvement, although a recent King's Fund publication refers to 'collective leadership', where all staff take responsibility for ensuring high-quality patient care and are accountable (West *et al*, 2014). It describes the cultural characteristics that underpin the delivery of continually improving high-quality care. The characteristic with the most influence on an improving quality culture is a leadership that operates at all levels within an organisation. The features of that leadership are described by Øvretveit (2011):

• envisions the future and inspires
• builds alliances for change
• spends time on improvement
• demonstrates commitment in different behaviours
• works persistently with others on a daily basis to raise the possibility of a better way
• creates systems
• changes procedures
• confronts poor performance.

Monitoring and measuring performance

In considering service improvement, it is important not to make changes blind. Measuring performance has not always been conducted well in psychiatry compared with other specialities, which could be a result of the challenges in obtaining good quality data in psychiatry.

Means of measuring service changes and improvements include use of the PDSA (plan–do–study–act) cycle, the lean model and Six Sigma, which, as detailed in Chapter 18, are useful vehicles for the benchmarking and continuous monitoring of service performance and efficiency. Participating in service improvement and modernisation projects is one way of bringing to life the use of service improvement tools and methodologies.

The psychiatrist can take a lead role in the inspection and analysis of data and consultants have an important role in contextualising data and exploring which interventions may work best for their patient group, ensuring team feedback meetings take place and assisting in the reflection on any results. Data can be used to ask questions, to know whether your service area conforms to a standard or is an outlier and then again to ask further questions.

Reducing variation as a means of ensuring quality and high performance

Jarman has highlighted the significant differences found in the productivity of individual clinicians as well as teams and organisations, and suggests these can be addressed by clinicians through ownership of and regular review of their data in order to improve individual practice and to explore both why their performance or outcomes vary and any differences in practice (Reinertsen, 2003).

Quality improvement approaches are focused more on improving processes and systems than on clinical practice. Variation can result in inefficiencies (waste) which relate to systems and processes. More importantly, it can result in harm, a reduction in patient safety and poor patient outcomes when there is deviation from established evidence-based best practice. Addressing variation can increase the reliability of care. Standardisation through use of protocols is one way of managing variation, although some variation is considered normal.

Clinician involvement in quality improvement

The key requirements for getting clinicians involved in quality improvement are a jointly owned vision and aims, collaborative working and engagement with front-line services. A useful Royal College of Psychiatrists framework for senior clinicians is illustrated in Box 19.2. *Kaizen* ('improvement') is a Japanese term taken from the business literature; an example of a *kaizen* project in mental health services is briefly described in Box 19.3, which highlights an integrative approach to service improvement.

291

Conclusion

The quality of services in the NHS has always been important, but with recent high-profile service failures the quality agenda has developed a new prominence in the delivery of healthcare services. The processes to ensure quality and safety of services and to improve the experience of stakeholders within services have been formalised, with changes to regulatory structures

---

Box 19.2   Clinical governance key standards

- Clinical team members understand their roles and responsibilities in relation to clinical governance – clinical teams meet regularly to discuss quality issues and review their progress

- Clinical audit
  - Staff and service users are involved in clinical audit
  - Clinical teams rather than individual members only
  - (All senior managers) Practitioners have received training in clinical audit

- Evidence-based practice (EBP) – all staff receive training in the following:
  - EBP
  - use of specific clinical guidelines and protocols agreed in their organisation (Trust)
  - critical appraisal
  - use of library, database facilities and search techniques

- *Revalidation / annual appraisal
  - 360 peer & patient feedback
  - Learning from complaints, serious incidents, compliments
  - Reflective practice
  - Personal development plan

- Clinical supervision and participation in peer group

- Multidisciplinary training

- Consultants promote quality improvement-focused culture
  - learning from mistakes
  - encourage and identify areas for improvement
  - awareness of the organisation's values, vision and quality strategy

- Positive feedback to staff

- Review patient feedback

- Prioritise participation in service area reviews to do with quality

- Identifying areas in own service area
  - Of concern
  - Quality / good practice

(Adapted from Worrall, 2001)

---

and a recognition that quality and safety are the responsibility of everyone working within an organisation, not just clinicians or those working at board level.

Box 19.3   A *kaizen* project for a community mental health team – an example of the importance of an integrated approach to quality work

A *kaizen* team event was undertaken by a London-based community mental health team (CMHT) in 2013 to generate ideas and areas for improvements in the team's working practices with the aim of achieving a 35% reduction (stretch target) in in-patient bed days for the team's patient case-load. This project was supported by trust senior leaders and 'lean greenbelt' training was given to the team's senior staff to promote the generation of ideas for improvement using lean principles. Possible improvements needed to be realistically achievable within the financial, practical and staffing resources available to the team.

Relatively small but significant changes were made to the team's working processes:

* biweekly senior leadership meeting
* biweekly steering group to report on progress and issues
* change from weekly to daily multidisciplinary team meetings to discuss patients of concern, with daily audit of the meeting process to maintain the team's focus on the improvement process and the quality of service delivery
* development of zoning criteria to identify clients in early stages of relapse and crisis, to facilitate early intervention after discussion in the daily multidisciplinary team meeting
* biweekly formulation meeting to review complex cases and recent admissions
* review of 'frequent flier' patients with multiple recent admissions and review of their management
* patient psychoeducation group initiated
* trial of mobile working (staff provided with tablet computers) to reduce time spent on administrative work, enabling additional time to be devoted to treatment and recovery-focused patient interventions.

After one year, a 25% reduction in occupied bed days had been achieved. However, this feedback on the team's performance was made available only after one year. The lack of feedback on the performance measures at an earlier point resulted in a drop in individual and team morale and high staff turnover within the team, due to a perceived impression that the changes implemented had made no impact on admissions and that the team was not performing as expected. This jeopardised the entire project and additional resources provided started to be removed by senior management. Although the trust had supported the team to make the changes initially, the lack of feedback on outcome information created a gap in the improvement process at a critical point.

This demonstrates the importance of information-sharing between teams at the front line of service delivery and at a higher organisational level during quality improvement (or other service change) initiatives.

References

Berwick D (2013) *A Promise to Learn – A Commitment to Act: Improving the Safety of Patients in England*. National Advisory Group on the Safety of Patients in England.

Committee on Quality of Health Care in America, Institute of Medicine (2001) *Crossing the Quality Chasm: A New Health System for the 21st Century*. National Academy Press.

Crerar LD (2007) *The Report of the Independent Review of Regulation, Audit, Inspection and Complaints Handling of Public Services in Scotland* (Crerar review). Scottish Government.

Department of Health (1997) *The New NHS: Modern, Dependable*. HMSO.

Department of Health (1998) *A First Class Service: Quality in the New NHS*. London, HMSO.

Department of Health (1999) *Supporting Doctors, Protecting Patients: A Consultation Paper on Preventing, Recognising and Dealing with Poor Clinical Performance of Doctors in the NHS in England*. Department of Health.

Department of Health (2000) *An Organisation With a Memory*. HMSO.

Department of Health (2004a) *National Standards, Local Action Health and Social Care*. Department of Health.

Department of Health (2004b) *The NHS Improvement Plan*. Department of Health.

Department of Health (2008) *High Quality Care For All: NHS Next Stage Review Final Report* (Cm 7432). TSO (The Stationery Office).

Department of Health (2010) *Healthy Lives, Healthy People: Our Strategy for Public Health in England*. TSO (The Stationery Office).

Department of Health (2011) *No Health Without Mental Health: A Cross-Government Mental Health Outcomes Strategy For People Of All Ages*. Department of Health.

Department of Health (2014) *Closing the Gap: Priorities for Essential Change in Mental Health*. Department of Health.

Francis R (2013) *Report of the Mid Staffordshire NHS Foundation Trust Public Inquiry. Final Report* (Francis report). Mid Staffordshire NHS Foundation Trust Public Inquiry.

General Medical Council (2013) Duties of a doctor. In *Good Medical Practice*. GMC.

Halligan A, Donaldson L (2001) Implementing clinical governance: turning vision into reality. *BMJ*, **322**: 1413–7.

ICSA (2011) *Mapping the Gap: Highlighting the Disconnect Between Governance Best Practice and Reality in the NHS*. ICSA: The Governance Institute.

Juran J (1951) *Quality Control Handbook*. McGraw-Hill.

Keogh B (2013) *Review into the Quality of Care and Treatment Provided by 14 Hospital Trusts in England: Overview Report*. NHS England.

Lohr KN (ed) (1990) *Medicare: A Strategy For Quality Assurance*. National Academy Press.

Monitor (2010) *Quality Governance Framework*. Monitor.

Monitor (2013) *Quality Governance: How Does a Board Know That Its Organisation Is Working Effectively To Improve Patient Care?* Monitor.

National Quality Board (2011) *Quality Governance in the NHS – A Guide for Provider Boards*. NQB.

NHS Leadership Academy (2013) *The Healthy NHS Board 2013: Principles for Good Governance*. NHS Leadership Academy.

Øvretveit J (2011) *Does Clinical Coordination Improve Quality and Save Money?* Health Foundation.

Palmer C (2002) Clinical governance: breathing new life into clinical audit. *Advances in Psychiatric Treatment*, **8**: 470–6.

Porter ME, Lee TH (2013) The strategy that will fix health care. *Harvard Business Review*, October.

Reinertsen JL (2003) Zen and the art of physician autonomy maintenance. *Annals of Internal Medicine*, **138**: 992–5.

Royal College of Psychiatrists (2013) *Driving Quality Implementation in the Context of the Francis Report: Key Principles for Quality Improvement*. RCPsych.

Scally G, Donaldson LJ (1998) Looking forward: clinical governance and the drive for quality improvement in the new NHS in England. *BMJ*, **317**: 61–5.

Scottish Executive Health Department (1997) *Designed to Care: Renewing the National Health Service in Scotland*. TSO (The Stationery Office).

West M, Eckert R, Steward K, *et al* (2014) *Developing Collective Leadership for Health Care*. King's Fund.

Worrall A (ed) (2001) *Clinical Governance Standards for Mental Health and Learning Disability*. College Research Unit, Royal College of Psychiatrists.

CHAPTER 20

Measurement of needs

Graham Thornicroft , Mike Slade and Koravangattu Valsraj

Defining needs

The American psychologist Maslow established a seminal hierarchy of need when attempting to formulate a theory of human motivation (Maslow, 1954). In Maslow's model, fundamental physiological needs (such as the need for food) underpin the higher needs of safety, love, self-esteem and self-actualisation. He proposed that people are motivated by the requirement to meet these needs, and that higher needs could be met only once the lower and more fundamental needs were met. This approach can be illustrated by the example of a homeless man, who is not concerned about his lack of friends while he is cold and hungry. However, once these physiological needs have been met he may express more interest in having the company of other people (Slade & McCrone, 2001).

Since the work of Maslow, several approaches have been developed for defining need with respect to healthcare. The sociologist Bradshaw (1972) proposed a 'needs taxonomy' with three types of need: (1) *felt* or *expressed* need that is mentioned by the user; (2) *normative* need which is assessed by the expert; and (3) *comparative* need, which arises from comparison with other groups or individuals. Such an approach helps to emphasise that need is a subjective concept, and that the judgement of whether a need is present or not will, in part, depend on whose viewpoint is taken. Other, somewhat more philosophical approaches to needs have also been proposed (e.g. Mallman & Marcus, 1980; Liss, 1990).

In the Medical Research Council (MRC) Needs for Care Assessment (NCA), a need is defined as being present when a person's functioning falls below, or threatens to fall below, some specified level, and when there is some remediable, or potentially remediable, cause (Brewin *et al*, 1987). Slade (1994) discussed the issue with respect to differences in perception between the users of mental health services and the involved professionals, and he argued that once differences are identified, then negotiation between staff and user can take place to agree a care plan.

Despite the common view that services should be based upon assessed needs, there is no consensus on how needs should be defined (Holloway,

1994) or on who should define them (Slade, 1994). Individual needs, for example, may be defined in terms of impairment or disability or of interventions.

The fact that a need is defined does not mean that it can be met. Some needs may remain unmet because other problems take priority, because an effective method is not available locally, or because the person in need refuses treatment. Furthermore, a need may exist, as defined by a professional, even if the intervention is refused by a patient.

A needs assessment is not intended to endorse the status quo. It is important to define need in terms of the care, agent or setting required, not those already in place. At the same time, a proper needs assessment should not lead to the imposition of an expert solution upon patients. A professionally defined need may remain unmet and have to be replaced by one acceptable to the patients. In addition, it is important to distinguish between need, demand and supply. Stevens *et al* (2001) state that:

- *need* is what people benefit from
- *demand* is what people ask for
- *supply* is what is provided.

A demand for care exists when an individual expresses a wish to receive it. Some demands are expressed in an unsophisticated form, for example 'something needs to be done'. The user should be involved in a negotiation as to what interventions should be provided for what problems. This will include an explanation of the options. The process should not be purely directed by experts or professionals.

In relation to supply, a distinction can be made between provision and utilisation:

- *Provision* includes interventions, agents and settings, whether or not used. Care coordination entails providing such a pattern of service after initial assessment and then updating the assessment regularly to assess outcomes and to modify the care if needs remain unmet. Overprovision is provision without need, such as providing food for patients who can cook for themselves. Underprovision is need without provision (unmet need).
- *Utilisation* occurs when an individual actually receives care, for example in-patient admission.

Need may not be expressed as demand; demand is not necessarily followed by provision or, if it is, by utilisation; and there can be demand, provision and utilisation without real underlying the need for the particular service used.

If need is defined as the ability to benefit, it also becomes important to distinguish need from efficacy, effectiveness and outcome (Stevens *et al*, 2001):

- *need* is the ability to benefit
- *efficacy* is the intervention's or care setting's potential to produce benefit in ideal (experimental) conditions

297

- *effectiveness* is the intervention's or care setting's potential to produce benefit in everyday conditions
- *outcome* is the benefit produced in the local setting.

Another approach to defining need has been proposed by health economists. Their contributions include, first, the proposal that 'need' refers both to the capacity to benefit from an intervention and the amount of expenditure required to reduce the capacity to benefit to zero; it is therefore a product of benefit and cost-effectiveness (Culyer & Wagstaff, 1992). Second, health economists have proposed that diagnosis-related groups are notably irrelevant for mental health services (McCrone & Strathdee, 1994). Third, they suggest that empirical data should guide operational needs definitions (Beecham *et al*, 1993). For example, there is an economic argument that services for people with schizophrenia should be improved (Andrews *et al*, 2012).

In the particular case of mental health services, needs have been described in terms of the gaps between the service needs of patients and of populations and the services actually provided. Lehtinen *et al* (1990) interpret needs as reflecting an inadequate level of service for the severity of the problem: patients with severe disorders who receive primary rather than specialised psychiatric care would therefore be rated as having unmet need. Similarly, for Shapiro *et al* (1985), unmet needs are defined as the combination of definite morbidity and lack of mental health service utilisation. A third view is that unmet needs represent insufficient provision of particular treatment interventions, and this approach is embodied in the three individual needs assessment instruments now described.

Measuring individual needs

In an ideal planning framework, a comprehensive needs assessment would be undertaken on all patients and the aggregated data would be used to plan the services. In practice this is seldom possible, but systematic assessment, review, and evaluation over months and years of contact should allow teams to work with their users to evolve services more appropriate to their needs (Brewin *et al*, 1987). Individual needs assessments for homeless people who are mentally ill, for example, exemplify these issues. In a study by Herman *et al* (1993), homeless people were asked if they needed 'help with nerves and emotional problems' and were independently rated by the interviewer. A quarter (24%) of the interviewees reported no need for mental health services when the interviewer rated them as having a need. In contrast, Mavis *et al* (1993) report a study of people seeking help for substance misuse, who were asked about specific areas of need. Two subgroups of the homeless were identified: 78% were 'economic homeless' people, with substantial employment and financial problems, and 22% were 'multi-problem homeless' people, with significantly greater problems also in physical health, alcohol/drug use, mental health, family and social life.

Over 800 clients were interviewed and the study showed the explanatory value of distinguishing the two subgroups of homeless people.

The issue of how best to make an assessment has taxed both researchers and clinicians, not least because their requirements differ. An ideal assessment tool for use in a routine clinic setting would be one which is brief, easily learned, takes little time to administer, does not require the use of personnel additional to the usual clinical team, is valid and reliable in different settings and across gender and cultures, and, above all, which can be used as an integral part of routine clinical work, rather than being a time-consuming extra. In addition, it should be sensitive to change, its interrater and test–rater reliability should be high, and it should logically inform clinical management (Thornicroft & Bebbington, 1996). The decision of which to use will depend on whether the approach is to focus on particular diagnostic or care groups, and on the balance to be struck between economy of time and inclusiveness of the ratings. Rating should cover a range of areas of clinical and social functioning. Individual assessments of need will now be summarised.

1. MRC Needs for Care Assessment

The NCA (Brewin et al, 1987) was designed to identify areas of remediable need. Need is defined as being present when: a patient's functioning (social disablement) falls below or threatens to fall below some minimum specified level; and this is due to a remediable, or potentially remediable, cause. A need is defined as being met when it has attracted an item of care which is at least partly effective, and when there is no other item of care of greater potential effectiveness. A need is said to be unmet when it has attracted only a partly effective or no item of care, and when other items of care of greater potential effectiveness exist.

The NCA has proved itself to be a robust research instrument, and there is a substantial body of research describing its use (Brewin et al, 1988; van Haaster et al, 1994; Lesage et al, 1996). However, it is probably too complex and time-consuming for routine clinical use, and difficulties have arisen when it has been used with long-term in-patients (Pryce et al, 1993) and homeless people who are mentally ill (Hogg & Marshall, 1992).

2. Cardinal Needs Schedule

The Cardinal Needs Schedule (CNS) (Lockwood & Marshall, 2001) is a modification of the NCA. It identifies cardinal problems which satisfy three criteria:

- the *cooperation* criterion (the patient is willing to accept help for the problem)
- the *co-stress* criterion (the problem causes considerable anxiety, frustration or inconvenience to people caring for the patient)
- the *severity* criterion (the problem endangers the health or safety of the patient, or the safety of other people).

299

The instrument involves the use of the Manchester Scale for mental state assessment, and the REHAB scale, as well as a specially designed additional information questionnaire. A computerised version known as AUTONEED is also available. Given the detail of this instrument, it is probably more suited to experienced researchers.

3. Camberwell Assessment of Need

The Camberwell Assessment of Need (CAN) is an individual needs assessment instrument for use with adults with severe mental illness. Four broad principles governed the development of the CAN (Phelan *et al*, 1995; Slade *et al*, 1999a).

- Everyone has needs, and although people with mental health problems have some specific needs, the majority of their needs are similar to those of people who do not have a mental illness, such as having somewhere to live, something to do and enough money.
- The majority of people with a severe mental illness have multiple needs, and it is vital that all of them are identified by those caring for them. Therefore a priority of the CAN is to identify, rather than describe in detail, serious needs. Specialist assessments can be conducted in specific areas if required, once the need is identified.
- Needs assessment should be both an integral part of routine clinical practice and a component of service evaluation, so the CAN should be usable by a wide range of staff.
- Need is a subjective concept, and there will frequently be differing but equally valid perceptions about the presence or absence of a specific need. The CAN therefore records the views of staff and patients separately.

The specific criteria that were established for the CAN are that it: has adequate psychometric properties; can be completed within 30 minutes; can be used by a wide range of professionals; is suitable for both routine clinical practice and research; can be learned and used without formal training; incorporates the views of service users, staff and carers about needs (Hancock *et al*, 2003); measures both met and unmet need; and measures the level of help received from friends or relatives as well as from statutory services.

There are four versions of CAN: CAN-R for research use, CAN-C for clinical use, CAN Short Appraisal Schedule (CANSAS) for routine use and CANSAS-Patient (CANSAS-P) for self-report (Trauer *et al*, 2008). All versions assess need in the same 22 domains of health and social needs:

1 accommodation
2 food
3 looking after the home
4 self-care
5 daytime activities

6   physical health
7   psychotic symptoms
8   information on condition and treatment
9   psychological distress
10 safety to self
11 safety to others
12 alcohol
13 drugs
14 company
15 intimate relationships
16 sexual expression
17 child care
18 basic education
19 telephone
20 transport
21 money
22 benefits.

The CAN requires updating in two ways. First, some domains have dated, such as the telephone, which is being increasingly replaced by internet access. Second, an exclusive focus on needs is not compatible with the more recent orientation towards recovery (Leamy *et al*, 2011), in which assessment of strengths is also part of a comprehensive clinical assessment. Strengths measures are available (Bird *et al*, 2012) and interventions using a strengths assessment are being evaluated (Slade *et al*, 2011). The next version of the CAN will update the focus of domains and also assess strengths.

Camberwell Assessment of Need Short Appraisal Schedule

The CANSAS (Slade *et al*, 1999a, 1999b) is a short (single-page) summary of the needs of a mental health service patient. CANSAS can be used in clinical settings, since it is short enough to be routinely used for review purposes. It can also be used as an outcome measure in research studies, especially when a number of assessment schedules are being used. CANSAS records the views of the patient, carers and staff about the needs of the service user. Questions are asked about each domain, to identify whether a need or problem is present in that domain and whether the need is met or unmet. On the basis of the interviewee's responses, a need rating is made: 0 = no serious problem (no need), 1 = no/moderate problem due to help given (met need), 2 = serious problem (unmet need), 9 = not known.

CANSAS may be used for at least three purposes:

- CANSAS data can be used at the level of the individual patient, by providing a baseline measure of level of need, or for charting changes in the patient over time. For example, one approach would be to use the CANSAS routinely in initial assessments of new patients, to identify the range of domains in which they are likely to require further assessment and (possibly) help or treatment.

- CANSAS data can be used for auditing and developing an individual service.
- CANSAS can be used as an outcome measure for research purposes, such as the impact on needs of two different types of mental health service, or the reasons why staff and patient perceptions differ.

Comparing staff and service user ratings of need

There is now strong empirical evidence that needs rated by service users, especially unmet needs, are more informative that those rated by staff (Slade *et al*, 2005). The comparison of these two perspectives on needs will be discussed now in relation to three illustrative studies, from England, Scandinavia and Italy.

The first example is the PRiSM Psychosis Study (Leese *et al*, 1998; Thornicroft *et al*, 1998). This staff–user CAN comparative project was nested within a larger prospective non-randomised controlled trial of two different types of community mental health team in south London. The needs of an epidemiologically representative sample of 137 patients from a catchment area psychiatric service in south London who had an ICD-10 diagnosis of a functional psychotic disorder were assessed cross-sectionally by patients and staff, using the CAN.

Staff were found to have rated patients to have on average 6.1 needs and patients rated 6.7 needs ($t = 2.58$, d.f. $= 136$, $P = 0.011$). This difference was accounted for by the staff rating of 1.2 unmet needs and the patient rating of 1.8 unmet needs ($t = 3.58$, d.f. $= 136$, $P < 0.001$). There was no difference in rating of total number of met needs. There was no difference in ratings in relation to any patient sociodemographic characteristics. There was moderate or better agreement on the presence of a need for 13 of the 22 domains in the CAN (Slade *et al*, 1998). There was moderate or better agreement on the presence of a need for 13 of the 22 domains, but while staff and patients agreed moderately about met needs, they agreed less often on unmet needs. The domains more often rated by staff were psychotic symptoms and safety to others. The items more often rated by the service users were: information on treatment, company, welfare benefits, sexual expression and transport. For example, there was most disagreement between staff and users on four key items, namely information (about diagnosis, treatment and prognosis), telephone, transport and benefits; staff rated a mean of 0.90 needs for these four domains while service users rated 1.57 (difference 0.66, 95% confidence interval 0.47–0.85). The study therefore found that although staff and users rated about the same number of needs as each other, and although there was agreement for many of the domains of the CAN on where needs existed, the most disagreement occurred not about clinical issues but primarily in relation to practical aspects of the everyday lives of the service users.

This finding underpinned a programme of research involving an increasingly sophisticated series of studies investigating the relationship between patient-rated unmet need and quality of life. The studies involved pre–post comparisons (Slade *et al*, 1999c) followed by graphical modelling (Slade *et al*, 2004) to the first multivariate time series analysis to show empirical evidence of a causal relationship (Slade *et al*, 2005). A second programme of work found a similar causal relationship between patient-rated unmet need and therapeutic alliance (Junghan *et al*, 2007). These empirical findings demonstrate a causal relationship between patient-rated unmet needs and important processes (therapeutic alliance) and outcomes (quality of life). In other words, clinical care planning should be based on assessing and then meeting unmet needs identified by the patient.

The second illustration of staff–user comparative assessments of need is the Nordic Multi-Centre Study (Hansson *et al*, 2001), which undertook a comparison of key worker and patient assessment of needs in patients with schizophrenia living in the community. Ten centres in five Scandinavian countries participated in this study (Denmark, Sweden, Finland, Iceland and Norway) and within a larger study of case management 300 matched pairs of staff and users used the CAN to rate needs. The authors found moderate or good agreement in 17 of the 22 domains, even closer than in the London study. On the other hand, there was more disagreement than in the earlier project on whether the right type of help was being given.

Domains that were more often rated by staff were psychotic symptoms, psychological distress and self-care. The item that was more often rated by service users was information on treatment, and overall there was relatively poor agreement in the domains of information about condition and treatment, welfare benefits and telephone. The authors also compared responses on whether the right type of help was being offered for the needs identified, and there was close agreement in only five domains. Staff and users were least likely to agree that interventions in the following areas were the correct form of treatment or care: physical problems, psychological distress, education, self-care and intimate relationships.

The third example of staff–user differences is the South Verona OUTPRO study (Lasalvia *et al*, 2000). Patients resident within a local catchment area of 75 000 were identified from a psychiatric case register, and included all those in contact with specialist mental health services. Within a larger study which implemented outcome measures in routine clinical practice, 247 staff–patient pairs used the Italian version of the CAN. While the patients had somewhat lesser levels of disability than the patients included in the Nordic study, the usual pattern of met needs exceeding unmet needs was found for those receiving care. The needs more often rated by staff were in the domains of: physical health, psychological distress, self-care and psychotic symptoms. Users more frequently rated needs in the domains of information on treatment, welfare benefits, safety in relation to self, food, intimate relationships, telephone, education and money.

The Verona group went further and identified predictors of high levels of need. High staff-rated levels of need were associated with higher levels of disability, unemployment and more service contacts, while high user-rated levels of need were associated with higher levels of disability only. Disagreement on the total number of needs was most strongly associated with a lower level of global clinical and social functioning. These results once again demonstrate the clinical/social difference in orientation typified in the studies discussed above.

International use of the CAN

The CAN is the most widely used needs assessment measure internationally (Trauer, 2010). It has been translated into 26 languages which are listed on the CAN website (http://www.researchintorecovery.com/can). In addition, independent psychometric evaluations of many of these translations have been published, such as the Danish, Dutch, German, Italian and Spanish translations of the European version of the scale (CAN-EU) (McCrone *et al*, 2000; Thornicroft *et al*, 2005).

It is in widespread use at national and large regional levels (Trauer & Tobias, 2004; Drukker *et al*, 2010). For example, in Ontario, Canada, there are more than 300 community mental health (CMH) agencies that, as a sector, identified 'the need to enhance the assessment process and make it more effective for both the consumer and CMH staff'. As such, from December 2007, the government-funded CMH Common Assessment Project (CMH CAP) was developed and is currently 'delivering on the sector's vision of a streamlined assessment process that will standardize current practices across the province'. Throughout, the main measure used was the Ontario Common Assessment of Need (OCAN), a modified version of the CAN that was chosen as the best measure to base this tool on from 80 candidate measures (Slade, 2012). A 2012 report detailed how all of the 294 CMH organisations eligible to implement OCAN would be doing so by the end of 2012, with, at that time, 20% of the organisations having completed all of their OCAN assessments.[1]

Another example is in the Netherlands, where the CAN is part of the Cumulative Needs for Care Monitor (CNCM) database, a psychiatric case register system developed to standardise and improve needs-based diagnosis in use throughout a defined catchment area in the south of the country (population 660000) (Drukker *et al*, 2010). Here, the CAN is described as 'the core instrument of the CNCM'. This project is producing clinical findings directly informing service development. For instance, they found that compared with a control region, out-patient care consumption in the CNCM region was significantly higher, regardless of treatment status at baseline (Drukker *et al*, 2011).

A further example is that CANSAS has been chosen for use in the Minimum Data Set of the Partners in Recovery (PIR) five-year national programme in Australia. This is a £343 million programme involving

---

1 See https://www.ccim.on.ca/CMHA/OCAN/Document/CMHProjectProfile_2012 0215_v1%206_CMHCAP-FINAL.pdf.

300 consortium partner organisations to provide coordinated support for 24 000 people with severe mental illness and complex needs. The aims are to facilitate better coordination, strengthen partnerships, improve referral pathways and promote a community-based recovery model.

The CAN is also recommended in a range of evaluation and policy documents in the UK. For instance, it was recommended 'for clinical use to identify need' by the National Institute for Mental Health in England's 2008 'Outcomes Compendium' (National Institute for Mental Health in England, 2008). In 2011 the Royal College of Psychiatrists published its *Outcome Measures Recommended for Use in Adult Psychiatry*; that document said that the CANSAS 'has the advantage of showing how a service improves a service user's proportion of met needs (versus unmet needs)' and that 'it may be especially important for rehabilitation services to evidence the degree to which they are addressing service users' complex problems' (Hampson *et al*, 2011).

Further afield, in 2012 the Mental Health Commission of Canada produced its Mental Health Strategy, one priority of which is to 'improve mental health data collection, research and knowledge exchange across Canada' (Mental Health Commission of Canada, 2012). It cites Ontario's CMH CAP, discussed above, as a best-practice example. It proposes the countrywide adoption of OCAN, adapted from the CAN, which it describes as 'the most internationally recognized and researched assessment tool available'.

The CAN is also widely used by non-governmental organisations (NGOs): 'of all the outcome measures, CANSAS has had the strongest uptake by NGOs' (Trauer, 2010: p. 165). For example, Neami National is an Australian non-government mental health organisation that provides support services within a recovery framework for 2300 consumers with a serious mental illness across five states. Since 2009, the organisation has adopted the Collaborative Recovery Model, which involves using CANSAS with all consumers as the basis for care planning (Oades *et al*, 2005).

Variants of the CAN have been published and are in widespread use for other populations, including:

- older adults (CANE) (Reynolds *et al*, 2000; Reynolds & Orrell, 2001; Orrell, 2003)
- people with learning or intellectual disabilities (CANDID) (Xenitidis & Bouras, 2001; Xenitidis *et al*, 2000, 2003)
- forensic patients (CANFOR) (Thomas *et al*, 2003, 2004; Harty *et al*, 2004)
- mothers and pregnant women with mental health problems (Howard *et al*, 2001, 2007, 2008)
- people in disaster relief situations, the HESPER scale (Semrau *et al*, 2012).

Specific applications of needs assessment in relation to other populations have also been discussed (Thornicroft, 2001), including children, ethnic groups, primary care settings, drug and alcohol misuse, eating disorders, and services in rural areas.

Measuring population needs for services

Measuring the population's ability to benefit from healthcare generates two very specific information requirements (Wing, 1992). First, top-down sources of information are needed, such as the local prevalence and incidence of disease, ranged by severity. Prevalence, the number of cases per unit population at a point in time, or over a period, is usually the appropriate measure for chronic disease; and incidence, the number of new cases per unit time, is usually appropriate for measuring acute disease. Second, it is necessary to know the efficacy of the care and care settings available or potentially available to cope with it.

In practice, several more detailed types of information are needed to assist judgements on how far mental health services meet need at the population level, especially resource costs and the number and characteristics of patients treated. Another potential approach is the measurement of diagnosis-related groups (Mitchell *et al*, 1987), which suggests that diagnosis is of little help in attempting to measure prospectively the resources required by individual in-patients. The relationship between individual-based needs assessment (bottom-up) and population-based information (top-down) is illustrated in Fig. 20.1. Bottom-up approaches, that is, the aggregation of individual-level data to give information about patient populations, are somewhat less common (Bebbington *et al*, 1996).

Traditionally, service-level needs have been approximated from service utilisation data, especially hospital bed use. This is often inaccurate because: in-patient care is a small and diminishing part of mental healthcare; in many respects in-patient care actually represents an alternative model of care to that practised (i.e. community-based care) for certain patients; the chronicity and episodic nature of mental illness means that episodes are often part of a longer sequence and are very varied in length and intensity; and there is a greater diversity of health professional contacts (i.e. psychiatrists, psychologists, community psychiatric nurses, and occupational therapists).

In terms of the needs for general adult mental health services for a defined population, Table 20.1 presents data from multiple sources and suggests that:

- the emphasis should be upon the number of places available rather than the number of beds
- a range of provisions should exist
- the number of places needed in each category depends upon the extent of provision in the other categories
- the overall requirement for services will correlate closely with the degree of socioeconomic deprivation experienced by that particular population (and therefore ranges of numbers rather than specific values are given for each category in Table 20.1).

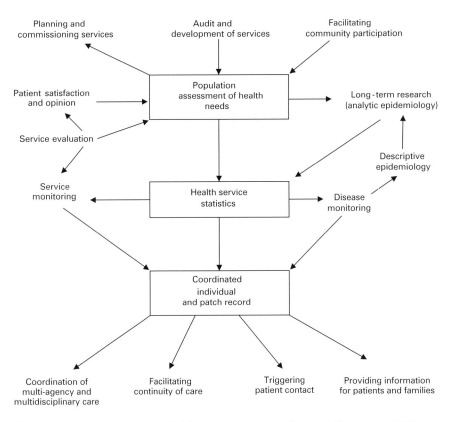

Fig. 20.1   Uses of mental health information systems (Fryers & Greatorex, 1992)

Conclusion

The assessments of needs for care and needs for services have been relatively recently developed. As yet, the issue of how service users participate in defining need is largely unexplored territory (Beeforth & Wood, 2001; Thornicroft & Slade, 2002). Just as formidable is the question – what are the consequences of conducting proper needs assessment (Goldman, 1999)? In assessing need, we are likely to confront previously inconspicuous layers of psychiatric morbidity and disability. This leads to two further questions: how shall we prioritise services, and is the pursuit of quality of life a reasonable proxy where staff are not able to provide a complete cure for mental disorders (Slade *et al*, 2004)?

Finally, it is sometimes helpful to step back from the detail of how to measure needs for healthcare and to ask *why* measure needs? Do needs reduce due to external factors, such as economic austerity leading to fewer available resources? In our view, an approach to health services that is fundamentally based upon need is in essence a moral choice. It is a view that

Table 20.1 Estimated need and actual provision of general adult (ages 15–64 only) mental health services (in-patient and residential care), places per 250000 population, estimated for England in 1992–96

Category of service	Wing (1992)	Strathdee & Thornicroft (1992)	PRiSM (1996)	Actual level of provision per 250000		
				Outer London (overall)	Inner London (overall)	Range in London
Medium-secure unit	1–10	1–10	5–30	8	27	0–58
Intensive care unit / local secure unit	5–15	5–10	5–20	8	16	0–41
Acute ward	50–150	50–150	50–175	73[a]	110[a]	48–165
24-hour nurse-staffed units/hostel wards/staff awake at night	25–75	40–150 for these 2 categories together	12–50	55	35	0–164
24-hour non-nurse-staffed hostels/night staff sleep-in	40–110		50–300	99	162	28–330
Day-staffed hostels	25–75	30–120	15–60	17	43	14–292 for these 2 categories together
Lower support accommodation	n/a	48–100	30–120	55	95	

For all estimates it is assumed that each category of service exists in the given appropriate range of volume. The Wing (1992) estimates include old age assessment places, and the Strathdee & Thornicroft figures apply only to general adult services for those aged 16–65. PRiSM (1996) estimated need levels based upon: London actual values, and an expected fourfold variation of need from least to most deprived parts of England, for most categories of service, with a far greater variation in medium-secure beds, and NHS Executive (1996) guidance for an average of 25 places in 24-hour nurse-staffed accommodation per 250000.

[a]Includes respite beds and supported self-contained flats. As not all agencies gave information on these categories, these estimates are conservative.

Sources: Glover (1996); Ramsay et al (1997); Thornicroft & Strathdee (2001).

attaches importance to the relief of suffering, whatever the circumstances of the person who is unwell, and which claims that a civilised society will offer services in proportion to the needs of those who may benefit from services. This sentiment has been more poetically expressed by Isabel Allende (1985), when she wrote 'They also forced me to eat. They divided up the servings with the strictest sense of justice, each according to her need'.

References

Allende I (1985) *The House of the Spirits*. Black Swan Books.

Andrews A, Knapp M, McCrone P, *et al* (2012) *Effective Interventions in Schizophrenia: The Economic Case. A Report Prepared for the Schizophrenia Commission*. Rethink Mental Illness.

Bebbington P, Brewin CR, Marsden L, *et al* (1996) Measuring the need for psychiatric treatment in the general population: the community version of the MRC Needs for Care Assessment. *Psychological Medicine*, **26**: 229–36.

Beecham J, Knapp M, Fenyo A (1993) Costs, needs and outcomes in community mental health care. In *Costing Community Care* (eds A Betten, J Beecham). Aldgate.

Beeforth M, Wood H (2001) Needs from a user perspective. In *Measuring Mental Health Needs* (2nd edition) (ed. G Thornicroft): 190–9. RCPsych Press.

Bird V, Le Boutillier C, Leamy M, *et al* (2012) Assessing the strengths of mental health service users – systematic review. *Psychological Assessment*, **24**: 1024–33.

Bradshaw J (1972) A taxonomy of social need. In *Problems and Progress in Medical Care* (Essays on Current Research, 7th series) (ed G McLachlan). Oxford University Press.

Brewin CR, Wing JK, Mangen SP, *et al* (1987) Principles and practice of measuring needs in the long-term mentally ill: the MRC Needs for Care Assessment. *Psychological Medicine*, **17**: 971–82.

Brewin CR, Wing J, Mangen S, *et al* (1988) Needs for care among the long-term mentally ill: a report from the Camberwell High Contact Survey. *Psychological Medicine*, **18**: 457–68.

Culyer A, Wagstaff A (1992) *Need, Equity and Equality in Health and Health Care*. Centre for Health Economics, Health Economics Consortium, University of York.

Drukker M, Bak M, Campo J, *et al* (2010) The cumulative needs for care monitor: a unique monitoring system in the south of the Netherlands. *Social Psychiatry and Psychiatric Epidemiology*, **45**: 475–85.

Drukker M, van Os J, Dietvorst M, *et al* (2011) Does monitoring need for care in patients diagnosed with severe mental illness impact on psychiatric service use? Comparison of monitored patients with matched controls. *BMC Psychiatry*, **11**: 45.

Fryers T, Greatorex N (1992) Case registers of service use and at risk groups. In *Measuring Mental Health Needs* (eds G Thornicroft, C Brewin, JK Wing). Gaskell.

Glover G (1996) Health service indictors for mental health. In *Commissioning Mental Health Services* (eds G Thornicroft, G Strathdee): 311–8. HMSO.

Goldman HH (1999) The obligation of mental health services to the least well off. *Psychiatric Services*, **50**: 659 63.

Hampson M, Killaspy H, Mynors-Wallis L, *et al* (2011) *Outcome Measures Recommended for Use in Adult Psychiatry* (Occasional Paper 78). Royal College of Psychiatrists.

Hancock GA, Reynolds T, Woods B, *et al* (2003) The needs of older people with mental health problems according to the user, the carer, and the staff. *International Journal of Geriatric Psychiatry*, **18**: 803–11.

Hansson L, Vinding HR, Mackeprang T, *et al* (2001) Comparison of key worker and patient assessment of needs in schizophrenic patients living in the community: a Nordic multicentre study. *Acta Psychiatrica Scandinavica*, **103**: 45–51.

Harty M, Shaw J, Thomas S, *et al* (2004) The security, clinical and social needs of patients in high security psychiatric hospitals in England. *Journal of Forensic Psychiatry and Psychology*, **15**: 208–21.

Herman D, Struening E, Barrow S (1993) Self-assessed need for mental health services among homeless adults. *Hospital and Community Psychiatry*, **44**: 1181–2.

Hogg LI, Marshall M (1992) Can we measure need in the homeless mentally ill? Using the MRC Needs for Care Assessment in hostels for the homeless. *Psychological Bulletin*, **18**: 321–3.

Holloway F (1994) Need in community psychiatry: a consensus is required. *Psychiatric Bulletin*, **18**: 321–3.

Howard L, Kumar R, Thornicroft G (2001) Psychosocial characteristics and needs of mothers with psychotic disorders. *British Journal of Psychiatry*, **178**: 427–32.

Howard L, Hunt K, Slade M, *et al* (2007) Assessing the needs of pregnant women and mothers with severe mental illness: the psychometric properties of the Camberwell Assessment of Need – Mothers (CAN-M). *International Journal of Methods in Psychiatric Research*, **16**: 177–85.

Howard L, Slade M, O'Keane V, *et al* (2008) *The Camberwell Assessment of Need for Pregnant Women and Mothers with Severe Mental Illness*. Gaskell.

Junghan UM, Leese M, Priebe S, *et al* (2007) Staff and patient perspectives on unmet need and therapeutic alliance in community mental health services. *British Journal of Psychiatry*, **191**: 543–7.

Lasalvia A, Ruggeri M, Mazzi MA, *et al* (2000) The perception of needs for care in staff and patients in community-based mental health services. The South-Verona Outcome Project 3. *Acta Psychiatrica Scandinavica*, **102**: 366–75.

Leamy M, Bird V, Le Boutillier C, *et al* (2011) A conceptual framework for personal recovery in mental health: systematic review and narrative synthesis. *British Journal of Psychiatry*, **199**: 445–52.

Leese M, Johnson S, Slade M, *et al* (1998) The user perspective on needs and satisfaction with mental health services: the PRiSM Psychosis Study 8. *British Journal of Psychiatry*, **173**: 409–15.

Lehtinen V, Joukamaa M, Jyrkinen E, *et al* (1990) Need for mental health services of the adult population in Finland. Results from the Mini Finland Health Survey. *Acta Psychiatrica Scandinavica*, **81**: 426–31.

Lesage AD, Fournier L, Cyr M, *et al* (1996) The reliability of the community version of the MRC Needs for Care Assessment. *Psychological Medicine*, **26**: 237–43.

Liss P (1990) *Health Care Need: Meaning and Measurement*. Linkoping, Studies in Arts and Science.

Lockwood A, Marshall M (2001) The Cardinal Needs Schedule – a standardised research instrument for measuring individual needs. In *Measuring Mental Health Needs* (2nd edition) (ed G Thornicroft). RCPsych Press.

Mallman CA, Marcus S (1980) Logical clarifications in the study of needs. In *Human Needs* (ed K Lederer). Oelgeschlager, Gunn & Hain.

Maslow A (1954) *Motivation and Personality*. Harper & Row.

Mavis B, Humphreys K, Stöffelmayr B (1993) Treatment needs and outcomes of two subtypes of homeless persons who abuse substances. *Hospital and Community Psychiatry*, **44**: 1185–7.

McCrone P, Strathdee G (1994) Needs not diagnosis: towards a more rational approach to community mental health resourcing in Great Britain. *International Journal of Social Psychiatry*, **40**: 79–86.

McCrone P, Leese M, Thornicroft G, *et al* (2000) Reliability of the Camberwell Assessment of Need – European Version. EPSILON Study 6. European psychiatric services: inputs linked to outcome domains and needs. *British Journal of Psychiatry*, **177** (suppl.): s34–40.

Mental Health Commission of Canada (2012) *Changing Directions, Changing Lives: The Mental Health Strategy for Canada*. Mental Health Commission of Canada.

Mitchell J, Dickey B, Liptzin B (1987) Bringing psychiatric patients into the medicare prospective payments system: alternatives to DRGs. *American Journal of Psychiatry*, **144**: 610–5.

National Institute for Mental Health in England (2008) *Outcomes Compendium*. NIMHE.

Oades L, Deane F, Crowe T, *et al* (2005) Collaborative recovery: an integrative model for working with individuals who experience chronic and recurring mental illness. *Australasian Psychiatry*, **13**: 279–84.

Orrell M (2003) *Camberwell Assessment of Need for the Elderly (CANE)*. Royal College of Psychiatrists.

Phelan M, Slade M, Thornicroft G, *et al* (1995) The Camberwell Assessment of Need: the validity and reliability of an instrument to assess the needs of people with severe mental illness. *British Journal of Psychiatry*, **167**: 589–95.

Pryce IG, Griffiths RD, Gentry RM, *et al* (1993) How important is the assessment of social skills in current long-stay in-patients? An evaluation of clinical response to needs for assessment, treatment, and care in a long-stay psychiatric in-patient population. *British Journal of Psychiatry*, **162**: 498–502.

Ramsay R, Thornicroft G, Johnson S, *et al* (1997) Levels of in-patient and residential provision throughout London. In *London's Mental Health* (eds S Johnson *et al*): 193–219. King's Fund.

Reynolds T, Orrell M (2001) Needs assessment in mental health care for older people. In *Measuring Mental Health Needs* (2nd edition) (ed G Thornicroft). RCPsych Press.

Reynolds T, Thornicroft G, Abas M, *et al* (2000) Camberwell Assessment of Need for the Elderly (CANE). Development, validity and reliability. *British Journal of Psychiatry*, **176**: 444–52.

Semrau M, van Ommeren M, Blagescu M, *et al* (2012) The development and psychometric properties of the Humanitarian Emergency Settings Perceived Needs (HESPER) Scale. *American Journal of Public Health*, **102**: e55–63.

Shapiro S, Skinner EA, Kramer M, *et al* (1985) Measuring need for mental health services in a general population. *Medical Care*, **23**: 1033–43.

Slade M (1994) Needs assessment: involvement of staff and users will help to meet need. *British Journal of Psychiatry*, **165**: 293–6.

Slade M (2012) An evidence-based approach to routine outcome assessment. *Advances in Psychiatric Treatment*, **18**: 180–2.

Slade M, McCrone P (2001) The Camberwell Assessment of Need (CAN). In *Measuring Mental Health Needs* (2nd edition) (ed G Thornicroft). RCPsych Press.

Slade M, Phelan M, Thornicroft G (1998) A comparison of needs assessed by staff and an epidemiologically representative sample of patients with psychosis. *Psychological Medicine*, **28**: 543–50.

Slade M, Thornicroft G, Phelan M, *et al* (1999a) *Camberwell Assessment of Need (CAN)*. Royal College of Psychiatrists.

Slade M, Beck A, Bindman J, *et al* (1999b) Routine clinical outcome measures for patients with severe mental illness: CANSAS and HoNOS. *British Journal of Psychiatry*, **174**: 404–8.

Slade M, Leese M, Taylor R, *et al* (1999c) The association between needs and quality of life in an epidemiologically representative sample of people with psychosis. *Acta Psychiatrica Scandinavica*, **100**: 149–57.

Slade M, Leese M, Ruggeri M, *et al* (2004) Does meeting needs improve quality of life? *Psychotherapy and Psychosomatics*, **73**: 183–9.

Slade M, Leese M, Cahill S, *et al* (2005) Patient-rated mental health needs and quality of life improvement. *British Journal of Psychiatry*, **187**: 256–61.

Slade M, Bird V, Le Boutillier C, *et al* (2011) REFOCUS Trial: protocol for a cluster randomised controlled trial of a pro-recovery intervention within community based mental health teams. *BMC Psychiatry*, **11**: 185.

Stevens A, Raftery J, Mendelsohn R (2001) The commissioners information requirements on mental health needs and commissioning for mental health services. In *Measuring Mental Health Needs* (2nd edition) (ed G Thornicroft). RCPsych Press.

311

Strathdee G, Thornicroft G (1992) Community sectors for needs-led mental health services. In *Measuring Mental Health Needs* (ed G Thornicroft): 140–62. Gaskell.

Thomas S, Harty MA, Parrott J, *et al* (eds) (2003) *The Forensic CAN: A Needs Assessment for Forensic Mental Health Service Users*. Gaskell.

Thomas S, Leese M, Dolan M, *et al* (2004) The individual needs of patients in high secure psychiatric hospitals in England. *Journal of Forensic Psychiatry and Psychology*, **15**: 222–43.

Thornicroft G (ed) (2001) *Measuring Mental Health Needs* (2nd edition). RCPsych Press.

Thornicroft G, Bebbington P (1996) Quantitative methods in the evaluation of community mental health services. In *Modern Community Psychiatry* (ed W Breakey). Cambridge University Press.

Thornicroft G, Slade M (2002) Comparing needs assessed by staff and by service users: paternalism or partnership in mental health? *Epidemiologia e Psichiatria Sociale*, **11**: 186–91.

Thornicroft G, Strathdee G (2001) Local catchment areas for needs-led mental health services. In *Measuring Mental Health Needs* (2nd edition) (ed G Thornicroft). RCPsych Press.

Thornicroft G, Strathdee G, Phelan M, *et al* (1998) Rationale and design. PRiSM Psychosis Study 1. *British Journal of Psychiatry*, **173**: 363–70.

Thornicroft G, Becker T, Knapp M, *et al* (2005) *International Outcome Measures in Mental Health. Quality of Life, Needs, Service Satisfaction, Costs and Impact on Carers*. Royal College of Psychiatrists.

Trauer T (2010) *Outcome Measurement in Mental Health: Theory and Practice*. Cambridge University Press.

Trauer T, Tobias G (2004) The Camberwell Assessment of Need and Behaviour and Symptom Identification Scale as routine outcome measures in a psychiatric disability rehabilitation and support service. *Community Mental Health Journal*, **40**: 211–21.

Trauer T, Tobias G, Slade M (2008) Development and evaluation of a patient-rated version of the Camberwell Assessment of Need Short Appraisal Schedule (CANSAS-P). *Community Mental Health Journal*, **44**: 113–24.

van Haaster I, Lesage A, Cyr M, *et al* (1994) Problems and needs for care of patients suffering from severe mental illness. *Social Psychiatry and Psychiatric Epidemiology*, **29**: 141–8.

Wing J (1992) *Epidemiologically Based Needs Assessment. Report 6. Mental Illness*. NHS Management Executive.

Xenitidis K, Bouras N (2001) Measurement of needs in people with learning disabilities and mental health problems. In *Measuring Mental Health Needs* (2nd edition) (ed G Thornicroft). RCPsych Press.

Xenitidis K, Thornicroft G, Leese M, *et al* (2000) Reliability and validity of the CANDID – a needs assessment instrument for adults with learning disabilities and mental health problems. *British Journal of Psychiatry*, **176**: 473–8.

Xenitidis K, Slade M, Thornicroft G, *et al* (2003) *Camberwell Assessment of Need for Adults with Developmental and Intellectual Disabilities (CANDID). A Comprehensive Needs Assessment Tool for People with Learning Disabilities and Mental Health Problems*. Royal College of Psychiatrists.

CHAPTER 21

Service users' expectations

Diana Rose

Patients are at the core of therapeutic encounters, yet often in psychiatric settings in particular they feel ignored. However, over the past few decades this has started to change, albeit far too slowly.

It is now a central plank of government policy that the NHS should be patient-driven, that there should be a high level of patient and public involvement in health services and that there should be a rapid expansion of choice. This represents a cultural shift and a rebalancing of power relations between patients and doctors. The Department of Health recognises that this is not easy, as doctors may not wish to hand over power to patients (Department of Health & Farrell, 2004). A further part of this cultural shift comes in the wake of the Francis inquiry into the failings of Mid Staffordshire NHS Foundation Trust. The report highlights the importance of the patient *experience* as of equal status to clinical outcomes (Francis, 2010).

In this context, there is a crucial dilemma for psychiatrists. The culture shift described above is supposed to be transferable to all medical disciplines and the mental health user movement has long struggled to bring this about in the psychiatric domain. It has to be said that there have been some successes here. The dilemma is that psychiatrists have the power to take all choice and control away from psychiatric patients by use of the Mental Health Act 1983. The 2007 amendments to the Act make the grounds for compulsory treatment wider and extended powers to compulsion in the community. Many psychiatrists were opposed to this, but it shows that government policy is pulling in two directions at once – more choice and involvement on the one hand and more control and coercion on the other.

In this chapter I will look at the mental health user movement, what it has achieved and what it has still to achieve. I will then look at research which has tried to determine what users want and do not want in terms of services, especially from psychiatrists. Much of this research has been user-led or carried out in collaboration with service user researchers. Finally, I will look at how the guidelines on the adult experience in mental healthcare from the National Institute for Health and Care Excellence (NICE, 2012) were formulated in collaboration with service users and focused on the patient experience, thus aligning with the more general concerns of the Francis inquiry.

The user movement

Campbell & Rose (2011) show how there have been protests by psychiatric patients since the days of Bedlam. At the end of the 19th century, John Perceval set up the Friends of the Alleged Lunatics Society to protest about the conditions in Victorian institutions. In the 1970s there were two small and very radical groups, the Mental Patients' Union (MPU) and the Campaign Against Psychiatric Oppression (CAPO). As the names suggest, they were highly critical of psychiatry and part of the radical culture of the time.

A new phenomenon that led to the rise of more user groups was the closure of the old asylums, with the re-provision of care in the community. A dozen user groups grew up across the country to make sure that that re-provision was working properly. These were mixed groups comprising users, carers and professionals. Later a 'user group' was taken to mean a group wholly made up of users or one where users held the majority in decision-making.

In the 1980s there were national user groups operating in the UK. The best-known was Survivors Speak Out, which campaigned for less use of medication, more information, non-medical crisis houses, more dignity for service users in hospitals and less stigma in society as a whole. The group drew up a patients' charter.

It is often said that the user movement is the child of consumerism – the market economies of Thatcher and Major, who took the view that people should stand on their on two feet and not rely on the 'nanny state'. Certainly the user movement grew exponentially at this time. In 1985 there were around 15 user groups but 20 years later there were over 700 (Wallcraft et al, 2004). The rise of local user groups saw the demise of the national radical ones and led to a much more practical approach, which we can call 'user involvement'. Where groups have funding, it often comes from statutory bodies and there is an expectation that the group will have some influence on the body. Whether this is real or window-dressing is a moot point; it is certainly complicated (Rose et al, 2014).

According to Wallcraft et al (2004) the commonest activity of user groups is self-help and mutual aid. The second most common activity is consultation with planners, policy-makers and mental health professionals. That users commonly consult with planners and policy-makers is a novelty worth commenting on and it is also not an easy process. Professionals may want to hear the authentic voice of experience but as soon as it becomes too authentic they pull back and relabel the person as ill. So, for today's user movement, what users expect from professionals, including psychiatrists, is to be listened to and have their views taken seriously, not only in their own care but sometimes at a strategic level. Consultation often takes the form of sitting on committees, and this can be intimidating for service users alone in such a situation. Use of jargon and acronyms makes proceedings incomprehensible and there always is the suspicion that decisions have been made already behind closed doors (or indeed in the canteen). Nevertheless, the fact that it has become possible for service users to occupy such high-status positions is a major advance. There is also some involvement at government level, intensified in the last 5 or 6 years by the emergence of the National Survivor and User Network (NSUN).

There are now active groups of patients in many medical specialties. But, as far as I know, the mental health service user movement was the first and remains the most sceptical, with the possible exception of young men living with HIV/AIDS (Epstein, 2000). This brings us back to the dilemma facing doctors described at the beginning of this chapter. For many service users in the field of mental health it is lack of power that prevents them having more influence. Power relations between psychiatrists and their patients are the most imbalanced in health services as a whole. From here comes the concept of 'empowerment', meaning that users themselves or in negotiation with their doctors need to take back control over their lives.

New understandings of mental health problems have been developed by the user movement and sustained through its various configurations. One such is the 'hearing voices' initiative, which began with the work of Romme & Escher (1993) in the Netherlands. These are organised as groups where people discuss their voices and are encouraged to come to terms with them. Many self-help initiatives now exist and align with the government's 'expert patient' programme, although they are often collaborations with professionals. A controversial idea is the self-harm network, which promotes 'safer self-harm' (Pembroke, 2005). Hearing voices and self-harm are regarded as serious problems by psychiatrists and it may seem odd to them that people in these situations can organise together to come to terms with their difficulties because they have not found traditional ways helpful. Perhaps it should be a lesson.

User-led research to produce evidence of what users expect from psychiatry

It is apparent that not all users are part of the movement described above. In fact, they are a small minority. In 2001, two reports were published that aimed to find out what 'ordinary' users want or do not want from services. These two reports came from user-led research teams based in large charities in London. The first was the Strategies for Living (S4L) team based at the Mental Health Foundation (Faulkner & Layzell, 2001). The second was the User-Focused Monitoring (UFM) team based at the Sainsbury Centre for Mental Health (Rose, 2001). Both these projects were user-controlled. Questionnaires or topic guides were devised by a group of users, which were then used as the basis for interviews with their peers. These service users were not experienced researchers. The coordinators of the projects taught them basic research skills, especially questionnaire construction and interviewing skills. The coordinators of the projects were also service users but in this case researchers as well. The difference between these two investigations was that S4L was largely qualitative while UFM was largely quantitative. In the following sections of this paper I will describe the issues that were most important to 'ordinary' service users.

Information

The single most important finding is that users want more information about and choice over a range of issues that affect their lives. One of these is medication, which I will discuss below. But users also want information about opportunities for work or leisure in their own localities. They want information about welfare benefits, which most are obliged to rely on, partly because of stigmatisation by employers which prevents them from securing jobs. The problem of welfare benefits and work is currently emotive in England, where there is a huge push to get people off welfare benefits and into work. Although many service users want to work, there are others who feel they cannot, especially in the current stigma-laden climate. These service users live in fear of officials deciding they must work and go to great lengths not to be 'found out'.

When in hospital and detained under the Mental Health Act, service users want more information about their rights. The first UFM team conducted site visits to four acute units and observed that there was scant information about the Mental Health Act or the Mental Health Commission on notice boards. Some of those interviewed said they had not had, or could not remember having, information leaflets about their section. Some users did not know whether they were voluntary or not, as practice in the units was applied universally, for example the right to leave. It did not seem to matter whether restricted leave was via section 17 of the Mental Health Act or not – everybody was subject to restricted leave. This mirrors the findings of the McArthur study, which showed that there was a discrepancy between actual coercion and perceived coercion in acute care (Lidz *et al*, 1995).

Medication

Users wanted more information and choice about medication, especially about dosage and side-effects. Those who received their medication from hospital pharmacies were the most frustrated in this respect, as they did not even receive an information sheet. Observation of hospital notice boards during UFM site visits revealed a lack of information leaflets about medication. Leaflets should explain what medication is for, the intended effects and the side-effects. Further, the S4L study found that users were ambivalent about taking medication. Many did take it but with misgivings about whether they really needed it or fear that withdrawal would be difficult. The UFM study found that when a doctor negotiated medication with a user, that person was happier overall with their mental healthcare. The most important aspects of this negotiation that were reported were what the medication was for and its side-effects. In the UFM study, 30% of people said they were overmedicated.

Medication has been an issue for activists for many years, and some psychiatrists have said that this is unimportant as activists are 'unrepresentative'. It is interesting, then, that the people in these two studies expressed the same concerns about medication that activists do and have done for a long time. The implication for psychiatrists is that they should provide full information about medication and negotiate with their patients about dosage and side-effects. Psychiatrists need to take account of a person's life circumstances. For example, it is counterproductive to ask someone to take highly sedative medication if they are in work and need to be alert for the working day. Psychiatrists should think carefully about dosage. Patients want the minimum effective dose and to avoid unwanted effects. It is alarming that nearly one-third of the participants in the UFM research felt overmedicated.

The Care Programme Approach

The UFM project found that most of the users interviewed were not aware of the Care Programme Approach (CPA), did not know who their keyworker was and did not know they had a care plan. Still less were they involved in drawing up their care plan or getting involved in setting up their review. Not a single person knew they could take an advocate to that review. The original UFM work was done in the late 1990s but more recent UFM work has had similar findings (Gould, 2012). This is despite a government review in 2008. The issue of involvement, in particular, seems intractable.

When presented at a workshop for rehabilitation workers who came from the more 'progressive' end of the profession, these findings did not come as a surprise. The participants said that patients were not interested in their care plan. When asked how long it had taken for them to learn about the CPA and then how long they had spent explaining it to their clients, the typical response was a 2- or 3-day course for the professionals. But some of them had not explained the CPA at all to their clients and the typical time spent on this discussion was 10 minutes. Such a discrepancy indicates an unhealthy and continuing power imbalance between professionals and their clients.

Involvement in individual care was covered by both the UFM and the S4L projects. Users did not feel involved in their care. However, the UFM work found that on the rare occasions when users were involved in their own care – drawing up care plans, arranging review meetings – they were more satisfied overall with their treatment.

Care coordinators generally see service users more frequently than users see their psychiatrist. Sometimes users see their psychiatrist only at CPA meetings and maybe once in between for follow-up. So this is an important occasion and the meeting should be taken very seriously, and should involve the service user as much as possible. He or she should not have to sign a care plan drawn up in advance of the meeting but should be asked about needs and preferences for care.

In-patient treatment

As already explained, the UFM project sometimes conducted site visits to hospitals or interviewed people about their experience of in-patient care. As with the questionnaires for community care, the questions for the site visits or interviews were drawn up by a group of service users. These service users had experienced in-patient care. Some of the questions they constructed were very basic indeed, but they came from the experience of people who had been in hospital themselves. For example, they asked whether people could get a drink when they wanted one and whether there was privacy in terms of sleeping areas. They also asked whether rights under the Mental Health Act had been respected and I have touched on this already in terms of information.

During site visits the team would observe the ward and also interview anyone who was prepared to be interviewed. The basic questions described above were discovered to be relevant. Kitchens were often locked and drinks provided at set times. Where there were water coolers they were usually empty and there were no cups. This is important, as the side-effects of medication can include a very dry mouth. In terms of privacy, many wards had dormitories with only thin and torn curtains between the beds. Staff were criticised for being inaccessible, staying in the office unless an incident occurred.

Perhaps the single most important thing that in-patients experience is crushing boredom. There is little to do, especially in the evenings and at weekends. Some units had gyms but patients could not use them as there was no one to staff them. A further feature of the boring nature of acute wards was the lack of access to fresh air. Even where a psychiatrist had given permission for someone to have escorted leave, the staff would say they did not have the capacity to provide someone to do the escorting. This sometimes meant that patients had to remain on stuffy wards for days on end with no access to fresh air.

These points are relevant for psychiatrists. Although trainees may spend more time on the wards, a large number of consultants generally come on the ward only once or twice a week for ward rounds. Psychiatrists may be unaware of what it is like to be on a ward in a routine way. They may not know that basic rights and dignity are not being respected, that patients have nothing to do or that the escorted leave agreed by the psychiatrist is not being carried out. In any event, many patients find ward rounds intimidating, especially in teaching hospitals when rounds are attended by students. In this context, service users may be reluctant to raise issues.

Moving on in research into in-patient care

The UFM work described above was conducted nearly 20 years ago. Have things changed? Anecdote says not. Although physical facilities may be better, there is still nothing to do and a 'them and us' culture prevails. To test an intervention that might improve in-patient care, an as yet unpublished study introduced therapeutic activities into the in-patient units of a metropolitan NHS mental health trust. The primary outcome measure used to test the effectiveness of the intervention was wholly patient-generated (Evans *et al*, 2012). This measure, called VOICE, is one of a suite of patient-generated patient-reported outcome measures (PG-PROMs) developed by the Service User Research Enterprise (SURE) at King's College London. PROMs are much talked about currently but the questions in routine PROMs are hardly ever devised by patients or service users: they are 'patient-reported' only in the sense that patients fill them in. The SURE used a participatory methodology to develop its PG-PROMs (Rose *et al*, 2011).

I will now briefly describe how VOICE was created, in order to demonstrate how the patient voice is put into research so that we know what users would like from services. The method is rigorous and also participatory. The process began with focus groups which met twice. All participants in the focus groups had been in acute wards in the local trust in the previous 2 years. One group was specifically for people who had been detained, although in the event all groups included participants who had experienced compulsory treatment. Of the two group facilitators, one had experienced in-patient treatment, including under compulsion (this was the current author), and the second was also a service user researcher. These researchers made use of their 'double identity' as both service users and researchers to facilitate a patient-generated and valued measure. On the basis of the focus group discussions, which were recorded and transcribed, a draft measure was constructed. This was then taken to 'expert panels', one drawn from focus group members and the second completely new but also made up of participants who had been in-patients in the previous 2 years. Quite a few changes were made, which is usually the case with PG-PROMs. The third stage is to run a feasibility study to find out whether the measure is easy to complete; this runs iteratively until we are sure we have a user-friendly questionnaire. The final stage of measure generation is psychometric testing. It is important to point out that we did the psychometric analysis for VOICE with acute psychiatric hospital in-patients, most of whom had a diagnosis of psychosis. This might be thought to compromise procedures such as establishing test–retest reliability. In fact, the standard psychometrics were better than is typically the case; for example, Cronbach's alpha was 0.9. This raises the question of whether the measure was user-friendly because it had been produced using a participatory, user-focused methodology. In addition, the measure had a different factor structure to a more mainstream measure, in that it contained a factor of 'security' while the mainstream one foregrounded the physical environment. Security and safety were of paramount concern in the focus groups and this was a factor in the final VOICE measure.

VOICE is very much a measure of the *experience* of in-patient care. It is about relations with staff, and safety and security, and the issues that arose are not new but they are more robustly developed. This is what the participants spontaneously produced.

Suffice to say that service user research has matured and now provides rigorous and rich material on which to make recommendations for practice. This was done in the NICE guidelines on adult mental health, to which I now turn.

NICE guidance on the service user experience

This guidance (NICE, 2011) was focused on the patient experience, of which I have made much. Perhaps the most interesting thing about it was the nature of its formulation, which was unique for NICE. The Guidance Development Group was evenly split between service users and providers and there were two chairs – one a service user researcher (the current author) and one a clinical academic psychiatrist. A 'generic' guidance document was prepared at the same time but although it had patient representation there was not equal representation as in the mental health one.

The guidance was structured around pathways to care and it included 15 quality statements. Most of these would not cost money to bring about; rather, they focused on attitudinal and cultural questions and the kind of dilemmas I discussed at the beginning of this chapter. They focused on issues such as dignity and respect and being treated in an atmosphere of optimism. It is perhaps salutary that this still needs to be said, as the need for such statements means that current care is falling short of providing for service users' basic human rights. Psychiatrists need to take note of this. However, the Guideline Development Group also recognised the powers of coercion that exist in psychiatry and the fact that there arise situations where dignity, respect and optimism cannot be maintained. Such would be control, restraint and rapid tranquillisation, for example. Recommendations were made for ameliorating this but in full knowledge that a sharp power differential could never be dissolved. Perhaps psychiatrists need to recognise when they write up prescriptions for intramuscular medications that the actual administration is traumatic for the patient. Many no doubt do so but they often are not present to witness what it is actually like. It can be traumatic for staff too, although some appear to be immune.

Finally, the Guideline Development Group recommended that service users should be involved in monitoring services and that service user research, of the kind discussed above, should be encouraged.

Conclusion

From the above discussion, and especially the findings of service user research, we can summarise what it is that users would like to see their psychiatrist providing. They would like more information and choice – about medication, financial matters and leisure opportunities. They also would like more information if they are detained under the Mental Health Act. They would like to negotiate with their doctor instead of being treated like passive subjects. They would like this negotiation especially in respect of medication and the CPA. They would like their psychiatrist to know more about what routinely goes on in the ward. The important elements are rights, dignity and safety, and relations with staff. My sense in writing this is that I have been writing it for over two decades now, so why does it still need saying? Something about psychiatric services seems intractable, at least at the sharp end. Personally I am not enamoured of the recovery movement in its professionalised form, but I could be wrong. I would rather see a rebalancing of power relations between psychiatrists and their patients and an acknowledgement that both parties have expertise. The impact of any NICE guidance is a moot question but perhaps the developments described above will facilitate this rebalancing of power.

References

Campbell P, Rose D (2011) Action for change in the UK: thirty years of the user/survivor movement. In *The SAGE Handbook of Mental Health and Illness* (eds D Pilgrim, A Rogers, B Pescosolido): pp 452–71. Sage.

Department of Health, Farrell C (2004) *Patient and Public Involvement in Health*. Department of Health.

Epstein S (2000) Democracy, expertise and AIDS treatment activism. In *Science, Technology and Democracy* (ed DL Kleinman): pp 3–32. State University of New York Press.

Evans J, Rose D, Flach C, *et al* (2012) VOICE: developing a new measure of service users' perceptions of inpatient care, using a participatory methodology. *Journal of Mental Health*, **21**: 57–71.

Faulkner A, Layzell A (2001) *Strategies for Living*. Mental Health Foundation.

Francis R (2010) *Independent Inquiry into Care Provided by Mid Staffordshire NHS Foundation Trust January 2005–March 2009* (vol. 375). TSO (The Stationery Office).

Gould D (2012) *Service Users' Experiences of Recovery Under the 2008 Care Programme Approach*. NSUN and Mental Health Foundation.

Lidz CW, Hoge SK, Gardner W, *et al* (1995) Perceived coercion in mental hospital admission: pressures and process. *Archives of General Psychiatry*, **52**: 1034.

NICE (2011) *Service User Experience in Adult Mental Health*. British Psychological Society & Royal College of Psychiatrists.

Pembroke LR (2005) *Self-Harm*. Chipmunka Publishing.

Romme M, Escher S (1993) *Accepting Voices*. MIND.

Rose D (2001) *Users' Voices: The Perspectives of Mental Health Service Users on Community and Hospital Care*. Sainsbury Centre for Mental Health.

Rose D, Evans J, Sweeney A, *et al* (2011) A model for developing outcome measures from the perspectives of mental health service users. *International Review of Psychiatry*, **23**: 41–6.

Rose D, Barnes M, Crawford, M, *et al* (2014) How do managers and leaders in the National Health Service and social care respond to service user involvement in mental health services in both its traditional and emergent forms? The ENSUE study. *Health Services and Delivery Research*, **2** (doi: 10.3310/hsdr02100).

Wallcraft J, Read J, Sweeney A (2004) *On Our Own Terms*. Sainsbury Centre for Mental Health.

CHAPTER 22

Clinical audit

Adrian James

Clinical audit is a central component of clinical governance and is the principal tool for providers and patients to find out if healthcare is being delivered to the required standard and continuously improves. It is defined by the National Institute for Health and Care Excellence (NICE) as:

> 'a quality improvement process that seeks to improve patient care and outcomes through systematic review of care against explicit criteria and the implementation of change. Aspects of the structure, processes, and outcomes of care are selected and systematically evaluated against explicit criteria. Where indicated, changes are implemented at an individual, team, or service level and further monitoring is used to confirm improvement in healthcare delivery.' (NICE, 2002)

Participation in clinical audit by hospital doctors was made mandatory with the publication of *A First Class Service* (Department of Health, 1998) and is a requirement of *Good Psychiatric Practice* (Royal College of Psychiatrists, 2009). Psychiatrists should 'participate in clinical audit to measure and improve clinical care provided by themselves and their team'. It is a prerequisite for revalidation (General Medical Council, 2012). Done well, it can lead to significant and sustained improvement in outcomes for users but at its worst it can be a time-consuming, demoralising waste, with no clear benefits, while diverting precious clinical time away from patients. The report of the public inquiry into Mid Staffordshire NHS Foundation Trust (Francis, 2013) marked a sentinel moment in quality improvement with a demand to put the quality of patient care, and especially patient safety, above all other aims; it reaffirmed the primacy of clinical audit in this process. Don Berwick asserted that mastery of quality and patient safety science and practices should be part of the initial preparation and lifelong education of not only healthcare professionals but also managers and executives (National Advisory Group on the Safety of Patients in England, 2013). He went on to highlight the 'most single important change' in the NHS would be for it to become 'a system devoted to continual learning and improvement of patient care, top to bottom and end to end'.

This chapter provides a framework to ensure that clinical audit is a worthwhile component of the quality improvement toolkit and meets the challenges set out by Francis and Berwick that will set the agenda for healthcare for the coming decade.

History

Clinicians have for millennia audited outcomes and it is reported that King Hammurabi of Babylon in 1750 BC instigated audit for clinicians with regard to outcome, with hazardous consequences for those not performing well (Copeland, 2005). Medical audit became part of mainstream practice in the NHS after the publication of *Working for Patients* (Department of Health, 1989); in recognition of the multidisciplinary nature of healthcare delivery, it became 'clinical audit' in the 1990s (Department of Health, 1997). Clinical audit can be considered the first pillar of clinical governance to be erected. It was a key component of the Commission for Healthcare Improvement's clinical governance reviews and continues to provide potentially important information that could trigger an inspection as part of the Care Quality Commission's inspection process.

Clinical audit in practice

Clinical audit is a cyclical activity that starts with the establishment of clear standards in healthcare; it then investigates these intended standards to see whether they are delivered in practice, investigates the performance gap, initiates change in practice and re-audits to ensure that real change happens. The audit cycle is illustrated in Fig. 22.1.

Several stages must be completed to carry out successful audit. These include:

- preparation – topic selection, identifying relevant individuals to carry out the audit, identifying technical support and ensuring those involved are appropriately trained
- criteria selection – identifying the process or outcome of care to be audited, ensuring that criteria are explicit, measurable and related to important aspects of care
- measuring performance – finding relevant sources of data, such as patient registers, collecting relevant data
- increasingly open publication of audit results – for instance cardiac surgeons have a public database of their individual results and mortality data (Royal College of Surgeons of England, 2014)
- making improvements – feedback of results to relevant individuals, dissemination in a variety of ways and agreement with key stakeholders (including users) as to what needs to be done to improve care
- sustaining improvement – continued monitoring and evaluation of improvement, setting up structures to ensure that improvements in care are integrated into clinical governance programmes.

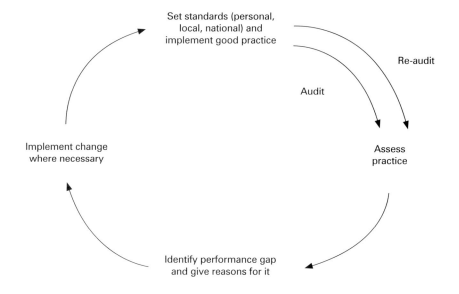

Fig. 22.1   The audit cycle

Organisation and resources

Clinical audit has a national structure. National Clinical Audit and Patient Outcomes Programme (NCAPOP) audits are commissioned on behalf of NHS England by the Healthcare Quality Improvement Partnership (HQIP). This includes more than 30 national audits. The National Audit and Governance Group (NAGG) provides a coordinating hub for regional networks and acts as the principal liaison with key stakeholders such as the Royal Colleges. The National Advisory Group for Clinical Audit and Enquiries (NAGCAE) is the main voice for clinical audit at NHS England and tries to provide a resource for NHS staff involved with clinical audit and generally to act as a bridge between the centre and the periphery.

The College Centre for Quality Improvement (CCQI) based at the Royal College of Psychiatrists runs the national programme of audits for mental health. Its current programme comprises:

- the National Audit of Psychological Therapies for Anxiety and Depression
- the National Audit of Dementia (care in general hospitals)
- the National Audit of Schizophrenia (NAS)
- the Prescribing Observatory for Mental Health (POMH-UK)
- the Memory Clinics Audit.

In response to the Francis report (2013), NAGCAE suggested that each healthcare organisation should have a board-level chief quality officer

---

Box 22.1 Membership of a clinical audit committee

- Chair/senior clinician
- User/carer representative
- Clinical audit leads from localities/directorates/services
- Representation from all disciplines
- Clinical audit manager
- Clinical audit facilitator(s)
- Information management and technology representative
- Training and development representative
- Social care representative
- Clinical effectiveness representative

(CQO), mirroring arrangements in the USA. The role of the CQO would be to provide oversight, vision, inspiration and leadership for quality improvement across the three domains of quality: effectiveness, safety and experience.

In order to progress clinical audit in a systematic way, healthcare organisations will need either a free-standing clinical audit committee, or have clinical audit as a major component within another committee such as that dealing with clinical effectiveness. The committee, in order to maintain a clinical focus, will need to be led by a senior clinician, and to have representation from across the organisation and across grades, be truly multidisciplinary and be supported by a clinical audit infrastructure. Suggested members are listed in Box 22.1.

It is essential to work with users and carers to ensure co-production and ownership of the audit process and programme as well as the actions following analysis of results. Good links with information management and technology and training departments are vital, and with the other areas of governance. Clinical audit must be seen as a methodology to be used by the other areas of governance and intrinsic to their workings.

A clinical audit programme will require both clinical leadership and effective management of clinical audit resources. It is usual to have a clinical audit manager, who may manage other areas of governance, with facilitators and audit clerks working as part of a combined department. Other models can include facilitators being embedded in directorates. This has the advantage of a closer link-up with the clinical interface but can result in isolation for the facilitators.

Each audit will need an identified lead, working with an audit project team which includes technical support, stakeholders who are involved in bringing about change and a range of people who fully understand the process of clinical care. The clinical audit department will need to arrange an ongoing programme of training, with set-piece training days that individuals from across health organisations can come to, but training within teams should also be provided.

It is essential that the clinical audit department has a budget. Each service and locality will need their own clinical audit lead.

Key tasks for the clinical audit committee include ensuring that audit is effectively supported. A priority should be to ensure that audit meets appropriate criteria, that performance monitoring is implemented and that feedback uses the Care Quality Commission's outcome standards as a framework. The production of a strategy, annual report and work plan, with clear actions and time scales, is also necessary.

Programme

In practice, nationally prescribed audits tend to dominate audit programmes. Organisation-led audits take second place and local teams often feel that bottom-up audits never see the light of day. It is best to find an equal balance between these three tiers and ensure that, whatever the origin, the process puts service users at the centre. An effective framework for prioritising audits is presented in Box 22.2.

Audit topics are inevitably dictated to some degree by the state of maturity of the audit environment within the organisation. While audit infrastructure is evolving, the selection of bottom-up straightforward audit by motivated staff can be prudent. As confidence, support and sophistication develop and the benefits of audit are plain for all to see, more ambitious topics can be taken on. Audit can be undertaken at various levels, from individual practice to team, service, trust and regional or national audits. Topics are suggested in Box 22.3.

A key aspect to all audits is the setting of standards for each topic, and audit should not be seen as merely a monitoring exercise. Care should be delivered according to the evidence of effective practice. Geddes (2005) suggests five stages in applying evidence-based practice:

Box 22.2 Priority areas for clinical audit

- Nationally prescribed topic
- Corporately mandated topic
- Topic identified by service users as an area of concern or where change is necessary
- Topic in an area where there is evidence of a serious quality problem
- Topic provides good evidence to inform standards (e.g. national clinical guidelines)
- Topic is concerned with risk to staff or users
- Topic addresses a high-cost activity
- Topic is linked to national priorities or guidance

Box 22.3 Clinical audit topics in psychiatry

- Record-keeping
- Care Programme Approach documentation
- Customer care (e.g. information for patients)
- Timeliness of interventions
- Critical incident/sentinel event audit (e.g. following suicide)
- Emergency readmissions
- Mental Health Act documentation (e.g. consent to treatment)
- NICE guidelines (e.g. on schizophrenia)

Box 22.4 Online sources of evidence in mental health practice

- Royal College of Psychiatrists, http://www.rcpsych.ac.uk
- Cochrane Library, http://www.cochranelibrary.com
- *Evidence-Based Mental Health*, http://ebmh.bmj.com
- *BMJ Clinical Evidence*, http://www.clinicalevidence.com/x/index.html
- National Service Framework, https://www.gov.uk/government/uploads/system/uploads/attachment_data/file/198051/National_Service_Framework_for_Mental_Health.pdf
- National Institute for Health and Care Excellence, https://www.nice.org.uk/
- Mental Health Partnerships, http://mentalhealthpartnerships.com/

- Ask a structured answerable clinical question.
- Find the evidence.
- Critically appraise the evidence.
- Apply the evidence to the clinical problem.
- Assess and improve the process.

Sources of evidence are listed in Box 22.4.

Making a difference

Clinical audit is a pointless and even damaging enterprise unless real improvements in patient care result. Problems often arise from not applying robust criteria for topics, lack of clear objectives and ill-defined outcomes. Achieving real benefit is often thwarted by lack of engagement with stakeholders, poorly conceived plans to change practice and failure to re-audit and review. Good examples of successful audits can be found in *101 Recipes for Audit in Psychiatry* (Oakley *et al*, 2011) and top tips are given in Box 22.5. Much depends upon creating the right environment, in terms of structure and culture, to allow audit to flourish. Good project design is at the heart of all quality improvement and this starts with effective strategy,

> **Box 22.5** Top tips for effective audit
>
> - Good project design
> - Preparation
> - Involving stakeholders in the audit and outcomes
> - Topic selection
> - Use of clinical audit facilitators
> - A venue to present audits to a wider stakeholder group
> - Action points from audits discussed at wider clinical governance meetings and regularly updated
> - User involvement
> - Information technology representation on audit committee and use of web space
> - End-of-year audit of audits to progress action points
> - Underpinning communication strategy

setting appropriate priorities and topic selection. A culture must be created where practice is critically examined and professionals feel able to say that they are getting it wrong. At the heart of all good audits lies user and carer involvement, along with the involvement of those whose practice is likely to change as a result of the audit, so that all key stakeholders buy into not only the audit itself but also the outcomes. Many methodologically sound audits flounder because not enough effort is put into communicating findings and achieving positive change. If action points entail just shouting at the system or mere assertion that certain practices must change, then little effective change is likely to happen. Education and training must underpin performance advancement.

Ethics

Ethical consideration should apply to all medical practice. However, audit is often excluded from the remit of research ethics committees. In order to avoid the minefield of ethical consideration, there is an ongoing temptation to label research as audit (Warlow, 2004).

Research investigates what should be done, whereas audit investigates whether it is being done. The reason for distinguishing between the two should not be to avoid appropriate ethical scrutiny. All clinical audit and quality improvement activities require ethical oversight by a group or individual firmly rooted in the governance of a healthcare organisation. The degree of ethical scrutiny will depend on the likely balance of risks and benefits and only rarely should reference need to be made to a formally constituted ethics committee. All healthcare organisations must have a policy in place on ethics and clinical audit. The Healthcare Quality Improvement Partnership (Dixon, 2011) gives helpful advice on the contents of such a policy.

> **Box 22.6** Circumstances requiring external ethical scrutiny of audit
>
> - Degree of conflict arising from competing interests of the investigator, clinician or other responsible party is great
> - Burden on the patient is great (time, effort and discomfort)
> - Risks are moderate to high
> - Potential benefit to the patient is likely to be small
> - Low likelihood of audit succeeding in its stated aim
> - Potential benefit for society is likely to be small

Box 22.6 lists some circumstances where clinical audit *is* likely to require external ethical scrutiny.

A further issue is confidentiality. If changes are to occur, then findings need wide dissemination. Patients' identifiable data must be anonymised or their specific consent obtained. Individual practitioners must be anonymised within findings unless they have agreed, in advance, to named dissemination to a wider audience. This is becoming much more accepted practice, especially in the surgical community. However, if data are clinician-anonymised, it is still important that the clinicians themselves are given individual feedback.

Future developments

The future for clinical audit depends upon the full implementation of both the Francis and Berwick recommendations. Clinical audit is likely to underpin all quality improvement processes. Much will depend upon mental health services' abilities to continue to develop robust standards and indicators, and to improve information management and technology, in order to provide both an effective tool in the quest for quality and a framework to bring about change. Quality improvement is at the heart of audit. As methodology and analysis become more sophisticated, the possibility has been raised for routinely collected hospital data and audit findings to be used to anticipate or predict poor performance on the part of individuals or services, so that wider interventions can be implemented before major harm is done (Harley *et al*, 2005). This is a fine aspiration but the Francis inquiry showed that much still needs to be done to develop robust systems to enable this to happen.

Many services are moving towards 'plan–do–study–act' (PDSA) cycles (see Chapter 18) as a form of rapid audit (and re-audit). This quality improvement methodology emanates from the Institute for Healthcare Improvement in Boston and was developed by Langley *et al* (2009) using the 'Model for Improvement' approach. It empowers small groups of front-line staff who manage direct healthcare processes to plan and implement change, study the results and swiftly modify processes where necessary, and to repeat the procedure several times to accelerate service improvement. It has transformed many areas of healthcare, particularly in high-risk areas, and is increasingly applied in mental health settings.

References

Copeland G (2005) *A Practical Handbook for Clinical Audit*. Clinical Governance Support Team.

Department of Health (1989) *Working for Patients*. HMSO.

Department of Health (1998) *A First Class Service. Quality in the New NHS*. Department of Health.

Department of Health (1997) *The New NHS: Modern, Dependable*. TSO (The Stationery Office).

Dixon N (2011) *Ethics and Clinical Audit and Quality Improvement (QI): A Guide for NHS Organisations*. Healthcare Quality Improvement Partnership.

Francis R (2013) *Report of the Mid Staffordshire NHS Foundation Trust Public Inquiry. Final Report* (Francis report). Mid Staffordshire NHS Foundation Trust Public Inquiry.

Geddes J (2005) Evidence-based practice. In *Clinical Governance in Mental Health and Learning Disability Services. A Practical Guide* (eds A James, A Worrall, T Kendall): pp 149–58. Royal College of Psychiatrists.

General Medical Council (2012) *Supporting Information for Appraisal and Revalidation*. GMC.

Harley M, Mohammed M, Hussain S, *et al* (2005) Was Rodney Ledward a statistical outlier? Retrospective analysis using routine hospital data to identify gynaecologists performance. *BMJ*, **330**: 929–33.

Langley GL, Nolan KM, Nolan TW, *et al* (2009) *The Improvement Guide: A Practical Approach to Enhancing Organizational Performance* (2nd edition). Jossey Bass.

National Advisory Group on the Safety of Patients in England (2013) *A Promise to Learn – A Commitment To Act. Improving the Safety of Patients in England* (Berwick report). Department of Health.

NICE (2002) *Principles for Best Practice in Clinical Audit*. Radcliffe Medical Press.

Oakley C, Coccia F, Masson N, *et al* (2011) *101 Recipes for Audit in Psychiatry*. Royal College of Psychiatrists.

Royal College of Psychiatrists (2009) *Good Psychiatric Practice* (CR154). Royal College of Psychiatrists.

Royal College of Surgeons of England (2014) *Measuring Surgical Outcomes*. Royal College of Surgeons of England.

Warlow C (2004) Clinical research under the cosh again. This time it is ethics committees. *BMJ*, **329**: 241–2.

CHAPTER 23

Confidentiality and management in healthcare organisations

Gwen Adshead, Roy McClelland and Mike Kingham

Leadership in organisations involves the management of boundaries between different people in different types of relationship. Many of the ethical dilemmas about confidentiality that arise for managers involve tensions between two different kinds of professional space (e.g. should what I learn in this space be told in another?) or tensions between conflicting professional obligations. In this chapter, we review some of these dilemmas and suggest ways of thinking about them.

There is limited guidance for psychiatrists on confidentiality, despite the range of guidance and training on information governance. The only national-level guidance is the advice produced by the General Medical Council (GMC, 2009) and the Royal College of Psychiatrists (2010, but under revision). There is also an NHS code of practice on confidentiality (Department of Health, 2003), which still has advisory force, and NHS England issued a policy statement on confidentiality. All of these are freely available online.

The GMC has advised that each discipline needs to develop guidance that deals in appropriately greater detail with situations of particular concern and relevance; for psychiatry, this would include concerns about reporting to multi-agency public protection arrangements (MAPPA) and multidisciplinary working. What we discuss here are the general ethical, legal and professional principles that underpin the management of personal information in the NHS across the UK (including Scotland and Northern Ireland). This chapter has no legal standing and if faced with a dilemma about sharing information, we advise discussion with senior colleagues, the Caldicott guardian and information governance staff.

Confidentiality: the ethical context

The principle of confidentiality has a lengthy history in medical ethics. The ethical duty to respect this principle is usually grounded in terms of the beneficial consequences of doing so. Keeping patient information confidential benefits the patient by promoting trust between doctor and patient, which is in the patient's interest because it promotes the type of frank discussion that is essential to any therapeutic encounter. If the patient does not feel able to trust the doctor with information, this may mean that the doctor's clinical opinion is compromised in a way that may harm the patient.

However, respect for confidentiality is also grounded in something of arguably more meaning than just the good consequences. In the age of the internet, social media and search engine monitoring, control of personal information that constitutes personal identity has never been more important. Now, for most of us, when we give away personal information, we are giving away something of ourselves. In the domain of healthcare, we make ourselves vulnerable when we give away our secrets to a doctor, especially in psychiatry, when we may be disclosing information that is shameful or traumatic. So the principle of confidentiality is as much about protection of the vulnerable as it is about the consequences of keeping confidences. The tradition of confidentiality probably arose in order to stop doctors gossiping, as much as to promote clinical dialogue.

The idea that patients entrust doctors with something precious when they disclose information about themselves finds support from the requirement that we get consent from patients before we share their information with others (i.e. it is not ours to do with as we please). Getting consent for disclosure is an act of respect for the autonomy of the patient, without which we do the patient a wrong, not just a harm. It is arguable that it makes more sense to conceptualise the whole discussion of confidentiality as really being about the process of getting consent to disclose information, and what professionals should do when patients refuse to disclose information: information that may help others or may prevent harm.

Lastly, vulnerability is a key issue in confidentiality because preventing harm to the vulnerable is the commonest justification for disclosing clinical information. The most obvious examples are the requirements of child protection legislation (GMC, 2012), where doctors are expected to disclose clinical information about their patients in the interests of children, as a matter of good practice. It is children's vulnerability to exploitation that justifies the breaching of the principle of confidentiality.

Confidentiality: law and policy

The common law in the UK assumes that doctors hold a duty of confidence to their patients. Most of the legal advice on confidentiality is based on cases that make up the common law, and not on specific statutes. Breach of medical confidence is a legal wrong in its own right but also may be evidence of clinical negligence.

The Human Rights Act 1998 allows individuals to pursue claims in UK courts for established torts such as breach of confidence or to bring an action against a public authority on the basis of the right to privacy under Article 8 of the European Convention on Human Rights. The Human

Rights Act underpins other legislation concerned with confidentiality – public authorities are required to construe the legislation under which they operate in accordance with the Convention and to ensure that their actions and those of their staff are consistent with it.

The Data Protection Act (DPA) 1998 gave effect in UK law to the European Union Directive 95/46/EC and introduced eight data protection principles that set out standards of information processing or handling. The term 'processing' includes the collection, use and disclosure of personal data. The DPA is now a central plank in the statutory framework underpinning confidentiality in the UK.

Clinical information management

The first data protection principle states that:

> 'personal data shall be processed fairly, lawfully and shall not be processed unless at least one of the conditions in Schedule 2 is met and in the case of sensitive personal data at least one of the conditions in Schedule 3 is also met'.

Schedule 2 requires that processing (use) is necessary for the exercise of functions of a public nature exercised in the public interest by any person. Schedule 3 requires that processing is with the consent of the data subject, or that:

> 'the processing is necessary for medical purposes and is undertaken by a health professional (or a person owing a duty of confidentiality equivalent to that owed by a health professional)'.

The term 'medical purposes' includes preventive medicine, medical diagnosis, medical research, the provision of care and treatment, and the management of healthcare services.

If processing takes place without consent, data controllers (doctors frequently) must be able to show that it will not be possible to achieve their purposes with a reasonable degree of ease without the processing of 'personal' data. The Information Commission is the independent authority for the UK set up to oversee and regulate information rights and data handling, including any queries about data handling and 'freedom of information' requests. It is led by the Information Commissioner. The Commissioner takes the view that when considering the issue of necessity, data controllers must consider objectively whether such purposes can be achieved only by the processing of personal data and whether the processing is proportional to the aim pursued.

There is an obligation on doctors who are data controllers to provide certain information to data subjects when they collect their personal data. This information is often referred to as 'fair processing information'. We should ensure that our patients are provided with the relevant information indicating the purpose or purposes for which their clinical information is typically used. For example, patients are likely to expect that basic information will be recorded on diagnosis and treatment. They may, however, by surprised to find that other information has been recorded, for example the circumstances surrounding an injury.

Patients require information as to specific disclosures. Given the sensitivity of medical information, a patient should be informed of any non-routine disclosures of their information. Patients must be given information as to whether any secondary uses or disclosures are optional. Where patients have choices, these should be brought to their attention. The Commissioner points out that patients who will have their personal data processed for additional purposes will need to be provided with this further information in order to satisfy 'the fair processing' requirements.

While the DPA does not provide any guidance on the meaning of the term 'lawful', the principle means that the data controller must comply with all relevant rules of law whether derived from statute or common law. In 2002, the then Information Commissioner, Elizabeth France, provided a comprehensive treatment of this issue. In relation to the requirement to process data lawfully, she writes 'The key issue for the processing of health data is likely to be the common law duty of confidence' (France, 2002: p. 11). Most relevantly, she stated that 'The duty of confidence is a common law concept rather than a statutory requirement' (p. 14). These excerpts suggest that common law, rather than the DPA, should be the basis for advice to doctor managers (see below). Indeed, it is the Commissioner's assumption that the processing of health data by a health professional is subject to a duty of confidence even though explicit consent for processing is not a requirement of Schedules 2 and 3 – based essentially on case law.

Disclosure of personal information

The default position is that no patient information can be disclosed to third parties without the patient's express consent. The usual basis for exemption is found in Schedule 3, namely that the 'The [information] processing is necessary for medical purposes'.

The DPA sets out how patients should be informed in a general way that their information is being disclosed and in what circumstances. Essentially, if patients are asked for their consent to disclose and they agree, there can be no breach of confidentiality.

Review of care, including clinical audit and case review of their own performance in caring for a patient, carried out by members of the care team and those supporting them, is for the purpose of improving the direct care of the patient. Such a purpose has sufficient connection with that direct care for the sharing of information to be justified on the basis of implied consent.

From a consent perspective, a clear distinction must be drawn between disclosures which are necessary for patient care and disclosures which are for secondary uses (i.e. that do not relate directly to patient care). While the informed cooperation of patients can provide a basis for inferring their consent to the use and disclosure of information for their care, there is no behaviour which clearly implies consent to other uses of the information.

There are concerns about the secondary use of health information for other purposes (such as commerce and technological development) and these will be discussed below. However, at this point, we focus discussion on the circumstances in which doctors disclose patient information to third parties, either in the absence of consent (i.e. without consulting the patient) or in the face of a refusal to allow disclosure.

Absence of consent

Where there is a statutory requirement

Doctors are required to disclose patient information under the terms of some specific legislation (e.g. in the case of notifiable diseases or under the Road Traffic Act). The ethical argument here is that disclosure of this information will help to prevent harm to the community. In these circumstances, consent is irrelevant: the patient may be informed that the information is being given (although this is not required, the DPA makes it good practice) but is not given a choice. In these circumstances, the breach of individual confidentiality is justified with reference to the public good.

Child protection legislation, the NHS code of confidentiality and the Crime and Disorder Act 1998 allow doctors to disclose under appropriate circumstances where there is concern that a crime may be committed and for 'the prevention of serious crime' (NHS England, 2013). These codes and laws do not *require* doctors to disclose but set out the conditions in which disclosure may be permitted; that is, they provide justification rather than obligation. Doctors may also be required by a court to disclose information about patients. Again, this breach of patient autonomy is justified by the public interest in ensuring that the judicial process is fair.

Secondary uses

Some uses and disclosures of patient information are for health service purposes not directly related to that patient's care, often referred to as secondary uses. Examples of secondary uses are: planning; financial management; commissioning of services; investigating complaints; auditing accounts; teaching; health services research; public health monitoring; registries; and reporting of infectious diseases.

Patient express consent is usually required for any proposed secondary use, unless the information is in a non-identifiable form. Nevertheless, situations arise where patient consent cannot practicably be obtained and de-identification is not an option, and yet there are clear public health interests at stake. Examples include disease registries for secondary uses, and administrative and financial monitoring. At present, legislation which exceptionally permits setting aside the common law duty of confidentiality exists in England and Wales (section 251 of the NHS Act 2006, formerly the 2002 NHS Act), but not in Northern Ireland or Scotland.

Refusal of consent

A more complex issue arises when the doctor perceives that particular patients present a risk to others because of their condition, and asks for consent to disclose this to appropriate third parties. If the patient consents, then there is no breach of confidence, and all is well. More commonly, however, the doctor may find that the patient refuses to give consent to the disclosure. The commonest examples are individuals with sexually transmitted diseases, who may be putting current sexual partners at risk, but who refuse to allow the doctor to share the information with anyone.

When this issue came before the GMC (especially when HIV was first identified as a cause of AIDS), it advised that doctors could breach confidentiality in these circumstances – that the prevention of harm to unsuspecting others justified the breach of patient confidentiality. Although overriding a competent patient's consent or refusal is a major insult to autonomy, the GMC clearly took the view that the prevention of harm to others justified this.

At the time of this advice, it was not suggested that it was mandatory for doctors to disclose, only that they would not be guilty of professional misconduct if they did. Since then, however, preventing patients harming other people has come to be seen as a medical duty, especially in mental health. The issue is sensitive for doctors, first because it makes them into agents of public order, which many do not like, but second, and perhaps more importantly, they lose their beneficent status with the patient. The patient's interests are no longer the doctor's first concern; in fact, the patient then knows that the doctor thinks that another person's interests are more important than the patient's claim to privacy. Further, disclosure of patient information may have negative 'personal consequences' for the patient (GMC, 2009); by disclosing such information, despite a refusal, the doctor appears to give a message to the patient that the doctor is not concerned about the consequences.

Because these issues are sensitive and complex to discuss with patients, many healthcare professionals avoid having the discussion with the patient altogether. Fearing that the patient may refuse consent to disclose, they instead debate disclosure of information in the absence of consent. It seems that many doctors would rather deceive the patient than have a painful discussion with them. Perhaps some doctors are fearful of conflict with patients, which in turn suggests a lack of communication skills. It is also true that doctors (especially psychiatrists) cannot guarantee that significant negative consequences for the patient will not arise as a result of disclosure of their personal information.

The ethical dilemma for doctor managers is between conflicting duties: the duty to the patient, the duty to the public interest and the duty they have to the organisation. A healthcare organisation may expect a manager to be committed to the aims of an organisation, and to protect its welfare, so it can continue to provide care. But it may be that protecting the organisation means overriding ethical obligations to patients; and this often takes the form of disclosure of clinical information.

Different types of disclosure

Disclosure to fellow professionals for direct care

The key message from the foregoing is that data protection legislation assumes that patients own their personal health data and, generally, have a claim to control it. All trusts must have data protection policies and staff to manage those policies. As there is a potential conflict between the need to use patient information for good clinical care and patients' expectations that their information will not be shared with others, each trust is expected to have an official whose task it is to monitor good practice. This person is called the 'Caldicott guardian' (named after Dame Fiona Caldicott, who chaired and authored the first review into information management in the NHS; Caldicott, 1997).

Health service managers will probably have most to do with policies and procedures relating to the ordinary management of patient information within an organisation, where the main tension is the one described in the first Caldicott review, of balancing privacy against the need of health services for good-quality information. The more recent 'Caldicott 2' review of the use of patient information emphasises the importance of sharing information, and comments that failure to share necessary information is just as harmful as needless disclosure (Information Governance Review, 2013).

There are two main ethical dilemmas faced by managers of mental health services in the context of disclosure to fellow professionals. First, many service users may not fully understand that their information is being used for audit and governance purposes. Second, doctor managers may come across information in their work that they know is clinically relevant to their ethical duties, but they are bound by professional duties to the organisation. The inquiry into practices at the Bristol Royal Infirmary criticised a doctor manager who did not disclose clinical concerns that came to his attention, apparently because it could have caused managerial difficulties for him (*Roylance v GMC*).

The GMC appears to take the view that the medical ethical role trumps other ethical duties to health service organisations; the doctor cannot serve two masters equally. The recent inquiry into failures of care at Mid Staffordshire Foundation Trust (Francis, 2013) also suggests that doctors have a duty to disclose clinical concerns and to act when they perceive hospital managers to be failing to act. However, this is problematic when those same managers are employers who may 'punish' doctors who speak out.

Doctor managers may also come across the problem that different professionals may have different understandings of their ethical duties and different perspectives about what counts ethically. The best example is of child health services, where social workers have a mandatory duty to disclose information that may prevent harm to children, whereas doctors have an interpretable duty of 'good practice' in disclosure. The manager may have to listen to both arguments and be able to understand and respect both perspectives. In addition, doctor managers may be uncomfortably aware that they are expected to take decisions that make their employing trust look good, and to do nothing that would make the trust look 'bad'. Trusts expect their doctor managers to put the interests of the trust first, but for those doctor managers, doing so may directly contradict the GMC's advice.

A kind of solution is to have agreed protocols between all relevant professionals working in multidisciplinary teams to cover different situations. The guidance produced by the Royal College of Psychiatrists suggests that awareness is key:

> 'Psychiatrists should seek to ensure that there is an agreed policy on confidentiality and the threshold for disclosure in different circumstances. Consultant psychiatrists must be aware of the variable boundaries around the core team, which may encompass temporary members, people from other agencies (e.g. education, housing and social services), students or managers, for particular functions (e.g. to discuss particular patients).' (Royal College of Psychiatrists, 2010: p. 13)

Disclosure to carers and the relevance of capacity

A significant feature of most accounts of bio-ethics is that they assume a two-person relationship between the patient and the doctor. Further, these accounts usually assume that the patient is fully autonomous and capable of acting autonomously within a medical relationship. In mental health, these assumptions fall short of the reality of service users' lives. All mental (and many physical) disorders compromise autonomy in various ways and for varying periods of time. Many service users live with the disability of mental illness in ways that mean that they live within a network of dependent relationships, so that the concept of autonomy becomes more complex. Agich (1993), writing about decision-making in old age, has described this as 'interstitial autonomy'; one may also think of it as 'relational autonomy', where a kind of autonomy emerges from the different relationships around one (as in adolescence; Sutton, 1997).

What is therefore relevant here is the capacity to make decisions about information disclosure. The principle of current legislation on capacity is that everyone should be assumed to have capacity to make decisions for themselves. Doctors are under a duty to respect the decisions of patients who have capacity, even if those decisions seem foolish or have uncomfortable consequences. Decisions about treatment include decisions about those to whom information is disclosed: therefore doctors are ethically and legally required not to disclose patient information to carers or relatives if a patient has expressly refused disclosure. The only exception to this is under Mental Health Act legislation where the 'nearest relative' (as defined in law) is entitled to information that will allow her or him to act in the patient's best interests: here, capacity is not relevant.

This is a complex issue in mental health, as people with mental disorders may have fluctuating capacity to consent or refuse disclosure. Clinically, recovery is often likely to be improved if family members and carers are involved in planning the care pathway and in decision-making. It may therefore be highly problematic if patients refuse to consent to their clinical information being shared with family members and carers. Clinicians may be uncomfortably aware that a patient's capacitous decision to refuse to share information with carers is clinically unwise and emotionally hurtful to those carers. However, if the patient has the capacity to refuse, then psychiatrists have to respect such decisions. The only circumstance in which this refusal may be overridden is if there is risk to the carer (see below).

Where patients lack capacity to consent to disclosure, relationships between professionals and carers are still somewhat complex, and duties are not always straightforward. Providing information to carers is often a way to provide good care for patients; but it is more than that. Sometimes a person's mental well-being will depend on the well-being of the carer, so that working with carers indirectly provides help for the patient. Alternatively, there are cases where the carers have a negative effect upon the patient, and where disclosure to the carer is not beneficial to the patient, even if there is policy and legal justification for such disclosure. Doctor managers may find that the demands of policies and trust procedures do not do justice to the ethical complexities of these relationships.

The Information Tribunal found that the duty of confidentiality should be maintained even after death. This issue arose following an appeal by Pauline Bluck in relation to her dead daughter's medical records, which were held by Epsom and St Helier University Hospitals NHS Trust (see Information Tribunal, 2007).

Disclosure of personal information without consent

A major source of tension about the limits of confidentiality relates to the extent to which patient information can be used without consent for the public good. In this section, the 'public good' refers either: to the benefits of research and service development or review in the NHS; or to the prevention of harm and reduction of risk of harm that may be achieved by disclosure of information.

Research and service development

There has been considerable debate about the extent to which personal patient information can be used without consent for research and audit purposes, with the current emphasis being on patient consent and privacy trumping the public interest.

Section 60 of the Health and Social Care Act 2001 (in England and Wales) created a power for the Secretary of State to make orders requiring the disclosure of patient data that would otherwise be prevented by a duty of confidence. This is intended essentially as a temporary measure until anonymisation measures or appropriate recording of consent can be put in place for some secondary uses. A major stimulus is the requirements of registries, particularly cancer registries. In England and Wales an independent statutory body – the Confidentiality Advisory Group of the Health Research Authority (initially the Patient Information Advisory Group, and subsequently the Ethics and Confidentiality Committee of the National Information Governance Board until March 2013) – oversees all applications for exemptions from the duty of confidence to use patient-identifiable information. Powers to set aside the common law duty of confidentiality are currently provided within section 251 of the NHS Act 2006 (formerly the 2002 NHS Act).

The Health and Social Care Act (2012) in England and Wales gave powers to set up a new NHS and social care data register (implemented by the Health and Social Care Information Centre, http://www.hscic.gov.uk). This register would upload patient data from general practitioners that could be used for research and service development. This proposal has caused some controversy as the proposal will be costly and there are concerns that identifiable patient data might be sold for profit to interested parties. (At the time of writing, plans had been put on hold.) In Scotland arrangements for de-identified data extraction from general practice records have been in place and working effectively across nearly all practices for several years, demonstrating the public health benefits and that patient confidentiality can be and is being both respected and assured.

Reduction of risk of harm to third parties

In contrast to the privilege approach taken with ordinary patient information, in cases where there is a presumed risk to the public, NHS policy appears to suggest that healthcare professionals should generally be quick to disclose information where this will result in the reduction of risks to others. For example, the Health Service (Control of Patient Information) Regulations 2002 support the use of identifiable patient information without consent in respect of communicable diseases that lead to a risk to public health.

Despite strong evidence to the contrary, a public perception persists that people with mental illness pose an increased risk of serious harm to others. Regulations and policies have been developed that commit healthcare professionals to disclosing personal patient information to third parties if they have reason to think this will prevent serious harm to others (e.g. MAPPA procedures). If a patient is referred to a multi-agency public protection panel (and even this decision obviously involves disclosure) then trusts (and trust employees) are required to cooperate with the MAPPA process. No mention is made of patient consent or even of a duty to inform patients, although this is good clinical practice.

Managers dealing with decisions about disclosure in relation to risk will find themselves having to deal with multiple policies and sources of procedural advice (including legal precedent), much of which conflicts in terms of issues like consent. NHS policy, the Data Protection Act and GMC guidance make it clear that patients have to be asked for their consent for disclosure of personal information, and need to be advised if their information is being passed to others, even if there are no personal consequences for the patient. However, the NHS code of practice on confidentiality (Department of Health, 2003) also states that NHS employees are expected to disclose patient information that will assist in the 'detection, prevention and prosecution' of 'serious crime'. Supplementary guidance (Department of Health, 2010) defines 'serious crime' as violence towards the person, but suggests that crimes like fraud will be left to individual judgement. It is assumed that persons in question have refused to give consent or cannot be asked for consent because they are suspects; however, it is not clear on what grounds it is assumed that even police 'suspects' lose rights to control over their personal health information. There will also be many cases where patients are not 'suspects' at all.

Disclosure of confidential information to third parties outside the NHS is usually justified with reference to the benefits achieved and/or the harms averted by disclosure. If failure to disclose information may expose others to risk of death or serious harm *and* there is a high probability that disclosure of information would lead to a reduction in that risk, then it seems ethically unremarkable to conclude that disclosure is justified. Such an approach was taken by the court in *Palmer v West Tees Health Authority* when it argued that health services could have no duties to protect unidentifiable subjects to whom they had no duty of care. By inference, therefore, if a healthcare provider identified a potential victim of a patient in its care, then a court might well argue that there was a duty of care to that named and identifiable victim, which could include advising her or him of the risk from the patient, and giving some limited information about the patient. In the case of *(T) v Mental Health Review Tribunal*, the Tribunal took the view that it was permissible to disclose to a previous victim information about a patient who was about to be discharged if it reduced that victim's anxiety. In *W v Egdell*, the Court of Appeal found that doctors could disclose clinical information in the public interest when the breach of confidentiality would be justified by the prevention of future harm.

Article 8 of the Human Rights Act provides for an individual right to a private life, which includes control over medical information. *Campbell (Appellant) v MGN Limited* emphasised the importance of people having control over their own lives, including information about themselves. However, any action under the Human Rights Act would probably be countered with reference to the right of national law enforcement to use reasonable measures to manage risk to the public. Essentially, people have the right to control their personal information, unless someone else sees them as a risk to others, in which case all bets are off.

Ethical concerns about disclosure and risk (of harm to third parties)

The ethical concerns here are considerable. The first concern is empirical: how is one to know if a named person is really at risk? The current risk assessment literature does not allow us to accurately estimate the likelihood of risk of harm to others, or the probability that disclosure will ameliorate the risk. In fact, there is evidence that risk assessment tools are largely inaccurate and provide *misleading* information about risk (Fazel *et al*, 2012). It is ethically unjustifiable to disclose information that may be inaccurate. It is also possible that disclosure of risk information will increase the possibility that patients will not disclose important information about themselves and their mental states and beliefs if they think others will be informed, and this will increase the overall risk.

Another ethical concern is that of justice. Given that professional disclosures about patient risk may affect that patient's liberty, there must be real concern that patients are not being treated *justly*. The disclosure of information about potential risk to others often has highly significant negative consequences for patients (such as deprivation of liberty), so respect for justice means that we need the best possible evidence to justify disclosure. However, decisions about risk are often made by anxious people, who have very particular perspectives on the situation. Risk assessment is not a simple algorithmic process: it is a human process, and because of that it is likely to be influenced by conscious and unconscious factors, both individual and group (Box 23.1).

Managers of teams, or organisations, will have to contain the anxieties of their teams or groups when dealing with risky situations. Managers, in particular, hold institutional or group memories, especially if they have been in post for some time; memories of previous disasters may hugely

---

Box 23.1 Hypothetical example of disclosure

Jim and Helen are patients on a ward. Helen accuses Jim of rape; Jim denies it. Jim is HIV positive. Helen refuses to let staff tell her husband about her rape allegation, which is the subject of a criminal investigation. Jim refuses to let staff tell Helen about his HIV status. This situation persists for a number of weeks. Eventually, Brian, who is a member of staff, decides to tell Helen's husband what is going on: about both the rape allegation and Jim's HIV status. Brian is disciplined under local management procedures. He claims that it was his professional duty to prevent harm to Helen's husband. Helen's husband sues the trust for failing to protect his wife. We do not know the outcome for Jim and Helen.

affect risk assessment decisions, and therefore decisions about disclosure. Managers in a trust which has not experienced a homicide inquiry may have a different take on risk from managers who have, so their decisions will be different, with different consequences for the patient.

Decisions, decisions: how to disclose sensitive information about risk of harm to third parties

Decisions to disclose patient-identifiable information outside the NHS are matters of judgement – judgements that may be finely balanced. Managers will often be the ones who have the final say in such judgements, which need to take into account the various legal responsibilities at stake, including the duty of confidence to the individual, and the public interest in the health service maintaining confidence. Consideration will need to be given as to whether the harm that could result from disclosure (e.g. the possible damage to the relationship of trust or the likelihood of non-compliance with a programme of healthcare intervention in the future) is likely to be outweighed by the benefit. The potential benefit would need to be soundly grounded on the expectation that disclosure would have the desired effect. All this will go to ensuring that the decision to disclose is a reasonable one.

We should note that many of these situations will require good communication and support to be available for patients whose confidentiality is to be breached. Whether a breach of confidence is justifiable in the public interest will depend to some extent on the scope of disclosure. When considering whether to disclose, the manager should also consider the extent of the information to disclose and to whom it is appropriate to disclose such information. The Royal College of Psychiatrists' guidance on confidentiality continues to advise disclosing the minimum amount of information to the fewest number of people. It also recommends that, wherever possible, consent be sought from the patient, and that there be an attempt to involve the patient in the risk management process, as a kind of therapeutic joint enterprise. The College's advice to doctor managers is this:

> 'Once a decision has been reached that it is appropriate to disclose patient information the usual procedure is as follows:
> - explain to the patient the reasons for sharing information
> - encourage the patient to inform the relevant authority (e.g. police or social services); if the patient agrees, you will require confirmation from the authority that such disclosure has been made
> - if the patient refuses, you should tell the patient that you intend to disclose the information to the relevant authority or person. You should then inform the authority or person, disclosing only relevant information, and make available to the patient the information that has been released.'
> (Royal College of Psychiatrists, 2010: p. 32)

Ultimately a court would take careful account of the opinion and guidance of professional organisations as to whether a decision concerning disclosure was one which fell within the reasonable practice of a responsible body of medical practitioners (*Bolam v Friern Hospital Management Committee*).

Conclusion

A key feature of dilemmas about confidentiality is that they arise at the boundary between different domains in a patient's life, and thus in different domains for professional action. A general practitioner may wonder whether to tell an employer about a patient's drinking habits; a psychiatrist may wonder whether to tell hostel staff that a resident is using cannabis. The clinician finds herself sitting on the disclosure 'fence', surveying the various foreseeable possible outcomes, and wondering uneasily what outcomes she has *not* foreseen. She may find herself thinking about her duties (ethical, legal, professional, personal) and becoming uncomfortably aware that she has duties to more than one person or persons, and that these duties conflict. She knows, above all, that she will have to come down from the fence and make a decision.

There has been a gradual shift in the priority for sharing information in the public interest – ranging from direct care (especially in the wake of the inquiry into Mid Staffordshire NHS Foundation Trust), exploiting the enormous health information content of NHS information repositories for research and beyond, to include public security and surveillance. The second Caldicott document (2013) introduced a new 'duty to share', and the Nuffield Council on Bioethics has recently held a public consultation on the linking and use of biological and health data.

Managers in mental health services find themselves on the boundary between different groups of people. They are always having to manage and negotiate human relationships at work from at least four perspectives: their own, their employer's, that of those they manage, and the patient's. As in any small group, there are likely to be tensions between different group members; and these are often most clearly expressed around ethical dilemmas.

The 'good enough' manager will try to bear all these perspectives in mind and to conduct discussions which facilitate the expression of everyone's views. It may not be possible to find a solution that everyone likes, and if that is the case the process of arriving at that conclusion is the 'good enough' part. There is evidence to suggest that decisions that involve many voices, especially dissenting ones, are the best-quality decisions; and quality of reasoning is essential for ethical decisions in management.

References

Agich GJ (1993) *Autonomy and Long-Term Care*. Oxford University Press.

Caldicott F (1997) *Report on the Review of Patient-Identifiable Information*. Department of Health.

Department of Health (2003) *Confidentiality: A Code of Practice for NHS Staff*. Department of Health.

Department of Health (2010) *Supplementary Guidance: Public Interest Disclosures*. Available at https://www.gov.uk/government/uploads/system/uploads/attachment_data/file/200147/Confidentiality_-_NHS_Code_of_Practice_Supplementary_Guidance_on_Public_Interest_Disclosures.pdf (accessed April 2016).

Fazel S, Singh JP, Doll H, *et al* (2012) Use of risk assessment instruments to predict violence and antisocial behaviour in 73 samples involving 24,827 people: systematic review and meta-analysis. *BMJ*, **345**: e4692.

France E (2002) *Use and Disclosure of Health Data: Guidance on the Application of the Data Protection Act 1998*. Information Commissioner's Office.

Francis R (2013) *Report of the Mid Staffordshire NHS Foundation Trust Public Inquiry*. TSO (The Stationery Office).

GMC (2009) *Confidentiality: Protecting and Providing Information*. General Medical Council.

GMC (2012) *Child Protection Guidance*. General Medical Council.

Information Governance Review (2013) *Information: To Share or Not To Share?* Department of Health.

Information Tribunal (2007) *Appeal Number EA/2006/0090: Freedom of Information Act 2000 (FOIA)*. Available at http://www.informationtribunal.gov.uk/DBFiles/Decision/i25/mrspbluckvinformationcommissioner17sept07.pdf (accessed May 2016).

NHS England (2013) *NHS England Confidentiality Policy*. NHS England.

Royal College of Psychiatrists (2010) *Good Psychiatric Practice: Confidentiality and Information Sharing* (2nd edition) (CR160). RCPsych.

Sutton A (1997) Authority, autonomy, responsibility and authorisation: with specific reference to adolescent mental health practice. *Journal of Medical Ethics*, **23**: 26–31.

Cases

Bolam v Friern Hospital Management Committee [1957] 1 WLR 583

Campbell (Appellant) v MGN Limited [2004] UKHL 22

Palmer v West Tees Health Authority [1999] EWCA Civ 1533

Roylance v General Medical Council (Medical Act 1983) [1999] UKPC 16 (24 March 1999)

(T) v Mental Health Review Tribunal [2002] Lloyd's Rep Med 324

W v Egdell [1989] EWCA Civ 13

CHAPTER 24

Patient complaints: every doctor's business

J. S. Bamrah

'Sometimes when you innovate, you make mistakes. It is best to admit them quickly, and get on with improving your other innovations.' (Steve Jobs, founder of Apple Inc.)

A complaint is any expression of dissatisfaction which requires a response. What every medical practitioner must appreciate is that behind every complaint, justified or not, is a patient who feels aggrieved. Good governance is required in order to ensure individuals and organisations deal with complaints in a timely fashion, and pick up any trends that might put patients or organisations at risk. Even vexatious or unsubstantiated claims must be dealt with effectively, in order to restore the confidence of the profession in the process, and to minimise the wastage of time and resources. This chapter deals with complaints about doctors from patients or their carers, although similar principles apply to complaints from other health professionals.

Patients are increasingly accessing healthcare to improve their lives, and to live longer, healthier lives. One unintended outcome of this is that doctors as well as others responsible for their treatment are likely to make more mistakes, sometimes with rather serious consequences. Despite the high profile that these cases might take, the practice of medicine is now more innovative, advanced and comprehensive than ever before. Perversely, it is also more risky in terms of causing harm to patients, because patients now have more complex problems, and many are older.

The issue of harm to patients from doctors is nothing new. Hippocrates referred to it nearly 2500 years ago in the oath that defined the ethical principles around the practice of medicine.

'Into whatever houses I enter, I will go into them for the benefit of the sick, and will abstain from every voluntary act of mischief and corruption; and, further from the seduction of females or males, of freemen or slaves.'

Of course, most doctors do not set out to harm their patients purposely, so when a complaint is made doctors tend to feel a range of emotions, especially when they might have gone that extra mile for the complainant.

Having an effective and robust complaints system ensures that justifiable lessons are learned not just by the doctors but by patients too, through the process, allaying some of the fears about patient complaints. Undoubtedly, analysing complaints has the prospect of enhancing patient safety (Reader *et al*, 2014).

A historical perspective on complaints

Despite the existence of the NHS since 1948, there was no overarching structure for handling complaints until 1996. Up until then, each trust or hospital had to set up its own system, with the result that there was considerable variation and fragmentation, and enormous dissatisfaction over the lack of national guidelines and agreed targets. Furthermore, the complaints procedure was regarded as not being sufficiently independent.

In 1996, the government introduced a complaints system throughout the NHS, in hospitals, community services and primary care. This was a culmination of long-standing dissatisfaction with the procedure and outcome of complaints and a growing ethos of consumerism within the NHS. There was concern about medical care, communication, and the behaviour and attitude of medical and nursing staff, but also an acknowledgement that the hotel services, such as food and cleaning, offered by hospitals were inadequate. The Patients' Charter made it possible to articulate some minimum standards of care expected by patients. The new service-wide system produced clear evidence that complaints were on the increase: in 2008–09 the NHS recorded 89 139 written complaints about NHS trusts and community health services; in 2009–10 there were 101 077; and in 2013–14 there were 174 872. This represents a 51% increase in 5 years. There are indications that this trend exists in private healthcare too; in 2011–12 there were 272 complaints against independent providers to the Parliamentary and Health Service Ombudsman (PHSO), a rise of 61% from the previous year. On average, the PHSO upheld 44% of complaints against acute trusts during 2013–14.

Investigations into and reports on high-profile failures – such as the Richard Neale case of botched gynaecological operations (2000), Clifford Ayling's sexual assaults on his patients (2000), the inquiry into the retention of children's organs at Alder Hey Children's Hospital (2001), the Bristol Royal Infirmary heart scandal (2002), the Shipman inquiry (2004) into over 200 alleged murders by a general practitioner (GP) and the Kerr/ Haslam report (2005) into sexual abuse by two psychiatrists – raised the anxieties of professional and patient groups on a variety of issues but principally standards of care and how complaints were not taken seriously. Possibly the most important landmark in relation to poor standards of care, high mortality rates and a blatant disregard of patients' complaints were highlighted in the inquiry by Sir Robert Francis into the Mid Staffordshire NHS Hospital Foundation Trust. Stafford Hospital was a small district general hospital where a systemic failure had led to an estimated 400–1200 patient deaths between January 2005 and March 2009. Francis (2013) made 290 recommendations, all of which have been accepted by the government. Of particular relevance to this chapter are the recommendations that every health organisation and its employees must have a duty to be open, transparent and truthful with patients and the public. This 'duty of candour' is now enshrined in how the NHS is regulated, with the expectation that there will be a cultural change in the care of patients. The report also recommended that 'gagging clauses' and non-disparagement clauses should be banned in cases where disclosure is in the public interest on patient care and safety, and that all complaints upheld and the trust's response should be anonymised and published on the trust's website.

While the Francis report was laudable in baring the fabric of a poorly run hospital and the consequences of sub-standard care, by contrast the Berwick (2013) report which followed this emphasised that patient safety problems exist throughout the NHS, not just at the Mid Staffordshire NHS Trust, that it is not justifiable to blame the staff of the NHS or to label them as uncaring, unskilled or culpable and that distorted priorities are dangerous. Berwick pointed out that warning signals must be heeded and that too often complaints from patients and carers are ignored, to their detriment and that of the organisation's reputation. In Berwick's opinion, the most important single change in the NHS would be for it to become more devoted to continual learning and improvement of patient care, unimpeded by fear, which he stated is toxic to both safety and improvement. He championed the case of 'zero harm', or 'harm-free care', which is central to the Health and Social Care (Safety and Quality) Act 2015,[1] which was enacted in the wake of the Mid Staffordshire scandal. It gives the Health Secretary the duty to introduce regulations to ensure that services provided in the carrying on of regulated activities cause no avoidable harm. It also gives further powers to regulatory authorities such as the Care Quality Commission (CQC), but it raises the possibility of raising fear among health professionals of the consequences of unintended harm caused to patients.

Another pivotal point for the NHS was the well-publicised complaint by the Labour MP Ann Clwyd against the Cardiff and Vale Health Board about the care of her late husband. She stated that her husband died 'like a battery hen' and that there was an almost callous lack of care. While most of her allegations were rejected, she did co-author a report detailing how complaints about care in NHS hospitals made by patients, their carers and representatives are listened to and acted on by hospitals (Clwyd & Hart, 2013). The review which produced that report was co-chaired by Professor Tricia Hart, Chief Executive, South Tees Hospitals NHS Foundation Trust, and commissioned by the Prime Minister, David Cameron, and Secretary of State for Health for England, Jeremy Hunt, after the Francis report into Mid

---

1 Available at http://www.legislation.gov.uk/ukpga/2015/28/pdfs/ukpga_20150028_en.pdf.

Staffordshire highlighted that complaints are a warning sign of problems in a hospital. The review received 2500 responses, the majority describing problems with the quality of treatment or care in NHS hospitals. The review panel also heard from people who had not complained because they felt the process was too confusing or they feared for their future care. Five key areas were identified:

- *lack of information* – patients said they felt uninformed about their care and treatment
- *lack of compassion* – patients said they felt they had not been treated with the compassion they deserve
- *lack of dignity and care* – patients said they felt neglected and not listened to
- *staff attitudes* – patients said they felt no one was in charge on the ward and the staff were too busy to care for them
- *lack of resources* – patients said there was a lack of basic supplies like extra blankets and pillows.

The recommendations in the report (Clwyd & Hart, 2013) covered:

- improving the quality of care
- improving the way complaints are handled
- ensuring the independence of complaints procedures
- whistle-blowing.

NHS complaints: the guiding principles

The NHS is one of the world's largest publicly funded bodies, and certainly the largest employer in the health sector in the UK. The NHS Constitution (Department of Health, 2009) sets out seven broad principles that define its roles and responsibilities:

1 The NHS provides a comprehensive service, available to all irrespective of gender, race, disability, age, sexual orientation, religion, belief, gender reassignment, pregnancy and maternity or marital or civil partnership status. The service is designed to diagnose, treat and improve both physical and mental health. It has a duty to each and every individual that it serves and must respect their human rights.

2 Access to NHS services is based on clinical need, not an individual's ability to pay.

3 The NHS aspires to the highest standards of excellence and professionalism – in the provision of high-quality care that is safe, effective and focused on patient experience.

4 The NHS must put patients at the heart of everything it does. It should support individuals to promote and manage their own health.

5 The NHS works across organisational boundaries as well as in partnership with other organisations in the interests of patients, local communities and the wider population.

6 The NHS is committed to providing best value for taxpayers' money and the most effective, fair and sustainable use of finite resources.

7 The NHS is accountable to the public, communities and patients that it serves.

The Constitution makes it necessary for all to understand that any erosion of duty or deviation from these principles might result in sub-standard care and the likelihood of dissatisfaction and complaints. The way in which these are handled has also been embodied in the NHS Constitution. Patients can expect:

- to receive an acknowledgement within three working days after a complaint has been received
- to be advised on the manner in which the complaint is to be handled
- to know the period within which the investigation is likely to be completed and the response sent
- to be kept informed of progress
- to know the outcome of any investigation into the complaint, including an explanation of the conclusions and confirmation that any action needed in consequence of the complaint has been taken or is proposed to be taken.

Patients have the right to take their complaint to the PHSO or Local Government Ombudsman (LGO) if they are not satisfied with the way their complaint has been dealt with by a trust, and to make a claim for judicial review if they think they have been directly affected by an unlawful act or decision by an NHS trust. The Constitution further states that in the case of negligence patients have the right to compensation. Patients also have the right to know that lessons will be learned to help avoid similar incidents occurring again.

The Constitution guides trusts to ensure that:

- patients are treated with courtesy and receive appropriate support throughout the handling of a complaint (it emphasises that just because patients have complained, this must not adversely affect their future treatment)
- when mistakes happen or if patients are harmed while receiving healthcare, they receive an appropriate explanation and apology, delivered with sensitivity and recognition of the stress they have experienced
- the organisation learns lessons from complaints and claims and uses these to improve NHS services.

Why do patients complain?

The NHS in England treats over a million patients every 36 hours, the vast majority of whom receive a good standard of care. In cases where the standard is inadequate or where there is malicious intent, it is in the interests of all that these are dealt with swiftly and justly, that lessons are learned and where sanctions are required that these are imposed quickly to ensure the care of other patients is not jeopardised. Broadly speaking, patients may receive poor care or suffer maltreatment due to the trust's processes and resources, or at the hands of individual practitioners. The assumption that psychiatric patients complain as a result of their illness has been challenged in one study where only 4% of complainants had psychotic symptoms (Pitarka-Carcani *et al*, 2000).

A review of the hospitals complaints procedure in 2012–13 (Parliamentary and Health Service Ombudsman, 2013) found simple themes around patient or carer dissatisfaction: 19% of complainants had received a poor explanation for their treatment, 18% did not get an adequate apology (rising to 28% in 2014–15) and 9% were inadequately compensated financially; in a further 7% of cases there were unnecessary delays in handling the complaint. Complaints about non-medical aspects of care are surprisingly high. Almost 30% of patients complain about poor communication and 20% about staff attitude.

Who can make a complaint?

Complaints may be made by patients, their legal or nominated representatives or any person(s) who may have been affected during the course of the patient's treatment. For the purposes of the Mental Health Act 1983 (as amended in 2007), the 'nearest relative' has considerable legal powers, which include being able to instruct another psychiatrist to assess the patient and to make a complaint on behalf of the patient.

The circumstances where the representative rather than the patient might make a complaint can include the following: the patient has died, is a minor, is physically handicapped so as not to be able to make a complaint, lacks mental capacity, or simply chooses for the representative to make a complaint on her or his behalf and has the capacity to do so. Where the patient has died or lacks capacity, evidence would need to be supplied on the authenticity of the representative before the complaint can be acted upon.

Then a test of suitability of the person is applied to demonstrate that the representative has 'sufficient interest' in the case. Where there are any doubts, that person will need to be notified in writing and given cogent reasons for the decision. If the patient has died, then it would be usual for the head of legal services to contact the coroner to assist the complainant, if it is appropriate. In the case of children, the representative may be a parent, a legal guardian or another adult who has been caring for the child, whether in a home setting or in an institution. In the case of the latter adult, the representative must have the authority of the local authority or voluntary organisation.

To whom can a patient complain?

The patient, relative or carer may complain to the trust directly by speaking to a member of staff, contacting the complaints manager or by seeking the advice and support of the patient advice and liaison service (PALS). The PALS provides advice and information to try to resolve concerns quickly and in liaison with the service where they originate. The supportive atmosphere of the PALS often assists in speedy local resolution of concerns. Alternatively a complaint can be made to either NHS England or clinical commissioning groups (CCGs). If they are not satisfied with how their complaint has been handled by the trust, patients have the right to report the matter to the PHSO, who will investigate the trust's handling of their complaint and the written response.

NHS complaints procedures

Complaints must be made within 12 months of the alleged incident(s), although if there are compelling reasons consideration should be paid to legitimate delays in making the complaint. The complaint should be connected with the services offered by the trust or individual.

All complaints must be dealt with in complete confidence. All trusts employ PALS, which is the point of liaison for patients or their representatives, and which can support complainants through the process. A further resource to the complainant is the NHS Complaints Advocacy Service, which is a free, confidential and independent service available through the local authority. There are two stages for dealing with complaints under the Local Authority Social Services and National Health Service Complaints (England) Regulations 2009.

Stage 1. Local resolution

The NHS encourages staff to resolve a complaint on the spot if it is possible. This tends to happen less often than one might imagine, resulting in a more formal approach being taken in cases where a simple apology would suffice. The idea is to make local resolution flexible, conciliatory, informal and non-bureaucratic. The General Medical Council (GMC) states very clearly what the duties are of a doctor in relation to complaints in its *Good Medical Practice* (GMC, 2013). The doctor must respond promptly, fully and honestly to complaints and apologise when appropriate. As mentioned above, often doctors will not apologise in a timely fashion because they might feel that this compromises their position, or they might fear some form of recrimination, or simply because they have an arrogant attitude. The GMC further recommends that any complaint must not adversely affect the care and treatment that the doctor has to provide or arrange.

Once a complaint is raised, the trust must acknowledge it within three working days. The length of time to respond to a complaint depends on the complaint itself and how complex it is. The NHS complaints regulations do not require complaints to be investigated within a set timescale but instead an individual timescale as agreed with the complainant and the services involved.

Following receipt of the results of the investigation, the chief executive must write to the complainant stating which complaints have been upheld and which have not, and set out any remedial actions.

The Health Care Commission, which previously handled complaints at stage 2, was abolished on 31 March 2009. Now, trusts are required to address each aspect of the complaint until local resolution is reached. If this process is exhausted only then may complainants take their grievance to the PHSO.

Stage 2: Parliamentary and Health Service Ombudsman

Complainants who are dissatisfied with the outcome of the local resolution can contact the PHSO. The PHSO investigates complaints that individuals feel have been treated unfairly and complaints that individuals have received poor service from government departments and other public organisations and the NHS in England.

The role of the PHSO is to help resolve complaints and help people get an answer to their concerns. The PHSO does this by liaising with complainants to determine what happened and what went wrong, how this affected them and what outcome were they seeking. The aim is to get complaints resolved quickly, without the need to investigate whenever possible. If there is a decision not to investigate, a clear explanation is given, and help and advice are offered to the complainant. In order to complete the assessment and to decide whether an investigation is warranted, the PHSO will contact the service provider for information about what has already been done to answer the complaint. Where needed, advice is sought from experts (e.g. from a medical professional or the PHSO's own legal team). The PHSO can look at other ways to resolve the complaint without investigating. This often involves talking to the complainant and the organisation to find an appropriate answer to their concerns and actions that help to put things right.

Should the PHSO uphold a complaint, recommendations are normally made in the final report as to what the organisation complained about should do in order to provide an appropriate remedy. These recommendations aim to remedy the injustice or hardship suffered, where possible returning complainants to the position they would have been in if things had not gone wrong. Additionally, the PHSO may make recommendations to put matters right for other people similarly affected and/or to ensure that the same mistakes do not happen again. These recommendations may include some or all of the following:

- an apology, explanation and/or acknowledgement of responsibility
- remedial action, such as reviewing or changing a decision on the

service given to the complainant, revising published material, revising procedures or policy to prevent the same thing happening again, or training or supervising staff
* financial redress for direct or indirect financial loss, loss of opportunity, inconvenience or distress (this may include a wider compensation scheme if more than one individual is affected by the maladministration or poor service).

Healthwatch

Healthwatch is a new independent consumer champion created to gather and represent the views of the public. It is designed to take the views of the public and patients into account through local Healthwatch branches, which report to the local authority. Healthwatch England, on the other hand, is funded by the Department of Health and although it has no direct responsibility for local Healthwatch branches, nevertheless it liaises closely with them, offering supervision and advice wherever possible. The Local Healthwatch was launched in 2013 with the responsibility to recommend to the CQC that action is taken where concerns are expressed about health or social services, and to advise the NHS Commissioning Board, English local authorities, Monitor (which regulates NHS foundation trusts) and the Secretary of State on any related issues. Local Healthwatch replaces Local Involvement Networks (LINks) and also represents the views of people who use services, carers and the public on the health and wellbeing boards set up by local authorities; it provides a complaints advocacy service to support people who make a complaint about services and reports concerns about the quality of healthcare to Healthwatch England, which can then recommend that the CQC take action. It is anticipated therefore that because of its wide remit Local Healthwatch will be a resource for patients making complaints about their treatment predominantly within primary care, but potentially in some cases at acute and mental health trusts as well.

The role of the General Medical Council

The GMC sets standards for doctors as well as regulating medical training and education. It is the role of the GMC to investigate and take action against doctors who may put patients' safety at risk, or doctors who risk compromising the public's confidence in the profession.

It seems that the public is increasingly aware of the powers of the GMC in sanctioning doctors. The public is the largest source of enquiries to the GMC, with 6475 enquiries during 2013, accounting for 66% of all contacts that year and an increase of 5% from the previous year and 43% since 2010. Although the highest numbers of complaints the GMC receives are about psychiatrists and general practitioners, the percentage who warrant a full investigation is relatively low. The three main reasons why patients complain to the GMC are misdiagnosis or treatment, communication failures and rude or arrogant behaviour. The first is a matter of clinical experience and knowledge, but the latter two are non-clinical behaviours which one could argue are basic bedside manners, which every doctor needs to have better training on, especially as these are also common themes in many complaints received about doctors to employing and regulatory authorities.

Confidentiality

The GMC sets out clear principles that govern the relationship of patients with their doctor. This is based on complete trust and there are very few circumstances in which this trust can be breached. All complaints must be dealt with confidentially by those involved and must be disclosed only on a need-to-know basis, unless access under the Data Protection Act 1998 and the Medical Records Act 1988 has been authorised.

All complaint records must be kept separately from clinical notes, although it may be necessary to record limited information clinically if it is justifiable. This must relate to the patient's health and not refer to the complaint.

Correspondence about complaints is not included in the patient's clinical records. Informal discussions about concerns can be documented in the clinical records. Where the complainant is the patient, consent to access information is not needed; however, in the event that the complainant is another legitimate party then it is essential to record the patient's consent, unless there are exceptions (see the above section 'Who can make a complaint?'). Any legal documents such as a will or lasting power of attorney, must be submitted as evidence before any information is accessed or disclosed. For administrative reasons, because the clock starts ticking when the complaint is received, if there is a delay in obtaining the required documentation, the complaint should be closed down and reopened when all necessary papers are resubmitted.

The only possible exception seems to be if a Member of Parliament complains on behalf of the patient. In these instances there is implied consent unless the complaint also identifies a third party. In the case where a vulnerable adult or child is subject to safeguarding procedures, there is a requirement to seek further information from the safeguarding lead.

In dealing with complaints, it is necessary for all documents to be labelled 'confidential' and for all emails to be anonymised. Any attachments to emails must be password protected.

Advice and support for the doctor

Receiving a complaint can be a distressing time for the doctor as well as the patient or patient representative. Trainees must enlist the support of their educational supervisor and tutor; for consultants and specialty and associate specialist (SAS) doctors this would be available from a variety of individuals, such as a colleague, the clinical director/lead consultant or peer group.

It is necessary in most cases to let a professional body such as the British Medical Association (BMA) or a medical defence organisation know of the details of the complaint so that legal advice is available through the complaint process. The NHS Litigation Authority (NHSLA) provides legal assistance for clinical negligence cases arising through NHS practice. It is common wisdom that the NHSLA does not cover all eventualities and so, for doctors at least, it is advisable to obtain negligence cover from a defence organisation.

The BMA offers a 'Doctor Advisor' telephone service for members and non-members, which runs alongside BMA counselling for doctors and medical students in distress or difficulty. It offers free, confidential advice from another doctor. The telephone Psychiatrists' Support Service is a free and confidential service for members, trainee members and associates of the Royal College of Psychiatrists through another psychiatrist. (See the organisations' websites for up-to-date details including telephone numbers.)

Quick tips on handling or avoiding complaints

Awareness

Astute doctors usually know when a clinical interaction has not gone well. It is best to try to remedy this then and there by understanding why the patient is dissatisfied and apologising if she or he has a point. Saying sorry is not an admission of guilt. Spending extra time will save hours and hours of work, and it could well result in a patient engaging even better in treatment.

Apology

An apology might be for something the doctor felt resulted in some harm to the patient. Conventional wisdom was that an apology will lead to a lawsuit, but there is evidence to suggest that a timely apology reduces the chance of this as well as the amount awarded in the case of liability. Indeed, it is the author's view that the doctor must declare what harm has been done and then seek to remedy it. The NHSLA advises that an apology is not an admission of liability and the GMC in its *Good Medical Practice* guidance states that 'an apology should be offered, but it is more important that the doctor explains fully and promptly what's happened, and what are likely to be the consequences both in the short and long term' (GMC, 2013).

Equally, it could be the case that what the doctor has done is correct, but the patient is nonetheless left distressed. So for instance, the doctor tells a patient that he has Alzheimer's disease and he becomes visibly upset. The doctor must not apologise for delivering the diagnosis but it is perfectly appropriate for the doctor to say she is sorry that the patient is distressed. It is important for a senior doctor never to apologise on behalf of a junior doctor or any other colleague, or for the lack of resources.

Accessibility

The meeting between the doctor and the patient (or a complainant acting on behalf of a patient) could be the most important part of the complaint process as far as the patient is concerned. This may also be true for the doctor, who may want to put the facts right, apologise or be relieved of the burden of a genuine error. Once the facts have been established, it is best for the doctor to meet the complainant at the earliest possible opportunity. The doctor should be accompanied by another member of staff. Any legal advisors should identify themselves; in most cases it is not appropriate to have a legal person there with one party and not with the other, as this detracts from the informal nature of this meeting. On rare occasions, the complainant may either want to make a recording, or might make a secret recording (as has happened on one occasion to the author). The object of such meetings is, as mentioned, to resolve matters in an informal fashion; therefore written notes on both sides should be permitted but visual or audio recordings must be a rarity and made only with the consent of all parties. Communication is key at these meetings so medical jargon must be avoided, or, where used, must be accompanied by an explanation in plain language. Doctors must be aware that complainants can become animated during these meetings and so any attributions must not be taken personally.

Writing a report

The most important issue in responding to complaints is to write the report within the given timescale. All too often this does not happen, which in a way is a false economy of time because that then results in further correspondence throughout the chain of the complaint, and could mean a rebuke from the Health Commissioner or the Ombudsman, and a fine. Reports must be concise, refer to the complaint in question and not peripheral issues, and be written in plain English. Where there are issues that are beyond the skill or knowledge of the doctor these must be acknowledged and no attempt made to address them. Once written, it is best to run the draft report by a colleague as well as either the BMA or a medical defence organisation.

Time constraints

- *Twelve months.* The complaint has to be made to the trust or commissioners within 12 months of the incident happening or being noticed.
- *Immediately.* The commissioner will usually immediately pass the complaint to the trust to deal with.

- *Three working days*. The complaints manager at the trust acknowledges the complaint with three working days.
- *No limit*. The length of time to respond to a complaint depends on the complaint itself and how complex it is. The NHS complaints regulations do not require complaints to be investigated within a set timescale but instead within an individual timescale as agreed with the complainant and the services involved.
- *No limit*. There is no deadline by which the PHSO must be contacted if the complainant is dissatisfied by either the trust's or the commissioner's response.

Case studies

An alleged assault on a woman with a borderline personality disorder

A woman with a borderline personality disorder was attending a therapy session at a mental health trust in the west of England. When she became distressed and went into a nearby room to lie down on the floor, a clinician called in two security guards to remove her. One of them allegedly kicked her. The trust took nearly a year to respond formally after the patient complained.

The PHSO's investigation uncovered serious flaws in the investigation. The trust had not taken statements from all key witnesses or obtained advice about calling in security guards. The trust apologised to the patient for the distress caused, paid her compensation, agreed that the executive board would consider the investigation report and agreed to commission an independent review into its complaint-handling function.

Withdrawal of donepezil

Mr S was seen by a consultant old age psychiatrist in May 2002 for poor memory and was prescribed donepezil for Alzheimer's disease. Monitoring by the community mental health team (CMHT) was intended, but this did not happen. In May 2003 his general practitioner re-referred him for an assessment of his deteriorating cognitive state. This was agreed, but monitoring by the CMHT was considered more appropriate than changing his anti-dementia drug. In January 2004 he was seen by a staff-grade psychiatrist for older people who stopped his donepezil and the patient was discharged to the care of the CMHT. At the time Mr S was living at home with care being provided by his neighbours and two adult sons. He continued to deteriorate so that in March 2004 he was admitted to hospital and in September that year he was transferred to a nursing home.

Mr S's son, Mr T, complained to the trust about a number of aspects of his care, mainly: the failure to inform the family and carers about stopping donepezil; the lack of a care plan after that; and that his condition had been allowed to deteriorate. Mr T was dissatisfied with the trust's handling of the complaint and so he referred the matter to the Healthcare Commission in October 2004. It told him to take matters up with the trust on details of the guidelines used to discontinue donepezil. In December 2005 Mr T took his complaint further, to the PHSO, who recommended to the Commission that it look at the complaint again. In February the Commission wrote to Mr T advising that the clinical care was adequate and the trust followed the guidance from the National Institute for Health and Care Excellence in stopping donepezil.

On reopening the case at the request of Mr T, the PHSO found that the trust: failed to communicate the withdrawal of donepezil; did not identify and plan for Mr S's deterioration after stopping the drug; and instituted inadequate monitoring after January 2004. In relation to the Commission, the PHSO found that: it had failed to take independent medical advice on two occasions; and it had failed to respond to the complainant in a timely manner. The trust apologised for the lack of communication over the withdrawal of donepezil before the PHSO's investigation, and made a number of other procedural changes in its care plans, follow-up and monitoring. Acting on the PHSO's report, the trust again apologised to Mr T and provided evidence that senior medical staff had been advised about the importance of monitoring and follow-up of patients when medication is discontinued.

Standards of care

Mr B was admitted to a hospital with chronic fatigue and tiredness but died a week later from a heart attack. His family complained about his clinical care, nursing care and deterioration.

The PHSO found that while Mr B received a good standard of care, there had been significant failings in recording and delays in the complaints process, and that the trust should apologise to the family and pay £250 to the family for the additional distress caused.

Failure to deal with a mental health crisis

Mrs C was receiving care from a CMHT and a psychologist who acted as the keyworker. The patient had a mental health crisis when the psychologist went on leave unexpectedly but despite seeking help several times she was not offered face-to-face contact. The trust's own investigation was robust. It made the recommendation that the CMHT improve its processes for dealing with crises and for appointing care coordinators.

However, the PHSO found that the trust had not put improvements in place to address the failings and asked it to demonstrate that there was a suitable process to assess the need for face-to-face contact and to highlight any escalation of a crisis.

Breach of the GMC's Good Medical Practice

Mrs C's daughter was referred to a consultant psychiatrist. Both attended the appointment but Mrs C's daughter's health deteriorated following this.

The PHSO found that the consultant's actions fell below the expected standard and were not in accordance with *Good Medical Practice*. There was a failure to undertake a robust assessment. A management plan had not been prepared and there was a lack of engagement, as well as a failure to engage the multidisciplinary team. Also, the patient was given inappropriate advice. The trust was asked to give a written apology, to arrange a face-to-face apology with the consultant psychiatrist and to put together an action plan to address identified failings.

References

Berwick D (2013) *A Promise to Learn – A Commitment to Act: Improving the Safety of Patients in England*. National Advisory Group on the Safety of Patients in England.

Clwyd C, Hart T (2013) *A Review of the NHS Hospitals Complaints System: Putting Patients Back in the Picture*. Department of Health. Available at https://www.gov.uk/government/publications/nhs-hospitals-complaints-system-review (accessed April 2016).

Department of Health (2009) *The NHS Constitution: The NHS Belongs To Us All*. TSO.

Francis R (2013) *Report of the Mid Staffordshire NHS Foundation Trust Public Inquiry. Final Report* (Francis report). Mid Staffordshire NHS Foundation Trust Public Inquiry.

GMC (2013) *Good Medical Practice*. General Medical Council.

Parliamentary and Health Service Ombudsman (2013) *The NHS Hospital Complaints System. A Case for Urgent Treatment?* Available at http://www.ombudsman.org.uk/__data/assets/pdf_file/0018/20682/The-NHS-hospital-complaints-system.-A-case-for-urgent-treatment-report_FINAL.pdf (accessed May 2016).

Pitarka-Carcani I, Szumkler G, Henderson C (2000) Complaints about care in a mental health trust. *Psychiatric Bulletin*, **24**: 372–6.

Reader TW, Gillespie A, Roberts J (2014) Patient complaints in healthcare systems: a systematic review and coding taxonomy. *BMJ Quality and Safety*, **23**: 678–89.

Further reading

Department of Health (2009) *Listening, Responding and Improving: A Guide to Better Customer Care*. Available at http://webarchive.nationalarchives.gov.uk/20130107105354/http://www.dh.gov.uk/en/Publicationsandstatistics/Publications/PublicationsPolicyAndGuidance/DH_095408 (accessed May 2016).

Local Authority Social Services and National Health Service Complaints (England) Regulations (2009) http://www.legislation.gov.uk/uksi/2009/309/contents/made (accessed May 2016).

Parliamentary and Health Service Ombudsman (2012) *Listening and Learning: The Ombudsman's Review of Complaint Handling by the NHS in England 2011 to 2012*. Available at https://www.gov.uk/government/publications/listening-and-learning-the-ombudsmans-review-of-complaint-handling-by-the-nhs-in-england-2011-to-2012 (accessed May 2016).

CHAPTER 25

Mental health review tribunals. Or, tribunals, and how to survive them

Nick Brindle

The Mental Health Act 1959 revised the procedures for admission to psychiatric hospitals and was intended to strengthen the rights and safeguards afforded to people with a mental disorder. In so doing the 1959 Act heralded the introduction of the Mental Health Review Tribunal (MHRT). The purpose of the MHRT was to independently review the cases of those patients detained under the Mental Health Act and subject to guardianship. What transpired was perhaps a less robust safeguard than was intended. Only patients admitted under the long-term provisions of the Act were eligible to apply to the tribunal; the onus was then on patients to demonstrate that they did not justify detention, and only unrestricted patients had the right of appeal; there were also other procedural issues which disadvantaged the patient. With the advent of the Human Rights Act 1998 the burden of proof is now no longer on the applicant (Mental Health Act 1983 (Remedial) Order 2001, SI 2001/3712) and although successive governments have arguably pursued an agenda of increased control of those with mental disorders, the concept of patients' rights and advocacy has received considerably more purchase with the Mental Health Act 1983 and Mental Health Act 2007.

Following on from this, there have been significant structural and procedural changes to the MHRT introduced by the Tribunals, Courts and Enforcement Act 2007. In November 2008 the MHRT became part of a new two-tier tribunal structure: the First-Tier Tribunal (FTT) and the Upper Tribunal (UT), which has appeal functions. In England the title for the MHRT is now the Tribunal Service (Mental Health), while Wales continues with the title Mental Health Review Tribunal for Wales, but for simplicity both will be referred to as 'the tribunal'. The rules governing the tribunal differ between England and Wales and are complemented by practice directions that set out what statements, information, documents and reports must be provided for cases.

In considering the role of the tribunal, the Care Quality Commission (2015) reported 58 399 uses of the Act in the year 2014/2015. This represented a 10% increase on the previous year, adding to the total number of people both detained under the Mental Health Act and subject to community treatment orders (CTOs). The reasons for this are complex but this increase has contributed to the receipt of more cases by the Tribunal Service, with more than 17000 hearings conducted in this timeframe.

Even aside from this increase in the use of the Mental Health Act, the workload for 'responsible clinicians', who are still mostly consultant psychiatrists, associated with tribunals has certainly increased. Several factors may have contributed to this, including: the increasing expectations of the tribunal in relation to the quality and stringency of responsible clinicians' reports; the upsurge in the use of section 2, with the requirement that the hearing for a section 2 appeal is heard within 7 (5 working) days; and an increased awareness of patients' rights and the use of advocacy.

With the advent of CTOs, the tribunal is no longer the sole purview of those consultants with in-patient responsibilities. For those working in in-patient settings or services with a high proportion of patients subject to CTOs, the tribunal is a frequent and unavoidable component of the day job. For others it will be a more occasional interruption, most likely for patients under a CTO or guardianship. Although the tribunal is supposed to be conducted in an inquisitorial rather than adversarial fashion it can feel awkward and challenging to navigate for those who have had less exposure. This chapter is not intended to provide an exhaustive account of tribunal law, practice or procedure but rather to give some guidance on the processes, requirements and issues that arise in relation to the tribunal for more experienced clinicians who are less well acquainted with tribunals. It will also provide an update for those who make regular attendances. Note that the content pertains to England and Wales only, although many of the observations may be relevant to other jurisdictions.

Powers and duties of the tribunal

The tribunal is the 'court' which convenes in the hospital or convenient community unit and is usually held in private. The primary purpose of the tribunal is to determine whether the grounds for detention under the Act continue to exist. The panel consists of three members, discussed below: the legal member, the medical member and the specialist member.

The scope of the tribunal relates to:

- those who are detained in hospital under a section of the Mental Health Act
- those who are conditionally discharged
- those who are subject to CTOs
- those who are subject to guardianship.

The sections relating to the powers of the tribunal are contained in Part V of the Mental Health Act (sections 65–79). Section 72 confers on tribunals the power to discharge patients from detention in hospital, from guardianship or from a CTO if they are not satisfied that the relevant criteria are met. For Part II detentions, the power of discharge applies to sections 2, 3, 4, 7 and 17A, and for Part III detentions to 37, 47, 48, 37/41 *but not* 45A, 47/49 or 48/49. In doing so, the tribunal is bound to consider all relevant circumstances and to have regard to the patient's history and the risk of deterioration in the person's condition if the patient is not subject to the relevant section.

The tribunal has the power to order immediate discharge of a detained patient. Or, if grounds for detention are not met but discharge should not be immediate the tribunal can defer discharge until after a further short period of detention, for example if the patient is awaiting implementation of a plan of aftercare.

The tribunal also has the power to make certain recommendations such as:

- consideration of leave of absence by the responsible clinician
- the patient's transfer to another hospital – for restricted and non-restricted patients (see below) this may be to a less secure facility
- consideration of a CTO by the responsible clinician
- the patient's transfer to guardianship.

Although these are just recommendations, the tribunal has the authority to reconvene and rehear a case if there is a failure to comply with its recommendations.

Briefly, the powers of the tribunal in relation to Part III patients are as follows. Some patients may be 'restricted' because they are subject to a restriction order made by a court. If relevant statutory criteria are not met the tribunal may direct either absolute discharge (effective immediately) or conditional discharge (which may be deferred) where it is satisfied that the patient needs to be subject to recall to hospital. There may be additional conditions imposed by the tribunal or the Secretary of State for Justice. A tribunal considering an application from a conditionally discharged patient may amend or remove the conditions or direct discharge. Another type of restricted patient is a transferred prisoner subject to a 'restriction direction'. The tribunal cannot direct the discharge of such a patient but can notify the Secretary of State of the suitability of an absolute or conditional discharge. The Secretary of State must take this advice into consideration but is not bound by it.

The tribunal also has a statutory duty to permit representations by a victim where a court has imposed certain orders, directions or a sentence for a violent or sexual offence. Submissions may be made in relation to the nature of conditions that may be imposed in the event of the patient's discharge (e.g. a prohibition of contact).

Applications and referrals

One application may be made by a patient to the tribunal in each eligibility period. These periods vary from section to section – see Chapter 6 of the Reference Guide to the Mental Health Act (Department of Health, 2015). If an application is withdrawn it is treated as never having been made and the patient can reapply within the same eligibility period. Where circumstances dictate, the hospital managers have a duty to refer to the tribunal for a hearing (section 68 of the Mental Health Act). For patients detained under Part II the nearest relative has no right to apply for an appeal unless the responsible clinician has issued a barring order in relation to a patient detained under section 3 or the nearest relative has been displaced by order of a county court on the grounds of unreasonable objection to admission or treatment or guardianship. The nearest relative may apply to the tribunal for patients under Part III and guardianship, although the stipulations vary between the different sections. The Secretary of State (or in Wales a Welsh minister) has powers to refer patients to a tribunal at any time.

The tribunal members

The legal member

The tribunal is presided over by the judge (England) or president (Wales). The legal member may be a senior solicitor, a circuit or higher judge, or a barrister. If the application to the tribunal is for a restricted patient the tribunal judge must be selected from a list of members approved by the Lord Chancellor. The legal member is responsible for ensuring that proceedings are conducted fairly and in accordance with the law and the Tribunal Rules. The legal member may advise on points of law and is required to draft the tribunal's decisions.

The medical member

The medical members are currently consultant psychiatrists, although it was the intention of the government in the consultation 'Transforming Tribunals' (2007) to reconsider this professional status. The Tribunal Rules (rule 34) direct that an 'appropriate member of the tribunal must, so far as is practicable (a) examine the patient and (b) take such steps as that member considers necessary to form an opinion of the patient's condition'. This will be the task of the medical member, who may examine the patient in private, have access to medical records and other documents and take notes or copies of records for use in connection with the proceedings. The inclusion of 'so far as is practicable' indicates that there is no absolute requirement for an examination to take place, presumably in circumstances where patients are uncooperative with the examination. The medical member presents the findings to other panel members prior to the hearing and he or she, or sometimes the judge, gives a summary of the pertinent points to the assembled gathering. Medical members contribute, with the other panel members, to the tribunal decision.

The specialist member

The specialist tribunal member will have significant professional experience in the health and welfare sectors, social care or other relevant sectors and may have a social worker, occupational therapy, psychology, nursing or other background. Specialist tribunal members will therefore provide an additional source of expertise, drawing from their experience in other fields.

The tribunal has established a child and adolescent mental health service (CAMHS) panel and ensures that at least one of the tribunal members has special expertise in dealing with cases where a child is subject to a section under the Act.

Other participants

The solicitor

Access to a court is a fundamental right guaranteed by Article 5 of the European Convention on Human Rights. The Human Rights Act requires that detained patients have effective legal representation provided by the state. The tribunal should also consider appointing a legal representative for an unrepresented patient, even where the patient has chosen not to be represented. The responsible clinician may be approached to make a statement as to the individual's capacity in this regard.

Solicitors are obliged to follow guidance and standards issued by the Law Society and must act in accordance with their client's instructions. The Solicitors Regulation Authority (SRA) has published a handbook that sets out all the SRA's regulatory requirements, along with the ethical standards that the SRA expects of law firms and practitioners (SRA, 2016). Furthermore, the Mental Health Lawyers Association (MHLA) has adopted a code of conduct which covers quality of service, making appointments, behaviour on the wards, disputes over representation, seeking clients, gifts and hospital procedures (MHLA, 2013).

Independent mental health advocates

The independent mental health advocate (IMHA) is appointed to help qualifying patients understand the legal provisions to which they are subject, and their rights and safeguards; they may also assist patients to exercise those rights. IHMAs can accompany patients to tribunals and hospital managers' hearings and may support the patient in the decisions that are made.

Before the tribunal

In order to comply with the Article 5 Convention requirement that detention be 'speedily decided by a court' the tribunal must hear appeals for section 2 within 7 days of receipt of an application; within 5–8 weeks for section 3 and 10–20 weeks for restricted cases. This is a challenge for the Tribunal Service and is logistically problematic for local Mental Health Act administrators to arrange. The relevant 'responsible authority' must send a statement of information and relevant reports to the tribunal or, where appropriate, the Ministry of Justice as soon as possible; other than for section 2 cases, this should be at the very latest within 3 weeks of receipt of the patient's application or reference. The 'responsible authority' is the hospital managers (essentially the board of directors of the hospital or trust) if detained in an NHS or independent hospital or if the patient is on a CTO, and is the responsible local social services if the patient is under guardianship.

Tribunals can be a significant interruption to a busy working schedule; however, when approached for availability the clinician should attempt to respond promptly and be flexible. If this is not done the clinician may find that the tribunal will issue a date that may be less suitable and with little or no opportunities to rearrange it. If anyone fails to comply with a direction, summons or order, the tribunal may take such action as it considers necessary. It may make an order requiring any defaulting party or any other person to produce any specified document or report; it may adjourn the case and make an order for wasted costs. At best, this is likely to cause unnecessary and avoidable stress and embarrassment.

With the increasing use of section 2 there may be limited time to garner all the information required to make the case for detention. For in-patients known to community teams, close working relationships and early dialogue between the teams may be required: to determine the natural history of the clinical predicament; to establish 'nature' or 'degree' criteria for mental disorder; to characterise the risks; to explore alternatives to hospital and detention under the Act; and to establish the purpose and likely clinical outcomes of admission. For patients not known to local services this may be even more exacting. However, given the personal and legal intrusion of detention under the Act, the clinical team must set about assembling the evidence without delay. The tribunal is unlikely to be sympathetic to medical evidence which comprises a series of unknowns.

The responsible clinician has a duty to consider whether statutory criteria for detention are met at all times and in approximately one-third of all detentions the section is discharged by the responsible clinician before the hearing (Care Quality Commission, 2015). Strong multidisciplinary team-working is key to good tribunal performance and working together increases the likelihood of getting the outcome the team is recommending, which may be, for example, in favour of continued detention if that is what is wanted, or, for restricted patients, the team may want conditional discharge.

If timescales permit, the clinician should arrange a care programming meeting before the tribunal or have one scheduled for soon after, in order that objectives can be clearly set and roles and timescales discussed. This is important evidence to include in the report if possible. Time should be spent thinking carefully about criteria and what it is that needs to be achieved clinically and why there are no alternatives to use of the Mental Health Act, as these will almost certainly form the basis of initial questions. Tribunals can be disconcerting and if clinicians do not rehearse these issues beforehand they may quickly feel underprepared and outmanoeuvred.

The responsible clinician also has a duty to examine a patient who is due for renewal of a section 3 order within the 2 months before the period of detention expires; similarly, there is a duty to examine a patient who is subject to guardianship or a CTO within the 2 months before the period expires and to determine whether the patient continues to meet the relevant criteria for detention. If a tribunal is then scheduled it is advisable that the responsible clinician examine the patient shortly before the tribunal so that up-to-date findings can be reported.

Tribunal reports

The responsible clinician's report forms an important element of the evidence considered by the tribunal in determining whether criteria for detention are met. It is therefore worthwhile spending time crafting the content to address *all* the issues that support the reasoning and even to highlight significant deficiencies – for instance, what information is missing and how any shortcomings will be addressed. Ignoring weaknesses will not make them go away and the clinician should assume that the solicitor will recognise and try to exploit them during the tribunal.

Practice directions have been made which specify the contents of reports submitted to the tribunal. The content of the responsible clinician's report will depend on the nature of the case but guidance is provided for five types of case: in-patients; guardianship patients; community patients; conditionally discharged patients; and patients under the age of 18. Common to all are the requirements that the report be up to date, specifically prepared for the tribunal, have numbered paragraphs and pages, and be signed and dated. The sources of information for the events and incidents described must be made clear and there is a requirement that the report is not an addendum to previous reports (nor reproduce extensive details from them), or recite medical records. Where circumstances allow the report to be prepared by someone other than the responsible clinician, it should be countersigned by him or her.

Although space does not permit reproduction of the practice directions in full, they are currently available at the Judiciary website (see under

'Online resources' at the end of the chapter) and it is important that they are followed. For example, for in-patients, the responsible clinician must briefly describe the patient's recent relevant medical history and current mental health presentation. There are 18 subheadings that *must* be included in the report. Not all may be relevant to any particular individual but it will inevitably mean that reports take some time to prepare. Judge Mark Hinchcliffe (Deputy Chamber President, First-Tier Tribunal) has expressed the requirements of the reports in the following way: 'What we need are succinct, stand-alone reports containing the required information, submitted on time' (Reports for Mental Health Tribunals – Practice Direction, Letter, November 2013). The tribunal can adjourn if it feels reports are inadequate.

The report must document the circumstances leading to detention and in particular give a clear justification that the criteria for detention are met. In so doing it can be helpful to include the wording of the relevant sections of the Act and set out specifically the basis and reasoning for which relevant statutory criteria are met. For example, for a section 2 order:

'In considering whether Mr M meets criteria for detention under section 2, the criteria are as follows:

(a) *He is suffering from mental disorder of a nature or degree which warrants the detention of the patient in a hospital for assessment (or for assessment followed by medical treatment) for at least a limited period...*

In the case of Mr M he appears to suffer from X disorder and it is currently the 'degree' of which warrants his detention for the following reasons...

There are also features of 'nature' which are as follows...

(b) *He ought to be so in the interests of his own health and safety or with a view to protection of others.*

In the case of Mr M it is predominantly for his own health that he requires detention for the following reasons...'

There is also the requirement to consider (and to have assessed and documented) the individual's mental capacity in relation to treatment and admission and whether or not the Mental Capacity Act (MCA) represents an alternative to detention under a section of the Mental Health Act.

Other notable highlights from the practice directions are the requirement for a summary of the patient's current progress, behaviour and insight, and any issues relating to compliance, risk and risk management. There are other issues that are important to communicate and which are less explicit in the practice directions but which may form the basis of questions from the panel or the patient's solicitor. These are as follows:

- What is the clinical team's plan and what is it they are trying to achieve?
- What are the anticipated outcomes and likely time course?

- For in-patients, what investigations or assessments remain to be conducted and are there positive aspects to detention under the Act (e.g. through the cautious use of section 17 leave in the process of rehabilitation) that may lead to a safer and better outcome for the patient?

If a CTO is being considered, the criteria for the underlying treatment section (section 3, 37 etc.) must still apply and the tribunal is bound to discharge if it is not satisfied that relevant statutory criteria are met. Therefore, the clinician should consider why the patient is appropriate for the CTO and what would need to happen for successful working of such an order. If the patient is already on a CTO, consideration should be given to what the plan would be that would lead to discharge (e.g. patient compliance with medication over a 12-month period).

Other issues which can be useful to reflect on are the patient's strengths or positive factors; the patient's own views; and, for in-patients, the resources available if the tribunal discharges the patient from detention and the patient leaves hospital. How are the principles of the Mental Health Act supported by the patient's continued detention?

Time spent in report-writing and including the pertinent information and balanced arguments may mean that the clinician can refer to written statements in the hearing. This can be easier to undertake for those who do not find the proceedings of the tribunal comfortable.

Finally, if the tribunal is not already aware, it may shorten the duration and facilitate smooth running of the proceedings if the report indicates whether the patient requires any additional support such as an interpreter, British Sign Language and/or a relay interpreter, as this will need to be arranged in advance.

Conduct of the tribunal

In general, the professionals who are present will be: the responsible clinician; a qualified nurse who has been directly involved in the patient's care; and the author of the social circumstances report. If someone is deputising for the responsible clinician, the Mental Health Act administrator should be notified in advance so that this can be agreed with the tribunal. For the purpose of the hearing, any party is entitled to representation. The responsible clinician may be asked if he or she is the nominated representative of the detaining authority. Under such circumstances the responsible clinician may call or cross-examine witnesses and sum up the case on behalf of the responsible authority but the tribunal must be notified prior to the hearing. This is very unusual and the responsible clinician is then entitled to (and should engage) legal representation. Ordinarily the responsible clinician will be a witness, not a nominated representative.

The legal member will start the proceedings with introductions and explanation. He or she may then summarise the preliminary discussions of the tribunal in relation to the patient's clinical state or invite the medical member to do so. There is some latitude as to the conduct of the hearing and the solicitor may wish the tribunal to hear evidence from the patient from the outset or wait until all the other witnesses have spoken. Tribunals are frequently a difficult time for patients and can carry a great weight of expectation. Some patients may still be acutely unwell and be unable to tolerate the proceedings and wish to leave. The solicitor (who usually expresses what the client wants) will therefore make a decision on how to present the case in a way that optimises the client's chances of success.

Proceedings are relatively formal and the responsible clinician, when attending as a witness, should speak when spoken to and resist the temptation to add to others' evidence. It is very common for the responsible clinician to give evidence first; as in a trial, the prosecution has to outline the case before the defence can answer the accusations. The starting point may be, for example, to provide an update since the report was written or provide a brief overview of relevant clinical issues to date. The clinician will then move on to examine whether the relevant criteria for detention are met and why. Questions are likely to be raised by all the tribunal members and the solicitor; moreover, they are likely to be probing and not always straightforward. The responsible clinician should state the case as clearly, honestly and in as balanced a fashion as possible. As discussed, this is easier to undertake effectively if all the issues are clearly articulated and argued in the report.

It can also be uncomfortable speaking with the required candour in front of the patient. If the patient continually makes interruptions, it is best to be sympathetic but it is the legal member who should manage the situation.

When the members of the panel have finished their questioning, if there is something of importance the responsible clinician wishes to contribute, permission to do so should be politely requested.

Factors which strengthen the case are good team-working and having a clear view of what it is that needs to be achieved. If a nurse is attending to report the views of the nursing team, it may help to resolve differences of opinion in advance. The solicitor will very likely exploit any divisions or lack of cohesion in the team to the client's advantage.

Once all the professional witnesses have been questioned, patients, if they wish, can make a statement or answer questions from their solicitor or the panel; if relatives are present they may also have something further to contribute.

Finally, the solicitor has an opportunity to sum up. This can all take time. There is a great deal of variation but the average tribunal can take upwards of 2 hours. Opinions vary but carefully consider the appropriateness of the responsible clinician delivering evidence and then asking to be excused because he or she is busy. At the very least one should be available in the vicinity, as further questions may arise. The tribunal has the authority to refuse such a request.

The tribunal may give a decision orally at the hearing, or written decisions must be sent within 3 working days of a section 2 hearing or 7 days for other cases.

Disclosure and non-disclosure of information to a patient

In the period between the receipt of an application and the tribunal itself, the responsible clinician will receive a request for access to medical records from the patient's solicitor. The response should be prompt in order that the solicitor has a reasonable opportunity to view the client's records. The Tribunal Rules provide that the tribunal may give a direction prohibiting the disclosure of information, reports or documents to a patient (or anyone else). Ideally, if there are points of controversy, hospitals, patients and/or their solicitors should come to an agreement regarding the documents that should be disclosed in tribunal proceedings.

However, if there are documents which it is felt should be withheld, the relevant material should be submitted and marked as follows:

'Not to be disclosed to the patient without the express permission of the tribunal.'

It is the tribunal's decision as to whether the criteria for non-disclosure are met. As there is a general imperative in favour of full disclosure, the onus is on the responsible authority to demonstrate the appropriateness of non-disclosure and it must provide the tribunal with full written reasons for the exclusion within 7 working days (3 working days for section 2 hearings).

The tribunal has to be satisfied that such disclosure would be likely to cause that person (or another person) serious harm and that it is proportionate to give such a direction. The threshold to withhold information is likely to be high. The Upper Tribunal (in *Dorset Healthcare NHS Foundation Trust v MH*) has issued guidance on how disclosure disputes can be managed.

Re-detention after discharge from a section

Following the tribunal's decision to direct the discharge of a patient, re-detention is not permitted except in very limited circumstances. Guidance on this is provided by Lord Bingham in the *R (von Brandenburg) v East London and City MH NHS Trust* judgment in the following way. The approved mental health professional (AMHP) in making an application must have 'formed the reasonable and bona fide opinion that he has information not known to the tribunal which puts a significantly different complexion on the case as compared with that which was before the tribunal'. The court gave a non-exhaustive list of examples where this may apply, paraphrased as follows. Has new information materialised in relation to an attempt on the patient's life that was not an issue during the course of the hearing? Has the patient reneged on the assurance of compliance with medication, thereby causing a risk to him- or herself or others, or has there been deterioration in the patient's condition not apparent when the tribunal made its decision?

Other grounds include whether the tribunal hearing was conducted in a way which was outside any reasonable court process (e.g. the responsible clinician was not permitted to speak). The hospital managers are not bound to accept the detention of a patient who has been recently discharged by the tribunal and if one is considering re-detention under these circumstances it may be advisable to seek legal advice.

Patient withdrawal and CTO hearings

A patient's application for appeal can be withdrawn only with the tribunal's consent. If the request is made in writing before the hearing date it is almost invariably agreed. Mandatory referrals cannot be withdrawn. A referral for a CTO tribunal can be disposed of without a formal hearing if the patient is 18 or over and either states in writing that he or she does not wish to attend or be represented (and the tribunal is satisfied the patient has the capacity to decide) or the representative states in writing that the patient does not want to attend or be represented. A report from the responsible clinician will still be required but the tribunal relies on the written evidence that is submitted and it is most likely that the clinician will not need to attend.

Conclusion

Tribunals, as all of us should, take very seriously the intrusion into a person's life of being detained or subject to a section of the Mental Health Act. Of 17 635 hearings in 2014/2015 only approximately 10% (1773) were discharged by the tribunal, so the odds are greatly in favour of continued detention. However, whatever the outcome, the key to a satisfactory tribunal performance relies on the responsible clinician having clarity of purpose in what it is that needs to be achieved clinically, having effective multidisciplinary team-working and communication with other agencies, and paying careful attention to the practice directions and the content of the report (setting out which statutory criteria are met, with meaningful examples and reasoning). It is helpful to read the written tribunal reasons as they often contain interesting insights or ways of phrasing.

For difficulties and questions in relation to tribunals or the Act, the codes of practice (there are separate ones for England and Wales) provide guidance on how the Mental Health Act 1983 should be applied. There are other published texts which may be helpful and mental health administrators can be a vital source of information and advice. There may be other local senior clinicians with formal or informal responsibilities or expertise who may be consulted and there may be the rare occasion when advice from the trust solicitors is sought (with prior approval). A final consideration is that if a psychiatrist finds that tribunal work is occupying a significant amount of time, it may be an issue for discussion in a job planning meeting.

References

Care Quality Commission (2015) *Monitoring the Mental Health Act in 2014/15*. CQC.

Department of Health (2015) *Reference Guide to the Mental Health Act*. TSO.

MHLA (2013) *Code of Conduct* (version 2). Available at http://www.mhla.co.uk/about/code-of-conduct (accessed April 2016).

Senior President of Tribunals (2012) *Annual Report*. Royal Courts of Justice.

SRA (2016) *SRA Handbook* (version 16). Available at http://www.sra.org.uk/solicitors/handbook/welcome.page (accessed April 2016).

Cases

Dorset Healthcare NHS Foundation Trust v MH (2009) UKUT 4 (AAC)

R (von Brandenburg) v East London and City MH NHS Trust (2003) UKHL 58

Other sources

Tribunal rules

England

The Tribunal Procedure (Amendment) Rules 2011
http://www.legislation.gov.uk/uksi/2008/2699/contents/made

Wales

The Mental Health Tribunal Rules for Wales
http://www.legislation.gov.uk/uksi/2008/2705/contents/made

Guidance for solicitors

http://www.lawsociety.org.uk/support-services/advice/practice-notes/representation-before-mental-health-tribunals/

Practice directions

https://www.judiciary.gov.uk/wp-content/uploads/JCO/Documents/Practice+Directions/Tribunals/statements-in-mental-health-cases-hesc-28102013.pdf

Part III

Personal development

Compassionate care: leading and caring for staff of mental health services and the moral architecture of healthcare organisations

Richard Williams, Verity Kemp and Adrian Neal

'Compassion (which is an element of loving-kindness) involves being open to the suffering of self and others, in a non-defensive and non-judgemental way. Compassion also involves a desire to relieve suffering, cognitions related to understanding the causes of suffering, and behaviours – acting with compassion. Hence it is from a *combination* of motives, emotions, thoughts and behaviours that compassion emerges.' (Gilbert, 2005)

As we write, the world is extremely concerned about the Ebola outbreak. Viral haemorrhagic fevers make carers' proximity to their patients dangerous and the protective equipment severely limits communication. The staff experience anguish because of the lethality of Ebola but also because very restricted personal contact with their patients limits their ability to express compassion and there are wide sociocultural impacts on western Africa and elsewhere (Ravi & Gaudlin, 2014). Perhaps there are lessons that could be learned from this awful epidemic and disasters generally about the nature of compassionate care and the care and support that staff require in order to sustain their work in more ordinary circumstances.

The staff of health services are renowned for their resilience and resourcefulness under pressure. Provided that resources are sufficient and the environment conducive, and they are well led, the quality of healthcare services is substantially related to the values and capabilities of the people who work in them. Public expectations are that staff consistently deliver effective, evidence-based care and interventions sensitively and compassionately, even if the environments in which they work are not optimal. However, there are, from time to time, lamentable lapses in the quality of care that patients receive and, despite an increasing focus on corporate and clinical governance over the last 20 years, there continue to be high-profile instances of catastrophic system failure in which organisations fail to deliver the minimum standards of compassionate care (Francis, 2013; Andrews & Butler, 2014).

This chapter focuses on the importance of providing staff within mental health services with effective leadership, support and care in order

377

to sustain them. It is our evidence-informed and values-based position that doing so is likely to enable staff to continue to consistently deliver compassionate care for their patients. We take the psychosocial resilience of staff as the anticipated position, but not as inevitable. We recognise that members of staff may find their experiences overwhelming at times, but, more importantly, also experience the effects of a slow accumulation of stressors. We contend that healthcare organisations must better understand the needs of their staff and provide appropriate care and support if they are to achieve continuity of compassionate, effective care for patients.

We identify the challenges and stressors that staff face, the roles of leaders and relationships, and provide a framework for managers at all levels to guide their work in sustaining the capabilities of healthcare staff. We assert the importance of balancing a sound organisational values base with evidence-based practice in creating capable, compassionate organisations. Thereby, we explore what a healthy workplace might look like.

We move between the experiences of staff and what we see as the opportunities and obligations that exist for employers to help them to be more effective and promote their achievements, emotional well-being, relationships and mental health. We recognise the foundational construct of moral architecture in healthcare organisations and the moral imperative it describes for strategists and leaders of healthcare to create a capable, sustainable workforce that is able to consistently deliver compassionate, effective care for patients.

The Royal College of Psychiatrists' College Centre for Quality Improvement has initiated its Enabling Environments Award as a 'quality mark given to those who can demonstrate they are achieving an outstanding level of best practice in creating and sustaining a positive and effective social environment' (College Centre for Quality Improvement, 2014). It defines enabling environments as places wherein:

- positive relationships promote well-being for all participants
- people experience a sense of belonging
- all people involved contribute to the growth and well-being of others
- people can learn new ways of relating
- the contributions of all parties in helping relationships are recognised and respected.

We draw together diverse constructs to illustrate these themes and illuminate the role of leaders in constructing enabling healthcare environments.

The context

Professional practice

Working with people who are in crisis or who are ill is a very unusual job, rich in social meaning and value. Compassion satisfaction describes the pleasure of being able to do this work well. It includes having positive feelings about helping others and contributing to the greater good of society (Stamm, 2002; Kemp *et al*, 2011). But the sense of not doing enough for patients and their families can create unpleasant feelings, including worthlessness, even when, objectively, staff know they have done everything possible to help their patients.

Working with people who are affected by illness and personal problems requires emotional labour, which has been defined as 'work done with feelings' (Hochschild, 1983). The notion of compassion gives voice to the importance of emotional labour. Yet, rarely, if ever, is this vital component of healthcarers' work acknowledged or recognised in their contracts. Our experience is that, without the passion, commitment, carefully positioned relationships and emotional labour of staff, the quality of the care of patients is unlikely to be optimal.

It is also important to consider that, too often, the context in which modern healthcare is provided is one in which mistakes are responded to with blame, resources are diminishing and expectations are high. These factors create ideal conditions for staff to feel increasingly vulnerable.

Healthcare organisations can take active steps to sustain healthcarers and support them in their emotional labour. These steps include refining the processes of managing and leading staff, recognising their emotional labour and providing them with social support in order to create and maintain organisational cultures in which attention to quality of care can flourish, and in which staff are sustained and developed so that they continue to gain satisfaction from their often emotionally difficult work and are available for future encounters. It is important to understand better how different working environments make different emotional demands on staff, and also what psychosocial factors underpin failures in compassionate care.

The UK policy context

The UK government's cross-government strategy for mental health for people of all ages establishes that mental health is everyone's business and is fundamental to our physical health, relationships, education, training and work and achieving our potential (Department of Health, 2011).

Policies in the UK show rising awareness of the importance of healthcare organisations as good employers and how this links to sustaining high-quality healthcare. The Chief Medical Officer (CMO) for England has made recommendations for positively changing the public's mental health that build on the importance of treating mental health as equal to physical health (parity of esteem). She said, 'Current evidence indicates that better psychological wellbeing of workers is associated with reduced sickness absence, higher productivity and, in the NHS, with lower staff turnover and higher patient satisfaction' (Department of Health, 2014).

Our summary of the reasons for ensuring that staff in mental health services are supported, developed and well led include:

- keeping them healthy in the face of their emotional labour and the risks for them, their patients and their colleagues posed by the challenging work that they do
- promoting and maintaining the psychological safety of working teams and the environments in which staff work
- promoting integrated values- and evidence-based practice (Williams & Fulford, 2007)
- recognising the importance of congruence between the values of organisations, the emotional needs of staff, the tasks that staff are asked to take on, and the values, preferences and needs of patients.

The NHS Constitution has outlined the values of the NHS in England (Department of Health, 2013). It includes four pledges that set out what staff should expect from NHS employers as part of the commitment of the NHS to provide high-quality environments for staff. Earlier, the National Institute for Health and Care Excellence (NICE) had recommended how organisations could improve their employees' well-being and exhorted managers to show respect for staff welfare (NICE 2009). In 2015, NICE published a guideline that focused on organisational culture and the role of line managers in the health and well-being of employees. NICE updated it in 2016 with recommendations for older employees (NICE, 2015/2016).

The challenges healthcare staff face

Primary and secondary stressors

In the course of their work, the staff of healthcare organisations face primary and secondary stressors.

Primary stressors are the sources of stress, worry and anxiety that stem directly from the tasks they do and events that they face at work and are inherent in healthcare. These include:

- caring for people with a range of diagnoses (acute and chronic conditions) who have a variety of natures of suffering and prognoses (rapid recovery to palliative and end-of-life care)
- exposure to patients', their relatives' and carers' experiences, needs and expectations in the context of the information age
- facing dangers at work, including being vicariously (re)-traumatised through the mechanism of empathy for suffering people (Stamm, 1999)
- dealing with difficult and confusing emotions while trying to care, including powerlessness, hopelessness, shame and anger.

However, leaders should be cautious before ascribing the stress that staff experience as necessarily resulting solely from what they witness and the work they do. Often, secondary stressors are hugely impactful.

Secondary stressors are circumstances, events or policies that are indirectly related to, or are not inherent in, the events, tasks and emotions that face staff but are consequential on them and concern the conditions in which staff work and live (Lock *et al*, 2012). Secondary stressors include the experiences that impact on the *psychological contract* between employee and employer (Rousseau, 1989). Breaches of this generally unspoken relationship often go unacknowledged, are difficult to repair and can reduce both staff morale and quality of care. Other secondary stressors include decisions that staff believe are morally and/or professionally unfair: notions of *organisational justice* can markedly influence their motivation and well-being (Latham & Pinder, 2005).

Box 26.1 summarises some of the stressors that are non-inherent to work (Sparks & Cooper, 1999) as well as more secondary stressors that staff of healthcare organisations face. Secondary stressors may persist over longer periods than do each of the tasks that make up the work of healthcare. Even though less visible than primary stressors, their impact may be long term and potentially devastating.

How staff can cope

We are repeatedly reminded of the time, energy and emotion that staff expend in trying to resolve non-inherent, secondary stressors. The majority of staff develop ways of coping and attend enthusiastically to the challenges

---

Box 26.1 Secondary stressors that staff face

Stressors that staff face that are not inherent to their work (Sparks & Cooper, 1999):

- Perceived job control
- Career development
- Workplace climate and culture
- Job and workload
- Home–work interface
- Role clarity
- Relationships at work

Other secondary stressors staff face:

- Arbitrary leadership and/or management practices
- Lack of materials to do their jobs
- Poor role definition and unclear expectations
- Poor organisation at work
- Lack of support at work
- Unnecessarily restrictive policies and practices
- Unnecessarily poor working conditions
- Poor scheduling of work
- Lack of skills or training to do their jobs
- Lack of opportunities for recreation
- Conflict and mistrust within and between teams
- Poor communication

work presents them through actively or passively deploying a range of coping strategies. Not all coping strategies are adaptive: some may be maladaptive and linked to unwanted behaviours that undermine compassionate care (e.g. avoidance and neglect). The employer's role in sustaining staff is an active process that calls for investment of time, effort and resources. Employers should not make assumptions about the extent of staff resilience, but, instead, begin by observing the true adaptiveness of coping methods that staff use, as well as those that employers deploy to help them.

The risk is that some staff may, often inadvertently, try to numb their feelings of empathy towards patients as a coping and preventive technique (Cicognani *et al*, 2009; Kemp *et al*, 2011). That risks them being experienced as cold, detached and dispassionate by the very people whose suffering they are trying to ease. Emotionally avoidant coping strategies not only block positive reinforcement from caring interactions but also the joy and satisfaction in a job well done, as well as support from colleagues (Brown, 2010). They deny the emotional nature of the human experience of trying to relieve the suffering of another. Behavioural and emotional avoidance (e.g. distraction) is commonly observed after serious events and is claimed to be associated with greater distress, burnout and compassion fatigue among ambulance personnel (Clohessy & Ehlers, 1999; Cicognani *et al*, 2009; Kemp *et al*, 2011). Furthermore, emotionally avoidant coping can quietly undermine staff's emotional well-being and plays a major role in maintaining mood and anxiety disorders. These paths are risky for both patients and staff.

The vicious cycle of distress avoidance can be perpetuated where blaming and shaming cultures are evident. The role of shame in organisational life is becoming better understood: it may have an important part to play in understanding how symptoms of disorders arise and how we deal with them (Clough, 2010). Staff who hold onto feelings are likely to have greater difficulty coping with traumatic experiences (Cicognani *et al*, 2009). Rarely are difficult feelings openly acknowledged and shared and people may put a lot of energy into hiding them, perhaps because of their perceptions of the consequences of being unmasked in front of others. In addition, some staff report being rejected when they try to share their experience of powerful emotions such as guilt, and this makes their sense of blame worse. They can feel rejected by their families and isolated from their closest social networks (Cicognani *et al*, 2009).

Long-term organisational stress and lack of support tend to go together. The former may stem from environments of low social and managerial support that inhibit the expression of emotional problems. Inadequate social support may contribute directly to the risk of staff developing mental disorders (Blanchard *et al*, 1995) and, indirectly, to staff being part of a wider dysfunctional work environment. The stress that ambulance clinicians face in their work as a result of aspects of organisational culture, for example, seems to be a bigger contributor to their levels of anxiety and depression than the traumatic incidents to which they respond (Bennett *et al*, 2005).

The risks of not caring for healthcare staff

The CMO for England has identified the benefits of staff well-being. Conversely, people who care for patients are more at risk of facing stress that creates problems for them than are many other people, on account of the nature of the work that they do and the expectations of them. We have identified that one of the risks of failing to care for healthcare staff adequately is an impact on the quality of care that they deliver.

We write as strategic leaders and managers whose current focus is on healthcare systems for disasters and conflict and the psychosocial and mental healthcare components of those services. Our experience indicates that there are lessons from disaster healthcare that also apply to more routine services. Research on humanitarian aid workers has shown, for example, that, on return from deployment, 40% reported that the mission was more stressful than expected and that this was due mostly to their working environments. One-third reported their health was worse on return than on leaving home (Dahlgren *et al*, 2009).

Box 26.2 Evidence on the risks of failing to attend to the needs of staff

- Compassion fatigue and burnout in the form of emotional exhaustion and sense of low personal accomplishment may occur (Figley, 1995).

- Professional healthcare responders in certain high-pressure roles and services may be more likely than the general population to take early retirement (Sterud *et al*, 2006).

- Exposure of health professionals who work in wards in which there is an average bed occupancy rate over 10% in excess of the recommended limit is associated with:
  - new antidepressant treatment among hospital staff who are so exposed for over 6 months
  - if they are so exposed during a 1-year period, twice the risk of sickness absence due to depressive disorders relative to colleagues working in wards with optimal or below-occupancy levels (Virtanen *et al*, 2008).

- A survey of 2608 doctors in the USA found that 87% of doctors who reported diminished enthusiasm for medicine ascribed this to inhibition of empathic care (Zuger, 2004).

- Burnout in health service staff (Schaufeli, 1999) is more likely in staff who:
  - are younger, with less work experience
  - have lower self-esteem
  - have less resilient personalities, more unrealistic job expectations, high dissatisfaction and increased intention to quit.

High-quality evidence on the morale of the mental health workforce in the UK is lacking (Johnson *et al*, 2012). Evidence on the impact on staff working in mental health services is fragmented, but what is available demonstrates that the emotional impact on staff is significant and occurs in all settings, including humanitarian, hospital and community services. Box 26.2 summarises recent evidence.

The number of medical graduates who accepted an offer of psychiatry training posts in England and Wales fell from 184 in 2009 to 158 in 2010 because, it is alleged, the specialism suffers from a poor reputation compared with other medical disciplines (Bhugra, 2013). Aarons & Sawitzky (2006) say, 'Staff turnover in mental health service organizations is an ongoing problem with implications for staff morale, productivity, organizational effectiveness, and implementation of innovation'. Their study examined models for the effects of culture and climate on work attitudes and the subsequent impact of work attitudes on staff turnover. They found that work culture influences work attitudes, which significantly predicted 1-year staff turnover rates. Conversely, clinicians' satisfaction with their relationships with patients can protect against professional stress, burnout, substance misuse and even suicide attempts (Shanafelt, 2009).

Sustaining healthcare staff

Our core theme is that helping to sustain staff calls for their employers to take active steps to recognise and understand their psychosocial needs, reduce the primary and secondary stressors bearing on them, and provide consistent access to good leadership, support, care and development.

Resilience

Resilience has been studied over a substantial portion of the last century. While the general construct is not without its critics, there is an increasing evidence base regarding psychosocial resilience. It describes how people, groups of people and communities may spring back to effective functioning after becoming distressed by perturbations, challenges and adversity (Ciccetti & Blender, 2006; Williams *et al*, 2014a).

Staff who are affected by problems at work as a result of their emotional labour and secondary stressors may become distressed. Psychosocial resilience is not a synonym for resistance to the impact of events, the absence of short-term distress after untoward events, or not suffering more prolonged distress if secondary stressors exacerbate it. Neither does psychosocial resilience describe absence of risk and it should not be inferred from: absence of distress; positive mental health; or absence of a mental disorder (Williams *et al*, 2014a,b). The corollary is that people who seem resilient after major challenges should not be assumed to be unaffected psychosocially.

Rather, the term refers to people's abilities to adapt to, and to recover and learn from, their experiences. Most people recover and cope well given social support from relatives, friends and colleagues. Thus, psychosocial resilience is a dynamic concept that describes interpersonal processes and the attributes of people by which they act singly and/or together to mitigate, moderate, and recover from the effects of stressful events through exercising adaptive capabilities. We identify three 'generations' of resilience (Omand, 2010):

- first-generation resilience – the ability to cope well with events and their immediate aftermath
- second-generation resilience – the ability to recover from events
- third-generation resilience – the ability of people to adapt in the light of lessons learned from events.

The adaptive capacities that comprise psychosocial resilience are of genetic, psychological, environmental and social origin (Amstadter *et al*, 2014; Wertz & Pariante, 2014). We support the views of Norris *et al* (2009), who define psychosocial resilience as a process linking a set of adaptive capacities to a positive trajectory of functioning and adaptation after a disturbance (Kaniasty & Norris, 2004; Williams & Greenberg, 2014). Box 26.3 lists our adaptation of the resilience factors that Southwick & Charney (2012) have identified.

The many environmental factors affecting healthcare staff include: their past, recent and contemporary experiences and relationships; situational factors; the levels and nature of the injuries and illnesses that their patients suffer; the community and hospital healthcare and social resources that are available; the levels of adversity within which they work; and their access to supportive colleagues and family members. Psychological factors may include their beliefs, attachment patterns, personality, relational style, sense of agency and tolerance of distress. Variations in these factors may well explain why the same people may respond differently in different circumstances (Williams *et al*, 2014*a*).

Box 26.3   Resilience factors

- Realistic optimism
- Facing fear
- Having strong guiding values
- Spirituality
- Social support
- Physical fitness
- Mental fitness
- Cognitive and emotional flexibility and the ability to improvise
- Creating meaning and purpose from events through personal growth

Adapted from the ten principles of Southwick & Charney (2012)

The quality of our relationships serves either to support or to undermine our resilience. Humans are highly adapted to function in groups. Social identity is the process by which we connect to others to form groups. Evidence from a multitude of psychotherapy trials points to the power of relationships as the vehicle for relieving distress. The social identity model, in particular, has shown the powerful influences on how people cope with adversity and ill health of their social identities, which are based on social relationships at home and work as well as with strangers at times of greatest need. These potentially positive influences provide the platform for the adaptive capabilities that influence resilience.

People who show better psychosocial resilience tend to perceive that they have, and actually receive, support. People's abilities for forming and maintaining relationships with others and accepting their support are key strengths. In this context, social support consists of social interactions that provide actual assistance, but also embed people in a web of relationships that they perceive to be caring and readily available in times of need (Haslam *et al*, 2012; Williams *et al*, 2014a,b). We emphasise its importance because of the emerging statistical evidence on its effect size (Haslam *et al*, 2012).

Within the professional world, relationships between managers and employees play a role in sustaining staff well-being (Black & Frost, 2011). Consequently, we emphasise the importance of leadership and advocate peer support as an important means for enabling staff. Research has identified its features (Varker & Creamer, 2011) (Box 26.4).

Box 26.4 Peer supporters

- Peer supporters should have clear goals, including:
  - providing an empathic, listening ear
  - identifying colleagues who may be at risk to themselves or to others
  - facilitating pathways to professional help

- Peer supporters should have definite roles. They should:
  - not limit their activities to high-risk incidents
  - maintain confidentiality

- Peer supporters should:
  - be members of the target population
  - be people who have considerable experience in the field of work
  - be respected by their peers
  - be trained
  - be looked after and have access to support
  - have their work evaluated

Based on Varker & Creamer (2011)

Teams, organisations, psychological safety and active coping

A recurring theme in this chapter is the power of interactions between individuals and groups of people, including: the people they work with; their families; and their employers. We focus now on the interface between staff members and their employers in achieving the goal of sustaining compassionate care.

A sense of self-efficacy increases with staff members' experience and levels of expertise. It is an important factor in reducing levels of distress (Regehr *et al*, 2003; Kemp *et al*, 2011) and is associated with compassion satisfaction and the use of active coping, rather than the avoidance techniques to which we referred earlier (Cicognani *et al*, 2009).

But, increasingly, the nature of planning and delivering healthcare is based on collaborative, coordinated team-working. The concept of 'collective efficacy' refers to what groups of people choose to focus on, the effort they put into it, and how groups perceive their abilities to accomplish their major tasks (Bandura, 1997; Kemp *et al*, 2011). Collective efficacy enhances job satisfaction and well-being (Jex & Bliese, 1999; Kemp *et al*, 2011). A sense of community at work among healthcare workers is important to them and feelings of belonging contribute to satisfaction (Cicognani *et al*, 2009). How each team copes with challenging experiences creates a series of assumptions and beliefs about the situations with which that group can deal effectively.

Staff of caring organisations report that it is possible to cope actively with the effects of traumatic experiences. Active coping includes techniques such as describing impressions and reactions in conversations with colleagues and other people (Cicognani *et al*, 2009).

Central to a group's ability to cope is the concept of emotional containment, as proposed by Bion (1961), whereby strong emotions can be held or contained by a group or system without members realising. This process can be supportive and foster exploration of other difficult emotions while making members feel safe. Groups that cannot hold or contain emotions do not support such expression, and leave people feeling unsafe, making the use of active coping techniques far less effective. This frames a vital challenge for leaders who wish to sustain the ability of their teams to deliver compassionate care.

The allied concept of psychological safety captures the degree to which people perceive their work environment as conducive to taking necessary interpersonal risks when doing their work. Edmondson says:

> 'in psychologically safe environments, people believe that if they make a mistake others will not penalize or think less of them for it … [and] that others will not resent or penalize them for asking for help, information or feedback.' (Edmondson, 2003: p. 257)

There is evidence that psychologically safe working environments are not only better for the well-being and welfare of the staff, but also less likely to result in errors of judgement or mistakes. Edmondson (2003) argues 'creating conditions of psychological safety is essential to laying a foundation for effective learning in organizations'. She says, 'Team leaders have a powerful effect on psychological safety' and 'The actions and attitudes of the team leader are ... important determinants of the team learning process'. She places the responsibility on leaders for creating working environments that are as psychologically safe as possible.

Leadership

Leadership is a complex array of values, attitudes, qualities, perceptive skills and transactional and translational capabilities that creates and communicates a vision of tasks (see Chapter 11). We have seen that leaders play important roles in fostering environments that contain their staff's emotions in realistic and safe ways, leaving patients' care enhanced and staff available and ready for fresh challenges. This requires team leaders to be acutely aware of team members' psychosocial capabilities and training needs and for the leaders to ensure the team members receive professional supervision, effective management and psychosocial support.

Research has shown that PhD students who had good leadership were 40% more likely to be in the highest category of job well-being and they had lower rates of anxiety, depression, and job stress and sick leave (Kuoppala *et al*, 2008). Evidence from research on military personnel shows that soldiers had significantly better mental health if they received psychoeducation before their deployments, perceived that they were well led and had good family support (Jones *et al*, 2014).

Leadership stands as one of the factors that are vital to keeping staff healthy and their work effective. The relationship between managers and staff has been identified as a predictor of both well-being and absence (Black & Frost, 2011). The other factors include providing sufficient resources, adequate peer support, adequate information about events, tasks and situational factors, and ensuring effective professional and managerial supervision.

There has been considerable debate around the ingredients that make up good leaders and two related factors have emerged: emotional intelligence (EI) and emotional literacy (EL). Emotional intelligence is the ability to monitor one's own and other people's emotions, to discriminate between different emotions and label them appropriately, and to use emotional information to guide thinking and behaviour (Goleman, 1995). Similarly emotional literacy relates knowing your feelings, having a sense of empathy, being able to manage your emotions, being able to repair emotional problems and sustaining emotional interactivity (Steiner, 1997). Both emotional intelligence and emotional literacy are well recognised correlates of good leadership, and may well form the conditions for staff to feel contained and safe. Whether these qualities can be trained or are innate is undecided, but they can be enhanced and supported in most people.

Creating and running psychologically safe teams and sustaining the resilience of healthcare staff requires leaders to:

- be accessible and supportive
- acknowledge fallibility
- balance empowering other people with managing the tendencies for certain people to dominate discussions
- balance psychological safety with accountability, safety and other components of strategic and clinical governance
- guide team members through talking about and learning from their uncertainties
- balance opportunities for their teams' reflection with action
- have the capacity for emotional containment/holding.

A strategic approach to caring for staff and sustaining compassionate care

We have recognised some uncomfortable pressures that fall on the staff of healthcare services. Generally, most staff cope and show enormous dedication to their work, which, all too often, they carry out in challenging circumstances. The science of understanding the impact of work on employees is in its infancy. But, just as we now appreciate the impacts of traditional industries and their work practices on physical health, so are we starting to understand the psychosocial impact of work. Often, staff are required to manage not only the stressors inherent in their exposure to patients but also secondary stressors, including pressure from peers, relationships, ever-changing organisational demands and the logistics of work. These pressures pose tasks for leaders and managers in developing the cultures and staff development activities of their organisations.

This is especially true when considering the industry of professional healthcare. While this is seen historically as low risk and benign, the implication of the themes in this chapter is that healthcare staff require effective, compassionate leadership, care and social support in their work if they are to continue to provide compassionate care for their patients.

We recommend that all policies and strategies should articulate not only *vision*, which comprises a statement of *intent* and a clear *direction* for actions to deliver the envisioned service, but also the *values* on which that vision is based, as well as a plan for developing and sustaining organisations and their staff. NHS Employers claims that 'performance is enhanced, patient care improves, staff retention is higher and sickness absence is lower' when NHS organisations prioritise staff health and well-being (NHS Employers, 2013). Organisations should attend to their *moral architecture* if they are to sustain their staff (Williams, 2000).

Moral architecture

The construct of moral architecture refers to the moral and human rights obligations that organisations acquire as employers and through their commitment to delivering high-quality services. In other words, we see employers as having moral as well as legal responsibilities to their staff. The moral architecture of organisations includes how well employers discharge these implied responsibilities, and recognising and attending to the implied psychological contract is one aspect.

Furthermore, we argue that it is difficult for healthcare staff to continue to provide compassionate, evidence-informed and values-based care for their patients unless they are supported by their employers; it will also be difficult if there is dissonance between the support, training and care for staff and the quality of care that they are expected to deliver (Williams & Fulford, 2007). This is especially so when employers ask staff to take more than minor risks in order to discharge their employers' roles.

These obligations should be reflected in organisations' policies, their design and delivery of services, and their corporate governance (Warner & Williams, 2005). This means that each organisation's visions, priorities, structures, activities, leadership, management and conditions of staff employment should be consistent with its stated roles and espoused values. Usually the ways in which organisations care for their staff tests their moral architecture (Williams, 2000).

One of us became interested in moral architecture some years ago (Williams, 2000). Subsequently, we came across the 'Living our values' initiative that the South Staffordshire and Shropshire NHS Foundation Trust in England launched in 2014. We were struck by the way in which the contents of this initiative resonate strongly with what we had written previously (Warner & Williams, 2005).

That trust identified five organisational values, which are that the staff and the organisation:

- are respectful
- are honest and trustworthy
- are caring and compassionate
- take the time to talk and listen
- work together and lead by example.

Senior staff of the trust say that simply having values in an organisation is not enough: the values have to be reflected in people's behaviour to make a difference. The organisational values were designed to ensure that, if they are embraced by staff within the organisation, they will, in turn, support delivery of the strategic objectives of the trust and the key areas for improvement.

During 2014, over 1000 members of staff of the trust, its partner agencies and service users and carers engaged in discussions around what it means to truly 'live our values'. This resulted in the trust's 'Living our values' charter and framework that the trust intends will be used in everything it does. We include the charter as Fig. 26.1 because the trust defines in it the responsibility of the organisation to its employees in respect of its values and the reciprocal responsibilities of the staff to help achieve sustainable quality improvements.

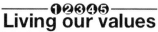

South Staffordshire and Shropshire Healthcare **NHS**
NHS Foundation Trust

A Keele University Teaching Trust

Our Charter

This is our Charter, it outlines how we, as an organisation will communicate our shared vision and has been developed in partnership with staff, service users, carers and partners. It defines the responsibilities of the organisation and the responsibilities of our employees to help achieve sustainable quality improvements, to improve the working lives of staff and thereby improve the quality of patient care and the interactions between staff and patients.

As an employee of South Staffordshire and Shropshire Healthcare NHS Foundation Trust you can expect:

- To be treated with **RESPECT** at all times and be valued for your individuality

- To work in an environment that nurtures **HONESTY AND TRUST**; even if the conversation is a difficult one

- To work with colleagues and managers who strive to provide a **CARING AND COMPASSIONATE** environment for all; demonstrating empathy in all working relationships, supporting others when things are tough and ensuring we get it right for our service users every time

- Everyone to endeavour to **TAKE THE TIME TO TALK AND LISTEN**, recognising the busy workloads we all carry, making sure there is time built in for 1:1 discussions and team meetings to help build a culture of positivity

- Development opportunities to enable people to **WORK TOGETHER** and feel valued and supported to build strong team working internally and communicate effectively with our external partners and stakeholders to ensure clarity of roles and objectives. Managers and team leaders will **LEAD BY EXAMPLE** and encourage decision making at the most appropriate level to make a real difference to service users

In Return we expect you as an employee to:

- Show **RESPECT** to everyone with whom you interact, ensuring service users and carers are respected for their individuality, that you respect your colleagues and managers at all levels, and recognise and embrace the value and contribution of others

- Adhere to any relevant job or professional standards and at all times demonstrate that you are **HONEST AND TRUSTWORTHY**

- Be committed to and show respect and empathy for your service users or colleagues and undertake your duties in a **CARING AND COMPASSIONATE** way at all times

- **TAKE THE TIME TO TALK AND LISTEN**, remember that if you only have time to say a few words, make them positive – make them count

- **WORK TOGETHER** help to break down barriers to effective service delivery, contribute to and participate in the development of your service, **LEAD BY EXAMPLE** and help your colleagues to feel valued and supported

Fig. 26.1 The charter produced by South Staffordshire and Shropshire NHS Foundation Trust (reproduced with permission)

We see this initiative as a good example of what is involved when organisations identify their values, work towards reducing the gap between what they offer staff and what they expect from them, and, thereby, endeavour to sustain compassionate care by harnessing the power of getting right their moral architecture.

A strategic stepped model of intervention

We propose a framework for how leaders and managers could organise their thinking and actions to create responsive services that offer leadership, psychologically safe teamwork, care and support in order to support them in delivering effective, compassionate interventions and care (Warner & Willliams, 2005; Varker & Creamer, 2011). A stepped strategic model is core (Department of Health, 2009) and ours is summarised in Box 26.5.

A more detailed version is presented as Annex A to this chapter, and Annex B provides an *aide-mémoire* for leaders listing actions that we recommend in discharging their responsibilities for staff of healthcare organisations.

Conclusion

We have considered the moral architecture of organisations and the components of working environments that make them more likely to enable staff to deliver compassionate and effective healthcare. We have drawn attention to organisational culture, enabling environments and the central role of relationships. We have introduced the concepts and significance of emotional labour, psychosocial resilience and psychologically safe teams, and pointed up the importance of providing resources, information, peer support, and professional and managerial supervision.

Box 26.5   The six-level, strategic, stepped model for staff development and support

Level 1. Strategic leadership and management

Planning, leadership, management and training sustain services and promote teamwork and therefore help to prevent unnecessary anxiety for staff by creating confidence in the plan.

Level 2. Operational leadership, service management and setting standards for practice

Translating plans into action requires excellent tactical management. Plans should be templates that are used to initiate services and later adjusted to fit better with events as they unfold. This requires good intelligence, leadership and review.

Level 3. Day-to-day leadership and management of staff and services

Ensuring the psychosocial welfare of all people involved, directly and indirectly, with delivering any service is a key part of that service. Risks to psychosocial well-being can be minimised by planning and implementing good leadership and management procedures and by ensuring that staff have adequate supervision, access to advice and support from colleagues and their families.

Levels 4–6. Psychosocial and mental healthcare for certain members of staff

Occasionally, some members of staff may develop distress that is usually short term but much less often is temporarily disabling or of longer duration. A much smaller number may develop more substantial problems with their mental health. Therefore, facilities should be available to support staff who are distressed or to enable access to mental healthcare according to need by providing appropriate psychosocial support and pathways to mental healthcare in the few instances in which it is anticipated that those services will be required. Such a stepped approach should include:

- measures that are based on the principles of psychosocial care (Williams *et al*, 2014a,b; Williams & Greenberg, 2014)
- surveillance, assessment and intervention services for people who do not recover from immediate and short-term distress
- access to primary and secondary mental healthcare services for people who are assessed as requiring them

Level 4. Offer psychosocial interventions based on the principles of psychological first aid

Level 5. Offer health assessment and intervention in primary care

Level 6. Deliver specialist mental health services for staff

Core to supporting people who are expected to consistently deliver compassionate care is ensuring that they are well led, well briefed, and offered sufficient peer and social support. Mols *et al* (2015) argue that people who promote 'lasting behaviour change need to engage with people … as members of groups whose norms they internalise and enact'. Central to this approach is leadership. Lilley (2014) says leaders:

- are visible, have a vision and share it often
- are brave
- set boundaries but realise boundaries are there to be porous
- are teachers
- lead by example
- need leaders around them
- need time
- are not perfect.

Lilley's opinion is that leaders deal with issues no one else can find a way into. One of those challenges is sustaining and developing compassionate care in a world in which governance procedures should be reviewed recurrently to ensure they reflect virtuous processes and, thereby, avoid perverse outcomes, and ensure that their effects are in harmony with the goals for which they were developed.

Annex A. The six-level framework of actions to support care for staff of healthcare organisations

Level 1. Strategic leadership and management

Planning, leadership, management and training sustain services and promote personal achievement and teamwork and, therefore, help to prevent unnecessary anxiety and strain for staff by creating confidence in the organisation. It is achieved by ensuring there is a psychosocial care plan for staff.

Strategic planning and preparation

Arrangements for strategic leadership and planning should be visible and integral to all services. Compassionate care for staff should be central to delivering the aim of all proposed developments. No general plan can be assumed to be appropriate to each situation. Development plans therefore need to include an explicit psychosocial care plan for staff and should be reviewed and adjusted to allow for the compassionate care of staff and to enable review and lessons for the future to be learned

Logistic and resource planning

Comprehensive planning, preparation, training and rehearsal of the full range of service responses that may be required should be undertaken and staff should be familiarised with the plans. This process should build their confidence in those plans, allow them to be engaged through suggesting changes, and build their resilience.

Developing models of care

Staff should have confidence in the models of care that are offered in their services. This involves reviewing services to ensure all the relevant providers of care and agencies work to jointly agreed models of care and case management. This includes working to minimise gaps and to develop clarity about mutual responsibilities.

Managing public and professional expectations

Planning and enacting a good public risk communication and an advisory strategy that involves staff, the public and the media and which provides timely and credible information and advice also supports staff confidence and psychosocial resilience.

Level 2. Operational leadership, service management and setting standards for practice

Translating psychosocial plans into action requires good tactical management. Plans should be templates that are used to initiate services that are adjusted subsequently to allow for development and delivery of services. This requires good intelligence, leadership and review.

Manage and lead expectations of practice and practitioners

Operational leaders and managers should manage the delivery of practice and the expectations placed on staff, and ensure that standards for practice and practitioners are realistic. This requires effective leadership, recognition of the potential impacts of day-to-day work as well as awareness that advancing science and developments in practice affect standards of care and negotiation of mechanisms for decision-making when services are under pressure.

Develop ethical and professionally acceptable care management frameworks and ethical frameworks for clinical and managerial decision-making

Care management systems should be based on the judgements of patients, their carers and professionals at preliminary, primary, secondary and tertiary levels. Staff should have confidence in the care systems that are put in place.

The NHS Constitution is an example of a framework for commissioners, services and practitioners that can be used as a reference point for underpinning compassionate care and decision-making. Each organisation is expected to develop and build on these values and tailor them to its local needs. The NHS values provide common ground for cooperation to achieve shared aspirations, at all levels of the NHS, and include:

- respect and dignity
- commitment to quality of care
- compassion
- improving lives
- everyone counts.

Educate, train and rehearse plans

The psychosocial plan to support staff and underpin compassionate care should be underpinned by training. Strategic advice on psychosocial and mental healthcare for patients and staff is required by planners when they design, test and implement their plans at strategic, tactical and operational levels.

Develop ethical guidelines and a staff competency framework

Commissioners, services and practitioners should adopt an ethical framework for planning and delivering services. Professional and general mangers should also be clear about the competencies required of practitioners, managers and others in caring for staff.

Level 3. Day-to-day leadership and management of staff and services

Ensuring the psychosocial welfare of all people involved in delivering mental health services is a key part of ensuring compassionate care. Risks to psychosocial well-being can be minimised by planning and implementing good management procedures and by ensuring that staff have adequate supervision and access to advice.

Provide accurate, up-to-date and relevant information about the situation

Staff must have confidence in the plans for day-to-day service delivery that are made, and this requires that they are fully informed about those plans and their anticipated roles in them. The feeling of being ill-informed can erode psychosocial resilience. Conversely, if staff are well-informed, consulted and involved, their confidence in the plans and their equipment is enhanced, their uncertainties are reduced and their psychosocial resilience is augmented.

Provide opportunities for operational, technical and personal discussions

Less-formal discussion about clinical experiences ordinarily occurs in work-places. In challenging circumstances, the support that comes from having access to team members, peers and others for discussion and advice and to share challenges and frustrations is invaluable. It is important to ensure that opportunities for informal peer support are valued and continue to be available, regardless of pressures on services. More formal peer-based reflection on and reviews of practice should also be encouraged.

Ensure staff take rests, adhere to duty rotas and have opportunities for recuperation

Staff (particularly senior staff with substantial responsibilities) must be enabled to take rests and work to realistic rotas to avoid them becoming overtired and 'burned out'.

Monitor practice and provide enhanced clinical advice and supervision

The work of staff should be monitored so that they have access to clinical supervision; this is likely to become more rather than less vital in stressful situations when critical and sometimes controversial decisions may have to be made.

Levels 4–6. Psychosocial and mental healthcare for certain members of staff

Occasionally, some members of staff may develop distress that is usually short term, but much less often temporarily disabling or of longer duration. A much smaller number may develop more substantial problems with their mental health. Therefore, facilities should be available to support staff who are distressed and to enable their access to mental healthcare, according to need, by providing appropriate psychosocial support and planned pathways to effective mental healthcare. Such a stepped approach should include:

- measures that are based on the principles of psychosocial care (Williams *et al*, 2014a,b; Williams & Greenberg, 2014)
- surveillance, assessment and intervention services for people who do not recover from immediate and short-term distress
- access to primary and secondary mental healthcare services for people who are assessed as requiring them.

Level 4. Offer psychosocial interventions based on the principles of psychological first aid (PFA)

The approach recommended here is based on an understanding that people who are affected by adverse events and ongoing pressures at work and elsewhere experience a broad range of reactions (physical, emotional, cognitive, behavioural and spiritual).

PFA is an approach and not a specific intervention that is used in disasters. It is intended to reduce people's initial distress in the immediate aftermath of events and to foster adaptive functioning. Its principles have currency in delivering care for staff in routine circumstances as well as after very challenging events and it is an approach that can underpin everyday practice. While PFA acknowledges that the majority of people who are affected emotionally by their circumstances and events are not likely to develop long-term difficulties in recovering, mental health problems or serious disorders, it is also a useful baseline for delivering clinical services if they are required.

Level 5. Offer health assessment and intervention in primary care

The care pathway should rely, initially, on support provided by people's families, communities and colleagues in workplaces, and then progress, according to need, to the primary or occupational health and social care services and voluntary agencies. Surveillance, assessment and intervention procedures should take account of local circumstances.

Level 6. Deliver specialist mental health services for staff

Despite estimates that the number of staff who will require referral is small, arrangements should be negotiated in advance for staff to have access to appropriate specialist healthcare, including mental healthcare according to their assessed needs.

Annex B. An *aide-mémoire* for leaders and managers of mental health services

A practical approach for leaders to caring for staff in mental health services is based on:

- effective leadership
- aligning staff to the realities of caring compassionately
- sound decision-making
- good teamwork
- clear and open communications
- clear awareness of situations and people
- providing support for the continuing welfare of staff.

Effective leadership

An effective leader will:

- be visible and available as a leader
- provide a conduit for communications for the team within the organisation
- provide practical day-to-day leadership for all team members
- ensure the flow of adequate and appropriate information
- signpost access to technical advice, support and supervision
- ensure access to an adequate peer-support service
- encourage reflective practice but not rumination.

Aligning staff to the realities of caring compassionately

Such alignment will involve the following steps:

- Prepare staff by aligning their thinking and expectations to the realities of what is important in caring compassionately for patients.
- Create and disseminate clear decision-making processes.
- Engage patients and staff in planning care programmes.
- Engage staff in decision-making.
- Support staff in their own decision-making.
- Recognise staff's emotional labour and provide support in conducting it safely and without withdrawing emotionally.

Sound decision-making

Sound decision-making requires people to:

- assess the situation accurately, effectively and rapidly
- take into account divergent views
- engage well with patients' relatives while respecting patients' privacy and their preferences for confidentiality
- make analyses of the risks and benefits of different courses of action.

This requires:

- Openness and transparency. Decision-making processes, including the evidence and arguments on which they rely, should be open to scrutiny.
- Inclusiveness. All parties who are affected by the processes and decisions should be able to express their views.
- Respect. Leaders' styles and practices should reflect respect for the needs and the human rights of each patient and member of staff. This means that staff members know how to assess what is in the best interests of each patient and are able to apply that knowledge.
- Proportionality. The approaches to making decisions must be proportionate to the needs of patients and any risks posed by each situation.
- Accountability. Each organisation is accountable for ensuring that staff members are trained to carry out the duties that they are asked to take on, and that the training properly equips them to assess risks proportionately and to match the techniques used to the risks presented in each situation.
- Reasonableness and lawfulness. Staff are able to justify against an ethical values framework each decision they make.
- Effectiveness and efficiency. The skills that staff use are effective and are compatible with compassionate care.
- Exercising a duty of care. Staff are trained in the skills to carry out with sensitivity, consistently and safely, the physical and psychosocial care of their patients and are supported in doing so.

- Reviews and complaints. Patients must have the confidence to use fair and credible complaints procedures. They should be given opportunities to use independent advocacy services to enable them to express their opinions and report their experiences with regard to how they are cared for and managed.

Good teamwork

Good teamwork requires:

- team-building
- ensuring staff are provided with training (both personal training and team training).

Clear and open communications

Clear and open communications are based on:

- listening actively
- providing an adequate and appropriate flow of background information
- briefing staff as situations and tasks change and develop.

Clear awareness of situations and people

Clear awareness of situations and people requires leaders to:

- attend to how tasks are allocated to staff
- enable staff to maintain a focus on what is involved in caring compassionately, sensitively and effectively for patients
- enable and support staff in their adapting reasonably well to changing situations
- provide staff with the means for ensuring their physical and psychosocial safety and a safe environment.

Providing support for the continuing welfare of staff

Supporting the continuing welfare of staff requires leaders to:

- use active listening skills
- offer staff access to a peer-support service
- provide adequate healthcare arrangements for staff, including access to an occupational health service
- actively monitor working environments, workloads and access to resources
- attend to events that impact on people's care and safety.

Acknowledgement

The authors are pleased to acknowledge the contribution of Steve Onyett. He is a psychologist who contributed thinking on the consequences of emotional labour to a paper that Kemp, Onyett and Williams wrote as a component of the Psychosocial Tools Project.

References

Aarons GA, Sawitzky AC (2006) Organizational climate partially mediates the effect of culture on work attitudes and staff turnover in mental health services. *Administration and Policy in Mental Health*, **33**: 289–301.

Amstadter AB, Myers JM, Kendler KS (2014) Psychiatric resilience: longitudinal twin study. *British Journal of Psychiatry*, **205**: 275–80.

Andrews J, Butler M (2014) *Trusted to Care: An Independent Review of the Princess of Wales Hospital and Neath Port Talbot Hospital at Abertawe Bro Morgannwg University Health Board*. Welsh Government. Available at http://wales.gov.uk/topics/health/publications/health/reports/care/?lang=en (accessed April 2016).

Bandura A (1997) *Self-efficacy. The Exercise of Control*. Freeman.

Bennett P, Williams Y, Page N, *et al* (2005) Associations between organizational and incident factors and emotional distress in emergency ambulance personnel. *British Journal of Clinical Psychology*, **44**: 215–26.

Bhugra D (2013) We can cure the mental health crisis. *Guardian* (Society), 24 September. Available at http://www.theguardian.com/society/2013/sep/24/cure-mental-health-service-crisis (accessed 3 December 2014).

Bion WR (1961) *Experiences in Groups*. Tavistock.

Black C, Frost D (2011) *Health at Work – An Independent Review of Sickness Absence in Great Britain*. Department of Work and Pensions.

Blanchard EB, Hickling EJ, Mitnick N, *et al* (1995) The impact of severity of physical injury and perception of life threat in the development of posttraumatic stress disorder in motor-vehicle victims. *Behaviour Research and Therapy*, **33**: 529–34.

Brown B (2010) The power of vulnerability. TED talk available at http://www.ted.com/talks/lang/eng/brene_brown_on_vulnerability.html (accessed April 2016).

Ciccetti D, Blender JA (2006) A multiple-levels-of-analysis perspective on resilience. *Annals of the New York Academy of Sciences*, **1094**: 248–58.

Cicognani E, Pietrantoni L, Palestini L, *et al* (2009) Emergency workers' quality of life: the protective role of sense of community, efficacy beliefs and coping strategies. *Social Indicators Research*, **94**: 449–63.

Clohessy S, Ehlers A (1999) PTSD symptoms, responses to intrusive memories and coping in ambulance service workers. *British Journal of Clinical Psychology*, **38**: 251–65.

Clough M (2010) Shame and organizations. *International Journal of Leadership in Public Services*, **6**: 25–33.

College Centre for Quality Improvement (2014) What is the Enabling Environments Award? Available at http://www.enablingenvironments.com (accessed April 2016).

Dahlgren A, DeRoo L, Avril J, *et al* (2009) Health risks and risk-taking behaviors among International Committee of the Red Cross (ICRC) expatriates returning from humanitarian missions. *Journal of Travel Medicine*, **16**: 382–90.

Department of Health (2009) *Pandemic Influenza: Psychosocial Care for NHS Staff During an Influenza Pandemic*. Department of Health.

Department of Health (2011) *No Health Without Mental Health: A Cross-Government Mental Health Outcomes Strategy for People of All Ages*. Department of Health. Available at http://www.dh.gov.uk/prod_consum_dh/groups/dh_digitalassets/documents/digitalasset/dh_124058.pdf (accessed 5 May 2011).

Department of Health (2013) *The NHS Constitution: The NHS Belongs To Us All*. Department of Health.

Department of Health (2014) *Annual Report of the Chief Medical Officer 2013: Public Mental Health Priorities*. Department of Health.

Edmondson A (2003) Managing the risk of learning: psychological safety in work teams. In *International Handbook of Organizational Teamwork and Cooperative Working* (eds MA West, D Tjosveld, KG Smith): ch 13. Wiley.

Figley CR (1995) Compassion fatigue as secondary traumatic stress disorder: an overview. In *Compassion Fatigue: Secondary Traumatic Stress Disorders from Treating the Traumatized* (ed CR Figley): pp 1–20. Brunner/Mazel.

Francis R (2013) *Report of the Mid Staffordshire NHS Foundation Trust Public Inquiry. Executive Summary* (HC 947). The Stationery Office.

Gilbert P (2005) *Compassion: Conceptualisations, Research and Use in Psychotherapy*. Routledge.

Goleman D (1995) *Emotional Intelligence*. Bantam Books.

Haslam SA, Reicher SD, Levine M (2012) When other people are heaven, when other people are hell: how social identity determines the nature and impact of social support. In *The Social Cure* (eds J Jetten, C Haslam, SA Haslam): pp 157–74. Psychology Press.

Hochschild AR (1983) *The Managed Heart: Commercialization of Human Feeling*. University of California Press.

Jex SM, Bliese PD (1999) Efficacy beliefs as a moderator of the impact of work-related stressors: a multi-level study. *Journal of Applied Psychology*, **84**: 349–61.

Johnson S, Osborn DP, Araya R, et al (2012) Morale in the English mental health workforce: questionnaire survey. *British Journal of Psychiatry*, **201**: 239–46.

Jones N, Mitchell P, Clack J, et al (2014) Mental health and psychological support in UK armed forces personnel deployed to Afghanistan in 2010 and 2011. *British Journal of Psychiatry*, **204**: 157–62.

Kaniasty K, Norris FH (2004) Social support in the aftermath of disasters, catastrophes, and acts of terrorism: altruistic, overwhelmed, uncertain, antagonistic, and patriotic communities. In *Bioterrorism: Psychological and Public Health Interventions* (eds RJ Ursano, AE Norwood, CS Fullerton): pp 200–29. Cambridge University Press.

Kemp V, Onyett S, Williams R (2011) Emotional labour: psychosocial aspects of the work of the staff of ambulance services. Available at http://www.healthplanning.co.uk.

Kuoppala J, Lamminpää A, Liira J, et al (2008) Leadership, job wellbeing, and health effects: a systematic review and a meta-analysis. *Journal of Occupational and Environmental Medicine*, **50**: 904–15.

Latham GP, Pinder CC (2005) Work motivation theory and research at the dawn of the twenty-first century. *Annual Review of Psychology*, **56**: 485–516.

Lilley R (2014) Roy Lilley's blog for NHS managers. Available at http://campaign.r20.constantcontact.com/render?ca=a201781c-3bf3-4423-88aa-de00e572c5fd&c=78ad62c0-b427-11e3-a94c-d4ae52725666&ch=798dfec0-b427-11e3-a988-d4ae52725666 (accessed April 2016).

Lock S, Rubin GJ, Murray V, et al (2012) Secondary stressors and extreme events and disasters: a systematic review of primary research from 2010–2011. *PLOS Currents Disasters*, October. doi: 10.1371/currents.dis.a9b76fed1b2dd5c5bfcfc13c87a2f24f.

Mols F, Haslam SA, Jetten J, et al (2015) Why a nudge is not enough: a social identity critique of governance by stealth. *European Journal of Political Research*, **54**: 81–98.

NHS Employers (2013) *Your Occupational Health Service*. NHS Confederation. Available at http://www.nhsemployers.org/~/media/Employers/Documents/Retain%20and%20improve/Your%20occupational%20health%20service%20-%20March%202014.pdf (accessed 3 December 2014).

NICE (2009) *Mental Wellbeing at Work* (PH22). NICE. Available at https://www.nice.org.uk/guidance/ph22 (accessed April 2016).

NICE (2015/2016) *Workplace Health: Management Practices* (NICE Guideline NG 13). NICE. Available at https://www.nice.org.uk/guidance/ng13 (accessed May 2016).

Norris FH, Tracy M, Galea S (2009) Looking for resilience: understanding the longitudinal trajectories of responses to stress. *Social Science and Medicine*, **68**: 2190–8.

Omand D (2010) *Securing the State*. Hurst.

Ravi SJ, Gaudlin EM (2014) Sociocultural dimensions of the Ebola virus disease outbreak in Liberia. *Biosecurity and Bioterrorism*, **2**: 301–5.

Regehr C, Hill J, Goldberg G, *et al* (2003) Postmortem inquiries and trauma responses in paramedics and firefighters. *Journal of Interpersonal Violence*, **18**: 607–22.

Rousseau DM (1989) Psychological and implied contracts in organizations. *Employee Responsibilities and Rights Journal*, **2**: 121.

Schaufeli WB (1999) Burnout. In *Stress in Health Professionals: Psychological and Organizational Causes and Interventions* (eds J Firth-Cozens, R Payne): pp 17–32. Wiley.

Shanafelt TD (2009) Enhancing meaning in work: a prescription for preventing physician burnout and promoting patient-centred care. *JAMA*, **302**: 1338–40.

Southwick SM, Charney DS (2012) *Resilience: The Science of Mastering Life's Greatest Challenges*. Cambridge University Press.

Sparks K, Cooper CL (1999) Occupational differences in the work-strain relationship: towards the use of situation specific models. *Journal of Occupational and Organizational Psychology*, **72**: 219–29.

Stamm BH (ed) (1999) *Secondary Traumatic Stress: Self-Care Issues for Clinicians, Researchers, and Educators* (2nd edn). Sidran Press.

Stamm BH (2002) Measuring compassion satisfaction as well as fatigue: developmental history of the Compassion Fatigue and Satisfaction Test. In *Treating Compassion Fatigue* (ed CR Figley): pp 107–19. Brunner Mazel.

Steiner C (1997) *Achieving Emotional Literacy*. Bloomsbury.

Sterud T, Ekeberg Ø, Hem E (2006) Health status in the ambulance services: a systematic review. *BMC Health Services Research*, **6**: 82.

Varker T, Creamer M (2011) *Development of Guidelines on Peer Support Using the Delphi Methodology*. Australian Centre for Posttraumatic Mental Health, University of Melbourne.

Virtanen M, Pentti J, Vahtera J, *et al* (2008) Overcrowding in hospital wards as a predictor of antidepressant treatment among hospital staff. *American Journal of Psychiatry*, **165**: 1482–6.

Warner M, Williams R (2005) The nature of strategy and its application in statutory and non-statutory services. In *Child and Adolescent Mental Health Services* (eds R Williams, M Kerfoot): pp 39–62. Oxford University Press.

Wertz J, Pariante CM (2014) Invited commentary on … psychiatric resilience: longitudinal twin study. *British Journal of Psychiatry*, **205**: 281–2.

Williams R (2000) A cunning plan. The inaugural lecture of Richard Williams. University of Glamorgan.

Williams R, Greenberg N (2014) Psychosocial and mental health care for the deployed staff of rescue, professional first response and aid agencies, NGOs and military organisations. In *Conflict and Catastrophe Medicine* (eds J Ryan, A Hopperus Buma, C Beadling, *et al*): pp 395–432. Springer.

Williams R, Fulford KWM (2007) Values-based and evidence-based policy, management and practice in child and adolescent mental health services. *Clinical Child Psychology and Psychiatry*, **12**: 223–42.

Williams R, Kemp VJ, Alexander DA (2014a) The psychosocial and mental health of people who are affected by conflict, catastrophes, terrorism, adversity and displacement. In *Conflict and Catastrophe Medicine* (eds J Ryan J, A Hopperus Buma, C Beadling, *et al*): pp 805–49. Springer.

Williams R, Bisson J, Kemp V (2014b) *Principles for Responding to People's Psychosocial and Mental Health Needs After Disasters* (Occasional Paper 94). Royal College of Psychiatrists. Available at http://www.rcpsych.ac.uk/usefulresources/publications/collegereports/occasionalpapers.aspx (accessed April 2016).

Zuger A (2004) Dissatisfaction with medical practice. *New England Journal of Medicine*, **350**: 69–75.

CHAPTER 27

How to manage committees: running effective meetings

Charles Marshall

Forming, running and managing committees is all about getting things done: committees, like any other team of people who are pulled together, are there to achieve a set of objectives. Far too often, committees exist for historical reasons: they meet at set times because that is when they have always met, they rarely revise their membership for fear of offence and their agendas suffer from a lack of focus and direction. They can quite often be an unwelcome intrusion into the day-to-day working lives of healthcare professionals or impose extra commitments for people beyond the scope of their everyday jobs.

It stands to reason, therefore, that committees and meetings need to be set up for a specific purpose and have substantial relevance for the people attending. It is not acceptable for people to leave meetings wondering why they were there in the first place and we will look at the responsibilities that need to be embraced by organisers and participants alike.

Before and after

There are certain ground rules which can be applied to running meetings, be they part of a committee structure or otherwise. These should be useful guiding principles in any meeting environment. Applying the ground rules established at the start is paramount to effective meeting control.

Make it necessary

Consider the information around which the meeting is planned. Is it necessary to call a meeting? If the meeting involves a large amount of one-way information transfer, it may be more practical to use other means, such as email or letter.

Even if there is an element of discussion to be had, then a telephone call may be sufficient. Where the dialogue involves more than two people, a teleconference should be considered, as these can be time- and cost-effective.

Set objectives for the meeting

If a meeting *is* seen to be the best way to meet the needs of the committee or group, it is important for that meeting to have a clear purpose and a structure. To help formulate this, complete the following statement: 'By the end of the meeting I want the group to...'. Write down several phrases and use them as your objectives. Having an objective will also help you to evaluate the meeting afterwards. It is important to assess how successful the meeting has been.

Provide an agenda

Use the objectives which have been decided upon to build the agenda. Also, take advice from the group on issues they want to discuss prior to the meeting.

Rather than have the agenda in the room when people arrive, send it out several days before meeting. The agenda should include:

- a brief set of objectives
- a list of topics, with an indication of who will address each and for how long
- time, date and venue
- any background information.

Once the agenda is in place – *stick to it!*

Assign preparation

For set topics it may be advisable to delegate preparation to individuals. This will save the committee chair a lot of time and has many benefits in terms of providing a wider range of thought processes. It can also act as a developmental process for certain members of the committee or team.

For problem-solving, make background information available to the whole group, as the solutions may be achievable only by utilising the strengths of the entire committee.

Ensure that everyone understands what is expected of them and that they have the resources to deliver the task.

Establish ground rules

Establish ground rules for the meeting.

- No one will be allowed to interrupt.
- Side conversations will be eliminated.
- A time-keeper will be used.
- Minutes or records will be kept.

In order to maintain this kind of process, a wide range of skills need to be utilised; these will be examined later. However, it is essential to establish a consistent process to save time at each meeting.

Assign action points

All points raised should have a resulting action recorded and, where appropriate, the name of the person whose responsibility it is to ensure the action is undertaken.

All objectives should meet the SMART criteria – that is, they should be Specific, Measurable, Achievable, Reviewable and Time-bound.

Examine the meeting process

Allocate a few minutes at the end of the meeting for a post-mortem examination: what worked well, what could be improved. All too often, committees and meetings waste time by repeating mistakes. Putting these right quickly can save time and a good deal of frustration. As a result of this analysis, formulate a plan of action for improvements in time for the next meeting

Structure

Meetings of any sort work better when they are structured properly. This is best done by allocating specific roles in the meeting to certain individuals. Some of these roles could be undertaken by the same person, but it could be argued that each role will warrant a separate individual.

The chair

This role will be expanded upon later; however, in broad overview the chair is responsible for the set-up, operation and follow-up of the meeting. The chair:

- decides on the why, what, where, when and who in relation to the meeting
- is responsible for publishing the agenda
- maintains adherence to the ground rules during the meeting
- controls the flow of the meeting
- ensures actions are assigned
- allocates follow-up to all the action points.

It is also important that the chair clarifies decisions and ensures they are published.

The presenter

Individuals might be called upon to present information or a project outline to the committee. There are then certain guidelines which they should be aware of prior to attendance.

- If they are not told exactly what is expected of them, they need to acquire an accurate brief for the topic and know how much time is allocated.

- On the day, they should provide the required information clearly and concisely, based on a thorough knowledge and understanding of the topic. There may be some unanswered questions and it is important that they are prepared for most eventualities.

- A good knowledge of the audio-visual equipment is important. It can be frustrating for other committee members if they have to waste valuable time waiting for the presenter to set up equipment.

- Keeping to time is also critical, as there will be other business to discuss. A good understanding between time-keeper and chair will help this process.

The recorder

An appointed committee member or dedicated secretary should be available to take minutes. It is a mistake for the chair to attempt to both chair the meeting and take notes. Remaining attentive is clearly important, as is the ability to condense the information into key points.

Decisions and actions should be documented and summaries provided as required during the meeting itself. This can help the chair stay on course and get a feel for what has been resolved and what has yet to be tackled.

Minutes from the meeting should be produced and distributed as soon as possible, pending the approval of the chair.

Time-keeper

The time-keeping role could be undertaken by the chair; however, it is useful to have a back-up as the chair can often get sidetracked into process issues and it is all too easy to lose track of time in a particularly intense situation.

Participant

'Participant' is a role which should be taken more seriously. Everyone who attends the meeting should feel that their attendance is both necessary and useful. Many committees are populated by individuals who attend because they feel they must or are coerced into doing so by others. Taking a more proactive attitude to attending is the duty of all participants and the responsibility rests squarely with them.

They have a duty to arrive on time and be well prepared. They should be able to remain attentive and alert throughout meeting, and contribute when appropriate. They should also be supportive of other team members, maintain respect, keep focused and avoid interruptions.

Environment

It is sometimes difficult to obtain a room that is ideal for the meeting, but the layout and size of the room can have dramatic effects on whether everyone can hear properly, on the energy levels of participants and on general comfort levels (it is hard to concentrate when uncomfortable).

Some opportunity for participants to move around should be built into the meeting and the layout should be suitable for the nature of what is being discussed. Boardroom style is the traditional approach, but for larger groups, cabaret style – with tables of four or five people – works very well, particularly if there is an opportunity for small-group work.

Process

Chairing the meeting

Leading and chairing meetings is a skill that can drastically affect the power and influence of a committee. In that context, the selection of the chair is critical. The person chosen should have demonstrable skill sets in the following areas.

Involvement

While there is an individual responsibility for participants to involve themselves proactively in the meeting, there will always be differences in how comfortable people feel about this. This will give rise to disproportionate contributions from certain individuals, creating an imbalance and potentially leading to animosity. It is essential, therefore, that the chair has the skill to encourage involvement from everyone, from the outset.

Some kind of warm-up procedure may be advisable for unfamiliar groups, whereas more established groups may feel comfortable engaging from the outset.

Impartiality

The temptation to steer the proceedings of the meeting or to input their own point of view is a real dilemma for chairs. Strictly speaking, they should resist that temptation and focus on the process rather than the content, although this is easier said than done. The main requirement is to ensure that all participants can express their point of view and ensure all delegates get the opportunity to contribute. There will be times when the chair needs to intervene to move things along, but this is very different from steering the meeting by using the position of chair to champion one's own cause.

Assertiveness

Assertive behaviour in chairing is one of the key skills required to ensure effectiveness. The line between firmness and overbearing aggression is quite fine but it does exist. Having sufficient respect for one's own point of view needs to be balanced by an equal respect for other people's views and their right to express them.

There will be numerous occasions when the chair needs to intervene, move matters along or clarify a point of understanding, and she or he needs to have enough confidence to do this without fearing the reaction of those in full flow. The chair may have to prevent certain individuals dominating and it is often those characters who resent it most, but it is essential that the chair can bring in all participants and 'protect' their contributions.

Stay on course

To enable this to happen it is important to allot time to each topic and stick to it.

It is quite acceptable to call further meetings if issues cannot be resolved; people's busy schedules can jeopardise this but if the issue is important enough, it is worth reconvening.

The group will often need to be pushed to reach a decision and it is important that this happens, otherwise discussions can become protracted and circular.

As part of the planning, enough time needs to be allocated for all topics to be concluded.

Summarising

Summarising is a useful technique, as it establishes the end of the discussion, promotes clarity and understanding, provides an impartial description of the discussion, and clearly sets out the next step. It also has the advantage of preventing the revisiting of decisions already made.

Facilitating the meeting

Facilitation is a unique process in itself and is fundamental to running meetings and committees successfully. To facilitate effectively, there are some core skills which should be recognised and practised.

Developing empathy and trust

Key to the building of empathy and trust is the employment of certain behaviours:

- knowing everyone in the group by name
- providing encouragement and acknowledging progress within the group
- intervening only when necessary
- being honest with the group (for instance, if the chair has suggested a method and it is not working, then a degree of flexibility and understanding is likely to gain far more respect than rigidly sticking to a course of action)
- involving the whole group and checking to ensure the group's agreement and support
- retaining a sense of humour (that is not to say that flippancy is appropriate, but a realistic sense of humour is important).

Questioning

Questions are the crown jewels of a good facilitator; they support the development of empathy and also encourage participation. They provide opportunities for clarification and will encourage people to be specific and more precise.

Good questions tend to be clear, appropriate, non-judgemental, open rather than closed, and non-threatening.

It is advisable to give the group some clear time to respond to questions and, needless to say, it is essential to listen to the answers.

Neutrality

Neutrality means suspending judgement. The chair must respect the right of everyone to their own opinion, no matter who they are and what their opinion happens to be. The chair should:

- be assertive, not aggressive
- reflect questions and comments back to the group
- ask other people's opinions
- treat everyone equally.

Observation

Looking out for signals within the group is a key skill in good facilitation. What is said is often the tip of the iceberg. Signals provide insight into certain key factors at play within the group.

Energy and activity levels

The group's effectiveness can be seriously reduced if the participants have become tired, bored or simply frustrated. A good facilitator should recognise these signs and introduce breaks or variations in activity to maintain good energy levels.

Emotional and comfort levels

A committee's role is to get things done and make things happen; it can fail to achieve its objectives if there are clear signs that members are unhappy or uncomfortable with decisions. These should be recognised and preferably resolved before the group can move forward.

It is not possible to please all the people all the time, but it is essential to be able to recognise when this is happening and to take action to minimise the impact.

Focus levels

Groups are renowned for straying off the point, not sticking to agendas, running over time and so on. The chair needs to be aware of the group moving outside its remit and must make a decision as to whether the diversion is appropriate or distracting. Assertiveness is required to move the group back on course.

Seating

The job of chair is made easier when he or she is able to see the rest of the group clearly. Control is difficult if eye contact is not achieved. Seating can also affect group dynamics (e.g. who sits near whom, whether there are subgroups within the main group). Limiting 'unofficial' conversations is important to the smooth running of the meeting.

Body language

Expressions and gestures can give the facilitator important insight into the reality of a situation. Picking up non-verbal cues is important and may enable the facilitator to ask clarifying questions when it appears that something is being felt but not necessarily expressed to the rest of the group.

Intervention

Intervention is an inevitable requirement of a good facilitator. Timing and appropriateness are key attributes to good interventions.

There are some specific points at which intervention is appropriate:

- setting the scene
- encouraging participation
- keeping on track
- time management
- clarifying issues
- helping the group reach consensus
- acknowledging feelings within the group
- monitoring energy levels
- challenging what is not being said
- dealing with individual behaviour
- feedback and review.

Dealing with problems

It would be ideal if every meeting ran smoothly, all participants played their role to perfection and the chair had merely to administer the process and keep everyone on track.

In the real world, however, personal agendas, organisational politics and vested interests tend to get in the way. We cannot ignore them, and anyone leading a committee or meeting needs to be prepared for them.

Having looked at the various principles concerned with structure and process, we now have to turn to the principles involved with managing people. This is an involved process over and above day-to-day management issues, as most of the people on the committee will not be directly responsible to the chair in their day-to-day jobs. Any authority must therefore be generated by the personality of the chair rather than that role in the committee.

It is a matter of gaining respect from other members. Utilisation of the skills already described will form a good foundation for this, but there will always be a need to handle all individuals, some supportive and some not: they are described here respectively as heroes and villains. Heroes, who are supportive of the chair, are driven by basically good intent. Villains are those who play games to undermine the process and disrupt progress.

Heroes

While heroes may be supportive on the whole, they also need to be 'managed' in order to get the most out of them and the rest of the group.

The creative inventor

Creative inventors display a creative genius and large ego. They are vocal, have a tendency to try to dominate and often come from a fairly obscure angle. It is sometimes difficult for the group to understand where they are coming from.

They need involvement, recognition and to be delegated to, as they have huge amounts of energy and enthusiasm. They will also need to be focused and controlled in order to stop them running away with ideas and initiatives.

The realist

Realists display focus, objectivity and attention to detail, and are very keen to apply and stick to a procedure or process. They can work against the creative inventor as they like concepts to be at least proven and realistic. They are pragmatists who need to have concepts expressed in a tangible setting.

They need the opportunity to input and have their views aired. They will also need time to apply more intangible concepts. They should be encouraged to be more flexible and less judgemental.

The facilitator

Facilitators display the ability to clarify, interpret and summarise; they are good at questioning and may have a tendency to try to 'out-chair' the chair.

They need to achieve some kind of team balance and thrive on support and encouragement. They can be indispensable when deadlock sets in, as they are good at cementing the group and working towards outcomes. Occasionally, their need for consensus can disrupt decision-making.

The mediator

Mediators display wisdom, experience and balance. Their behaviour is driven by a need for team spirit, harmony and non-confrontation with their peers.

While their intent is clearly supportive, it may be necessary to suppress their tendency to trivialise issues, which they may do to avoid confrontation or embarrassment.

411

The supporter

These people display encouraging behaviour; they are positive, enthusiastic and have a good deal of energy. They need harmony, team balance and involvement in order to thrive.

The shy one

These individuals are on the border between heroes and villains, depending upon their motive. If they are genuinely shy, they feel discomfort when pushed into a situation where they have to contribute. They prefer a lack of involvement and a quiet life.

To bring them out of their shell they need space, eye contact, direct questions and support. It is important that they realise, however, the fact that a degree of responsibility rests with their position on the committee and that a significant contribution will be expected of them, as befits the role.

The villains

The monopoliser

Monopolisers display a tendency to interrupt, ramble, repeat themselves and generally take over the commentary.

They are best dealt with by waiting for a suitable space in the proceedings, acknowledging the point they are making and then perhaps bringing in another participant into dialogue.

It is also worth making the point that, as chair, it is important that you give everyone on the committee a chance to express their opinion.

The distracter

These people tend not to be involved in the process of the meeting. They are attention-seeking and tend to make continual irrelevant and verbose side comments. This may be a consequence of their attention span, the relevance of the topic or a deliberate attempt to undermine the chair. As a result, a fairly direct intervention is required: halt them firmly, restate the objective or topic and ask them a specific question in relation to the topic.

The sniper

Snipers are characterised by their use of side comments, again, trying to undermine the chair and put him or her on the spot.

There are several ways to deal with this. It may be helpful to ask snipers to share their comments, rebound their question if it is deliberately misleading or ask the rest of the group for their thoughts and comments.

The sceptic

It is sometimes difficult to separate the sceptic from the realist. It is mainly to do with motives. Sceptics tend to be critical, negative, unhelpful and resistant to change, whereas realists need things putting into perspective.

Sceptics can be turned into realists by gaining their support. Ask for solutions not problems; apply objectivity to their cynicism.

Judgement

Chairing meetings, managing committees and running groups are all bound by the same basic set of rules and processes. What characterises an effective chair is the ability to make interventions and apply the principles at the right time, with the correct emphasis. This needs experience and it is important to be prepared to make mistakes.

Trial and error will help you to develop good judgement and the confidence this brings can make the whole process an enjoyable and stimulating experience.

As a postscript, here are some scenarios that might occur in a meeting or committee situation. Have a look through them and using the information from this chapter and your personal judgement, make some decisions about what you would do. There are no right or wrong answers, but some actions may produce better outcomes than others!

- Your meetings normally involve about 20 professional people and the seating is horseshoe or boardroom style. The outputs from the meeting are often poor, in terms of both keeping to the agenda and follow-up.
- The meeting has been broken into subgroups for part of the agenda; attendees have been given their discussion assignments and asked to report back at a specific time. After the meeting, everyone separates. One attendee approaches you and says that he cannot stay in the group to which he was assigned because of a personality conflict with one of the other members.
- As you begin your meeting, you sense a great deal of hostility in the room. The attendees' arms are folded in a defensive style and they respond only when called on. This continues even after the agenda has been outlined and the attendees asked for comments.
- You are one-third of the way through your meeting and you are summarising the previous discussion. An attendee blurts out, 'I disagree. You are totally out of touch with the real world. That's great in theory but it won't work here.'
- During your meeting, several attendees engage in side conversations. This is not the first time they have done so. You have so far ignored the situation, hoping they would stop on their own, but the situation seems to be getting worse.
- The entire group begins talking among themselves, sidetracking the discussion you are trying to lead. In fact they seem to be attempting to take control away from you.

CHAPTER 28

Presentation skills

Greg Lydall and Judith Harrison

This chapter will help you prepare stimulating and effective presentations. This is an essential skill in getting your ideas across to your audience at a conference, job interview, the hospital board, or colleagues, students and patients. Candidate presentations in particular are now an established feature of selection and assessment for many roles within medicine.

In the first part of this chapter we draw on the rhetorical model of public speaking, used by great orators. We examine the process of developing arguments (invention), how to organise arguments for best effect (arrangement), how to present arguments (style), use of the voice and body (delivery) and the use of memory. In the second part we consider the science of persuasion: the use of visual aids, common pitfalls. In the third part we explore two approaches to improving performance and managing performance-related anxiety. In so doing, we expect to improve the reader's understanding, enjoyment and application of these skills in delivering memorable presentations.

The rhetorical model

Rhetoric, the art of speech-making, has been studied for thousands of years. Aristotle wrote a treatise on the subject. This model of communication has been applied to medical discourse (Haber & Lingard, 2001). Aristotle's 'five

---

Box 28.1   Aristotle's five canons of rhetoric

1   Invention: the process of developing arguments
2   Arrangement: organising the arguments for best effect
3   Style: determining how to present the arguments cogently and artistically
4   Delivery: the gestures, pronunciation, tone and pace used when presenting persuasive arguments
5   Memory: the process of learning and memorising the speech and persuasive messages

---

canons of rhetoric' (Box 28.1) serve as a guide to creating and delivering compelling speeches (Cline, 2006: p. 29).

Invention

Message

In the preparation phase of any planned message, consider answering three key questions first:

- Why am I communicating?
- How should I do so?
- What do I communicate?

- Why: to inform a conference, to inform colleagues, to get the job?
- How: simple language, technical language, written, spoken, visual?
- What: structure and content – background, problem/hypothesis, analysis, conclusions, recommendations.

Then draft an outline of your content. You may wish to use a spider diagram (Fig. 28.1) to map out your ideas. Refine your draft, aiming to cover only the most relevant areas and to reduce the content by at least a third. It is better to make a few points clearly than lots of points hurriedly; if you try to include too much your audience will 'switch off'. Consider what your 'take-home message' is.

A sense of structure and narrative is important: all presentations should at least have a clear introduction at the beginning, evidence to support and refute the argument, and a summary at the end. Consider repeating key points to improve understanding. It is often helpful to specify the objectives for the talk at the beginning, proceed through your arguments, recap those

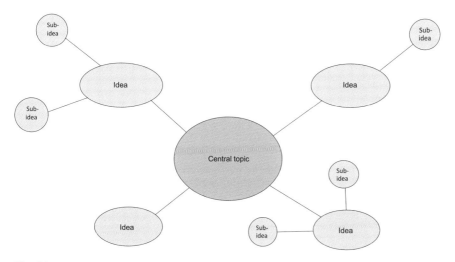

Fig. 28.1 Spider diagram

at the end, and then offer an opportunity for questions and answers. As with school essays, one should always: say what you are going to say; say it; then say what you've said.

Audience

Good speech writers emphasise the importance of 'knowing your audience'. The size of the group, their level of knowledge of the topic, professional and personal backgrounds, and preconceived ideas should all be considered. Consider their reasons for attending, objectives, fears, issues and attitudes. If possible, check the names of attendees and whether they might have specific areas of expertise or agendas. Ask yourself: What is their perception of you and your institution? What are their questions likely to be? What is personally at stake for them? How much detail do they need? Aim to make your talk highly relevant to the group, using examples that they will be familiar with. Understanding your audience will also help you prepare for the questions they may ask you.

Purpose

You may be presenting in a teaching, academic or leadership setting. You might also be asked to present for a job interview, a debate or even a 'dragons' den' pitch of a proposal. Common to all of these is selling both yourself and your ideas. Depending on the setting, ask the following questions. Is there a particular reason you were asked? Is there a question they would like you to answer or topics they want to cover? Who is speaking before and after you? Is there a theme for the day or session? Ultimately, what impact do you want to make? What will the audience feel, believe and do after hearing your (life-changing) talk?

Occasion

Consider the broader context of your talk. Does the subject relate to current news stories? Is it controversial? Are you speaking on a national awareness day or relevant anniversary? If so, you should acknowledge this in your presentation. Where will your presentation be delivered? The dynamics of a large conference venue, a lecture theatre, a board room and a small teaching room are very different.

Arrangement

Enhancing attention

The average attention span of an audience is 15–20 min, with best retention in the first 5 min (Burns, 1985). If you are speaking for longer than that, you could consider the use of props or models, and concentration breaks or 'change-ups' if appropriate (Middendorf & Kalish, 1996). This approach also fits well with Kolb's experiential learning model, which recommends providing opportunities for reflection, connection with existing knowledge and experimentation, in addition to content presentation (Kolb, 1984).

Box 28.2 Ideas for concentration breaks

- 'Now I would like you to turn to the person sitting next to you and, for 2 minutes, discuss the last presentation you gave: what, where, when and how it went.'

- 'Now I would like you to take 1 minute to write down the three best speakers you have heard and what they did that was so great.'

Concentration breaks should be brief and with clear instructions to do a specific activity, usually with a partner or in a small group for a defined length of time. Examples are suggested in Box 28.2.

Timing

You must not exceed the time you have been offered; to do so is encroaching on other's time. If you use PowerPoint,[1] you should allow one slide per minute of your talk. Time your presentation when you practise it to ensure it is reliably within your allocated time. You should allow extra time for questions at the end if the organisers have not already allowed for this. It may be helpful to use a stopwatch or mobile phone app, and an ally in the audience to ensure that you keep to time. If you are presenting at a conference, the session chair will also give timing prompts. To quote Dorothy Sarnoff: 'Make sure you have finished speaking before your audience has finished listening'.

Style

Audiovisual material

The use of electronic presentation software like PowerPoint is almost ubiquitous, but it may not always be the best medium, especially for teaching. Flipcharts and dry-wipe boards work well for small audiences. Remember that PowerPoint is a visual aid and not the speaker. If you are using PowerPoint or similar, you should aim to apply three principles: big, simple, clear (Fig. 28.2). Consider the relative impact of the layout and content of the two slides in Figs 28.2 and 28.3.

Remember that technology may fail, so always bring back-up copies of your presentation in different storage formats. Email your presentation to the organisers beforehand and bring a paper printout of the slides. Consider use of back-up materials like overhead projector slides if visuals are critical to your presentation.

Practical preparations

Remember that technology may fail, so always have back-up copies of your presentation in different storage formats, such as on a USB stick and

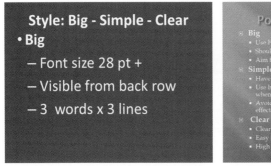

Fig. 28.2 Slide style guide: a big, simple, clear layout

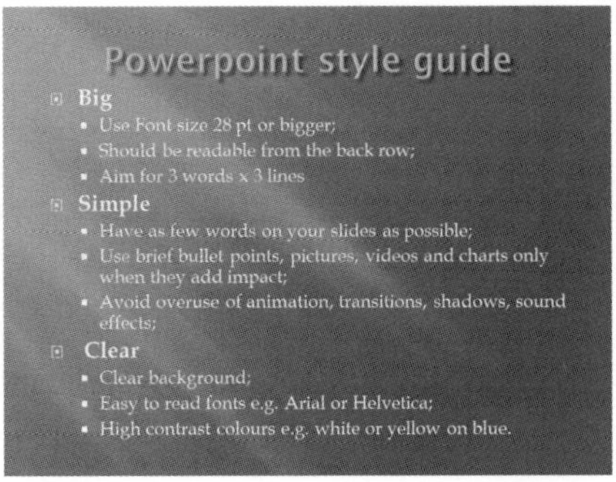

Fig. 28.3 Slide style guide: an overcrowded slide

saved online. Check the file formats you are using are compatible with the equipment provided, and that any videos work. Lastly, give yourself an easy ride by checking that you are not unintentionally straying into contentious waters, or are well prepared if that is the intent (Box 28.3).

Determine how to present yourself

Consider your appearance, position and posture. If you want to be seen as a rising leader or an aspiring academic, you should dress the part. Stand up even if a chair is provided: you will appear more authoritative.

Delivery

When rehearsing, pay attention to your voice and body language. Bear in mind that communication is considered to be up to two-thirds non-verbal (Hogan & Stubbs, 2003). However, even the most engaging body language may be undone by a soporific voice in the session after lunch. When using your whole body for communication, pay attention to the factors in detailed in Table 28.1.

Practise with a friendly audience who will give honest critical feedback. This will help you judge the pace and impact of your talk, identify any major issues, and enable improvements to increase your confidence.

Memory

You do not need to memorise every word of your talk. Your slides should jog your memory. Avoid using prompt cards or notes as these can be distracting and suggest a nervous speaker who is not master of the subject. If you are prone to performance anxiety, the third section of this chapter offers some techniques to help.

Box 28.3 Handling awkward audience moments

The first four points below are quoted from Brammer (2008), who gives the excellent advice in her article in *BMJ Careers*; we have add two further points of our own (on heckling and social media).

Random interruptions

'If someone asks a question in the middle of your presentation, make a decision whether it would be appropriate to deal with it now or later. Don't be forced to change your structure unless you believe it is really necessary. Acknowledge the question and reassure the person that there will be opportunities to discuss that later. Equally, if it is an unrelated or irrelevant question remember to acknowledge it but make it clear that such a topic isn't going to be dealt with on this occasion. You can always offer to research that question for them at a later opportunity.'

Audience looks bored

'Many people feel they are poor presenters because their audiences can look distracted or even bored. The key thing here is to ask yourself if they are actually bored or whether they are just presenting you with a professional and impartial expression. In your clinical work you need to be able to focus on a task and not be distracted by personal emotional considerations or anxieties; this is no different. Treat the presentation as a professional exercise and move on.'

Someone is talking to someone nearby

'Depending on your audience (senior consultants or medical students, for example) you may want to vary your specific response to this. However, a good technique with any audience is to pause in your delivery, look at the culprits while smiling, and wait for their attention before you start again. This is an effective (and non-aggressive) way of acknowledging that they are distracting both you and the rest of the group. That is usually all it takes to get their full attention. However, if they are persistent offenders maintain your professionalism and carry on regardless.'

Questions you can't answer

'Sometimes the dread of the questions at the end of a presentation can overshadow the whole experience. Avoid this by framing your question-and-answer session with a reassurance that you'll do your best to deal with any questions now and will guarantee to follow up any additional questions after the session. If you are asked a reasonable question which you genuinely can't answer, remember that part of good medical practice is to know your limits and work within the parameters of your knowledge; it sounds far more confident and impressive to admit you can't answer a question fully at this moment, rather than try to cobble together a poor answer and pretend you know. You could turn the question back to the audience, asking for their answers. This is ideal when teaching, or if it is a subjective matter and you wish to encourage debate.'

Heckling

Sometimes an audience members are unable to help themselves and the speaker may be drawn into an argument. Most of the audience will not appreciate this. Despite anticipating any hot topics and avoiding sensitive subjects, there may be heckling, unfair criticism or negative feedback. We suggest the following techniques:

- Clarify the question
- Try to address the question, remaining attentive and neutral.
- Never argue with an audience member.
- Keep answers brief and move on (e.g. to a 'friendly face' in the audience).
- Be honest if you don't know the answer.
- Ask the session chair to intervene if necessary.

Social media

Many conferences and meetings encourage attendees to share the remarks of speakers on social media in real time. Be aware that what you say can be quoted and shared on Twitter to an audience far beyond the auditorium.

Table 28.1 Guidelines on voice and body language in giving presentations

Voice	Body
Vary your tone, volume, rate, pitch and emphasis	Smile
Audibility: project your voice to the back of the room	Maintain eye contact with the whole audience
Pace: neither too fast nor too slow	Use open body language (no crossed arms or hunched posture)
Clear articulation and pronunciation	Own the space: don't stay in one spot
Use pauses for impact and pacing	Convey confidence
Avoid overuse of jargon and stock expressions	Use natural gestures
Avoid substandard grammar	Breathe deeply to remain calm

The science of persuasion

The first part of this chapter covered the Aristotelian rhetorical model, adapted for modern speech-makers and audiences. This second part builds on that model to enhance the impact of your presentation. For Aristotle, rhetoric is more than the content, structure and style of a speech. He considers it a science of persuasion, and identifies three types of rhetorical proof (Cope, 1867; Nichols, 1987; Rapp, 2010):

- ethos – the perceived credibility of the speaker
- pathos – inciting an emotional responses
- logos – using logical, reasoned arguments.

Ethos

The perceived credibility of a speaker influences audiences' views of the arguments he or she espouses. This could be influenced by the position of the speaker as an acknowledged expert in the field, or friend or acquaintance who has personal experience of it. Three factors are believed to contribute: perceived intellect, reputable character and affability.

What does this mean for your presentation?
- Introduce yourself and explain your background in the subject you are speaking on.
- Speak as clearly and confidently as you can.
- Dress smartly.
- Smile and be friendly.

Pathos

Inciting an emotional response from the audience can alter their views. Using metaphors can create an emotional response or motivate your listeners. Storytelling is very effective, especially when the audience can identify with the individuals described in the narrative.

What does this mean for your presentation?

- Draw comparisons with things that your audience will be familiar with.
- Give examples from your own experience, including anonymised case vignettes, which you feel the audience will be able to relate to.
- If appropriate, have a patient/service user contribute to your talk. They can make your points more credible and poignant with the authority of their lived experience.

Logos

Approaching the subject in a rational and objective way can be persuasive. The use of statistics drawn from the peer-reviewed literature is an example.

What does this mean for your presentation?

- Quote relevant high-quality research, national reports and surveys.
- Reference all data, tables and charts and give your reference list at the end of the presentation.

Despite your skills in the art of persuasion, there are still potential areas of difficulty. Try to avoid sensitive topics (politics, religion, race, gender) and be aware of the perils of immediate quotation on social media. Even the best-prepared and most confident orator may encounter awkward audience moments. We have suggested some ways around these in Box 28.3.

Get in the zone: cognitive reframing and creative visualisation

In this third part of this chapter we explore two approaches to improving performance and managing performance-related anxiety, based on modern psychology: cognitive reframing and creative visualisation. The first uses cognitive–behavioural techniques to recognise our less helpful thoughts (cognitions) and reframe them in a more helpful way (Box 28.4).

Visualisation techniques, also referred to as 'creative visualisation', 'sports visualisation' and 'creative imagery', are commonly used in sports psychology. They can improve performance (Weinberg, 2008) and have been shown to be effective in combating performance-related anxiety (Vado *et al*, 1997). It is the process of creating a detailed schema of the desired outcome and visualising it repeatedly. Some suggest the process is similar to developing muscle memory. For example, a golfer may visualise the perfect stroke to rehearse the sensations associated with it. In addition to learning the physical feelings and sequences involved in a task, athletes

421

Box 28.4 Some unhelpful cognitions and how to reframe them

'If I don't put everything I want to say on the slides I will forget things.'
I know my subject and have practised; therefore I won't forget anything important.
If I do, I can always make the point later on in my talk.

'If I don't stick to my script exactly people will know and I will look stupid.'
My audience doesn't know what I am going to say or when, so if I say things in a
slightly different way or in a different order on the day it won't matter.

'If I hesitate or pause I will look stupid.'
Some of the best speakers appear to hesitate. It demonstrates that they are thinking about what they are saying. Politicians often hesitate intentionally to seem
more genuine. Deliberate pauses are used by famous orators to emphasise their
points.

'If I speak too slowly I will run out of time.'
I have refined my presentation to include only the most important material and
timed it carefully. I must speak slowly and clearly to allow my audience to listen.

'I have to tell them I am standing in at short notice for someone more important.'
I will not apologise for anything at the start of the presentation. The presentation
I am about to give is interesting and relevant to my audience.

---

practise the cognitions associated with it. Coaches use this method to
prepare their athletes psychologically the day before a competition. We
believe that the same techniques can be used to enhance your presentation
skills and minimise the anxiety associated with oral presentations, as in
the two examples below.

Example 1

A 10 000 m runner visualises a race. With eyes closed, she imagines:

- What can she see? The final lap of the track; the finish line ahead; no
other runners in sight – she is in the lead.
- What can she feel? The ground hard under her feet; the wind on her
face; her heart pounding.
- What can she hear? Gasped breaths and the footsteps of other runners
behind her; the sound of her own trainers hitting the ground; the roar
of the crowd as she approaches the finish-line.
- What can she smell? Sweat.
- Her thoughts. 'Dig deep now. You can do it.'
- Outcome. She visualises sprinting past her opponents and over the
finish-line in first place.

Example 2

You are presenting at a conference. You have prepared carefully but you are quite nervous. If you can, find out the size and layout of the room you will be speaking in and whether you will be on a stage or behind a podium. As a golfer visualises the perfect stroke and a runner imagines sprinting to the finish, you should practise imagining your presentation going smoothly. Close your eyes and think about a moment during your presentation:

- What can you see? A large room in a hotel conference suite; 200 people, sitting in rows. They look at you attentively – what you are saying is interesting – your presentation is going smoothly. You make eye contact across the room. The session chair is smiling and occasionally nods in agreement as you talk.
- What can you feel? Cool, air-conditioned air on your skin; the laser pointer in your hand; your suit jacket sits evenly around your shoulders; your heart beats steadily – you feel in control of the situation.
- What can you hear? The quiet hum of the air-conditioning; a cough; a shuffle; from the next room, a quiet clatter of cups as the staff prepare for the coffee break.
- What can you smell? The starch on your shirt; the aroma of the coffee from the other room.
- Your thoughts: 'I have time to speak deliberately and clearly. This is going well. What I am saying is relevant to everyone here.'
- Outcome. Visualise your finish-line. You give a clear, confident conclusion and invite the audience to ask you questions. You receive a round of applause and smiles of approval from members of the audience.

On the day

- Arrive early and go to the room where you will be speaking.
- Ensure slides are loaded on to the computer (if using PowerPoint).
- Familiarise yourself with the position of the projector and computer screens.
- Make sure videos, slide changers and laser pointers work.
- Stand where you will be giving the presentation, close your eyes and visualise your presentation going well.

Conclusions

This chapter has explored the process of developing, organising, delivering and memorising a scintillating and persuasive presentation. We have detailed the science of persuasion, the use of visual aids, how to avoid common pitfalls and methods for managing performance anxiety. We anticipate that by applying these principles, readers will find themselves well prepared, confident and enjoying the art and science of presentation. As W. B. Yeats said, 'I always think a great speaker convinces us not by force of reasoning but because he is visibly enjoying the beliefs he wants us to accept'.

Take-home messages

- Plan ahead.
- Know your audience.
- Slides: big, simple, clear. Less is more.
- Say what you are going to say; say it; then say what you've said.
- Allow time to get in the zone before you start.
- Stick to time.
- Enjoy!

Acknowledgements

Pat H. Wilson AMEB, MSc (http://patwilson.com.au); Laura Brammar, Senior Careers Consultant, The Careers Group, University of London (http://www.c2careers.com); Tony Lydall, Facilitator/Trainer, TLConsulting SA.

References

Brammar L (2008) Presentation skills: plan, prepare, phrase, and project. *BMJ Careers*, at http://careers.bmj.com/careers/advice/view-article.html?id=3048 (accessed April 2016).

Burns RA (1985) Information impact and factors affecting recall. At http://eric.ed.gov/?id=ED258639 (accessed April 2016).

Cline AR (2006) *Rhetorica: A Rhetoric Primer*. Missouri State University.

Cope EM (1867) *An Introduction to Aristotle's Rhetoric*. Macmillan.

Haber RJ, Lingard LA (2001) Learning oral presentation skills. A rhetorical analysis with pedagogical and professional implications. *Journal of General Internal Medicine*, **16**: 308–14.

Hogan K, Stubbs R (2003) *Can't Get Through: 8 Barriers to Communication*. Pelican Publishing.

Kolb DA (1984) *Experiential Learning*. Prentice-Hall.

Middendorf J, Kalish A (1996) The 'change-up' in lectures. *National Teaching and Learning Forum*, **5**(2): 1–2.

Nichols MP (1987) Aristotle's defense of rhetoric. *Journal of Politics*, **49**: 657–77.

Rapp C (2010) Aristotle's rhetoric. *Stanford Encyclopedia of Rhetoric*. Available at http://www.science.uva.nl/~seop/entries/aristotle-rhetoric (accessed April 2016).

Vado EA, Hall CR, Moritz SE (1997) The relationship between competitive anxiety and imagery use. *Journal of Applied Sport Psychology*, **9**: 241–53.

Weinberg R (2008) Does imagery work? Effects on performance and mental skills. *Journal of Imagery Research in Sport and Physical Activity*, **3**: 1–21.

CHAPTER 29

Time management

Jill Sandford

'Time goes, you say? Ah no!
Alas, Time stays, we go'
Austin Dobson, *Proverbs in Porcelain* (1877)

Time and its management have become familiar components of management books and the self-improvement movement as a whole. The sense of powerlessness we have at the march of time (reflected in the epigraph) and the increasing pace of life mean that often people feel that they are managing their time 'badly'.

Myers–Briggs types and time management styles

Attitudes to time vary from culture to culture and person to person. In the West we tend to have a linear, 'time is money' attitude. We are a product of our cultural upbringing. Your own attitude to time will also be affected by your personality preferences. You may be familiar with the work of Jung and the personality types that can be explored and defined by the use of the Myers–Briggs Type Indicator. The very notion of time management appeals to certain of these type classifications. It can be a useful starting point for you to consider how you manage your time and why this may, or may not, be important to you. The Myers–Briggs Type Indicator identifies whether you take in information with a sensing or an intuitive preference, make decisions with thinking or a feeling preference, and organise your life by judging or perceiving (some detail is given in Chapter 36). It also identifies levels of extraversion and introversion – but this is less relevant in time management. Judgers tend to respond to ideas of structure and planning and perceivers want more of an open-ended free flow of events, with less structure. For the purpose of time management, I will summarise the styles.

Sensing/judging types

Such individuals are often good at time management. They are very grounded in reality but can be rigid when plans have been fixed. They find it hard to relax and the judging preference can make them stressed and time anxious. They will push for a decision to be made and for plans to be clearly established. They like things to be planned in advance, not last minute.

Sensing/perceiving types

Such individuals can meet immediate needs well and they are less anxious to push for a decision or closure. Their efforts can be scattered. They may get caught up in the moment. They are flexible and can handle schedule change. They are more last minute. They will often procrastinate about planning for the longer term, as they are more grounded in the here and now.

Intuitive/feeling types

They are sensitive to the needs of others. They may find it hard to say no and neglect their own needs. To them, time is useful to find one's life purpose. They are generous with their time.

Intuitive/thinking types

Time is a concept to these people. Once they have thought it through, they may not think it necessary to take action. Time is a tool to them, but they may ignore people's needs. They sometimes need to ground their goals in practical plans with deadlines.

Understanding your own time management style in this way can help you to overcome your shortcomings and to identify strengths upon which to build. This chapter offers you the opportunity to do this.

A process for managing your time effectively

What is effective time management? It must be 'getting the desired results in the time available'. Focusing on the bigger picture – the outcome of your role – is one way of managing your time more effectively. The nature of managerial work is that it is frequently unbounded and does not always lend itself to a clearly defined set of tasks. The demands, particularly when there is an enhanced level of responsibility for people and services, can be great. We can easily feel that we have too much to do. Interestingly enough, having too little to do can cause as much stress as being overwhelmed. Time is to some a concept, to others a precious gift, or a horse galloping ahead that we can never catch – always getting away from us. How we think about time and the attitudes we have about it are complex and deep rooted.

This chapter, however, is essentially a practical and pragmatic set of activities and ideas for you to consider. It offers a framework (with some activities) to help you. The stages it outlines are as follows:

1 Identify your own use of time and your strengths and weaknesses (your style).

2   Identify your purpose and main goals in life, and consider how to plan to achieve these. What is really important to you? What do you want to do more and less of?

3   Develop strategies for more effective and satisfying uses of your time – ones that assist you in achieving your goals.

Identifying your own use of time

This is the diagnostic stage. Its purpose is to indicate how you use your time at the moment. This sounds relatively easy, but we often delude ourselves that things are better or worse than they actually are. I usually recommend keeping a time log for a few days to monitor how you are actually spending your time. This may seem tedious but it is worthwhile. You might want to use a time log, an example of which is given in Fig. 29.1. You can also get apps for your phone or tablet to help you record your use of time.

Date				
Activity	Start time	Finish time	Planned	Imposed

Fig. 29.1   A format that might be used for a time log

How to complete a time log (be honest!)

Make a note of each activity and how long you were engaged in it. If you were interrupted, enter each stage as an activity and note that you were interrupted. If you get a lot of interruptions, it is important to be aware of the scale of these.

Which activities were planned? These might be meetings, training, a ward round or a clinic. 'Imposed' means an interruption or an unexpected task given to you by someone else – or even yourself! Travel, eating and even walking from one place to another all need to be noted as activities. Do not forget thinking time – even if it is in the car. To what extent you wish to draw a firm line between work and home, I leave up to you. If you find work spills over into home and leisure time, then you may wish to log this.

It is worth keeping this log for several days. It is not always necessary to wait for a typical day – but it is obviously not a good idea to complete the log when you are on holiday.

Reviewing your log

- Is there a pattern emerging in any of the columns? For example, are many of the activities imposed?
- Are you able to complete a task without being interrupted?
- Are you giving adequate time to current activities and to planning future activities?

- Who are you spending most time with? Are these the people you ought to be spending time with?
- If you have someone to delegate to, are you doing this sufficiently often?
- How do you deal with interruptions and emergencies? Do you defer these until tomorrow so that you can execute today's plans? Is this always possible?
- Are you spending a lot of time on certain aspects of your job to the detriment of others? What is the right balance?

This should result in an analysis of how you utilised this precious resource over a few days. The purpose of the log is to provide a baseline to come back to in stage 3 (developing strategies). It all depends on what you think you should be doing with your time in the first place. Unless you are clear about this, then you will not be sufficiently motivated to change anything about your personal time management style. Keep the log and your conclusions to one side for the moment and let us move to stage 2.

Identifying purpose, setting goals and establishing priorities

Your role defines your purpose at work. It establishes what you are there to achieve, with whom, for whom and on what timescales. You will work within frameworks and guidelines in order to do much of this. You may have a reasonable degree of autonomy and control over how you execute the tasks that enable this.

If you were to define your role or your purpose as a medic or a manager in one or two sentences, how would you do so? Write down a statement:

- My role/purpose is to ...

It often helps to start this activity by listing the verbs that best express what your role is fundamentally about. You might advise, provide psychiatric diagnosis and treatment for a specific patient group, deliver education and training for junior staff, or research and develop new approaches. You might want to have some words like 'prevention' in it too. These are just suggestions to help you get started. Once you have some key words you are happy with, frame them into a sentence. Once you start listing tasks then you usually find you have gone too far down into the *how*. A role or purpose statement is about the *why*.

Identifying and allocating tasks – achieving the *why*

The secret of effective time management is to focus on the important tasks that directly contribute to the successful implementation of your role. I would like to introduce you here to the work of Stephen Covey, *The 7 Habits of Highly Effective People*. Covey focuses on being 'on purpose' and the successful fulfilment of things that are important to you. His time management strategies build on the identification of the important tasks, quality time with people, and looking after yourself and your health and development as a professional. The last is what he calls 'sharpening the saw'. Essentially, he says there is no such thing as time management – only self-management. He categorises how we spend our time and energy as indicated in Table 29.1.

Prioritising and planning

The first task is to understand what is urgent and cannot wait, even if it is not important to you. Clinical matters will come into play here.

It is important to spend time with other members of the team to understand their strengths and weaknesses, so that when it comes to delegation you can do that appropriately. If Table 29.1 is viewed as four quadrants, the ideal is to get out of the other quadrants and into the top right quadrant (quadrant 2) as much as possible – important non-urgent tasks. The more time spent doing these key tasks, the more everything else will take care of itself. So a starting point is to plan your time in weeks, not days. To do this, you have to keep an over-arching perspective, thinking first of your purpose in life and work. Time spent planning and scheduling is never wasted. Allocate slots of time to do the quadrant 2 things. Ensure you have sufficient time to react to situations that need your attention, but develop an approach that says 'I will spend only so much time on this activity'. Take control of your time and decide what you are going to spend it on.

By now, you should have some insights into your own time management and its strengths and weaknesses. Covey also suggests that it is important to look after yourself. When you have busy weeks ahead, try to set some time aside for you. It is easier said than done but is very important.

Developing strategies for more effective and satisfying use of your time

Better time management falls into two main areas: organisational skills and interpersonal skills.

Table 29.1 Covey's categorisation of how we spend our time and energy

	Urgent	Non-urgent
Important	Dealing with crises and deadlines	Prevention, relationship building, recognising new opportunities, strategic thinking, planning, prioritising, long-term processes, recreation, self-development, thinking
Not important	Interruptions, some emails, some meetings	Trivia, time-wasters, some emails and calls, displacement activity such as playing electronic games

Adapted from Covey (1989).

Organisational skills

The following areas are all worth considering:

- *Planning and organising work activities* – being clear about what needs to be done and when. Establish lists and use a diary or time management system if this might work well for you. Break down the big jobs into smaller tasks and put a timescale against each one.
- *Gathering and using information* – being able to find out the right information and apply it appropriately. Ensure you have the information you need in order to complete tasks.
- *Keeping records simple, accessible, up to date.* If you forget things (as I do!), then write lists and keep notebooks (paper or electronic). You can use an app on your phone or tablet that will record activities and alert you to appointments (see also Box 29.1).
- *Evaluating demands* – creating short- and long-term plans for work and being flexible in the short term but focused in the long term. Covey calls this 'keeping the end in mind'. Do not lose sight of your goals. Ask yourself, 'Will doing this take me towards my goals or not?'
- *Managing and allocating resources* – making the best use of materials and operating within financial constraints.
- *Assessing the effects of change* – adapting and revising plans in response to change, in terms of both changing needs of individual patients and developing local policies.
- *Managing your environment.* Consider what is the best time of day for you to do the tasks that demand all of your attention, and the location that is best for you to work in.

Interpersonal skills

A good leader and manager needs to work with and in teams. Thus, awareness of the strengths and weaknesses of various team members is critical. Good leaders should surround themselves with those who are unlike them and can cover and provide support for overcoming the weaknesses the leader may have. Interpersonal skills involve communication that is clear and concise without any ambiguity. The leader should be able to monitor the team as well as take action when needed (Hill, 2007).

The model also includes both internal and external leadership actions. Hill (2007), using the McGrath (1986) model, suggests that managing teams and interpersonal connections depends upon both monitoring and executive actions. Hill (2007) suggests that decision-makers need to be aware of whether they should meet task or relational needs and inevitably this has a major impact on time management.

Teal (1998) highlights that integrity in management means being responsible, communicating clearly, keeping promises and knowing oneself. Teal (1998) reminds us that good managers have obligations to the institution and also have a moral imperative. Thus, prioritisation becomes a matter of great importance in managing time and tasks.

Working effectively with others

Establish working relationships that are effective and where you can share solutions and good practice with colleagues. This is helped by knowing individual team members' strengths so that they can have the right tasks and right degree of delegation and freedom.

Communication

Communication can be verbal or written, and involves both listening and talking. Be clear at all times. This includes being assertive and saying 'no' in an appropriate way when you need to, especially if you find yourself being distracted from those important quadrant 2 activities. Clear communication without any ambiguity is crucial in achieving targets set within and for the teams.

Valuing colleagues and other professionals

Show appreciation and respect for others and their time. When delegating it is important that it is clearly communicated that work is being delegated not because the task is unpleasant or the person to whom the task is being delegated is being punished.

Being flexible and responsive

Be open to change, and adapt and make changes to plans when you need to. Good managers and leaders are open to suggestions and change. Listen freely and respond accordingly. Some of the best ideas come from junior members of the team, because they may be more willing and able to look outside the box.

Managing paperwork (this includes electronic communication such as email)

There are three ways to deal with paperwork (the three 'D's):

- Read it and deal with it (*deal*).
- Read it and pass it on (*delegate*).
- Put it in the bin (*ditch*).

Sounds too simple?

Read it and deal with it

How many times have you picked up a piece of paper or re-read an email and thought 'I must deal with that'? A novel approach is to put a dot on the paper each time you move it around – just see how many dots it gets. Once it looks like a bad case of the measles, you will have wasted a lot of your time. A really brave approach is to cut the top 2 cm off the paper each time you pick it up or move it! More seriously, I am trying to encourage you not to put off dealing with the perhaps boring and unpleasant tasks.

> **Box 29.1** Bring forward
>
> This is a clever little folder which is divided into days of the month. I simply place letters, documents, maps, presentations and so on into the appropriate date. I can then find what I need before the meeting. I can remind myself to reply to a communication on a certain date too. In conjunction with a diary, I can keep a busy life organised and ensure I do not let people down. You need to remember to look in the 'bring forward' folder each day. If I want to read something in advance, I simply pop it in the section for the day before. If you are lucky enough to have a PA, then encourage him or her to practise this system on your behalf. You can use the Outlook Express diary to run a 'bring forward' system electronically if you prefer.

It may be the sheer volume of paperwork that makes it daunting. I find an initial sort into the three piles I have indicated above really does help. I deal with the first category straight away by replying or actioning. You can flag emails and come back to them if you need to think about how to respond. I keep an 'electronic filing cabinet' and move emails into the appropriate section (see also Box 29.1). I flag whether I want to come back to it or read it properly later. Do not be tempted to rush off a response – unless it is urgent! Email has a tendency to be experienced as immediate and urgent – it frequently is *not*.

Read and pass on

Is this item 'just for information'? If so, read it quickly and pass it on to whoever needs it. Copy and keep in files if necessary. I find my reading file tends to get quite big sometimes and often it is ideal train reading!

Put in the bin

This pile is often easy to deal with. If you are not brave enough to bin it, then put in the bottom drawer of a desk or filing cabinet. Clear that out every 3 months. I wager you will not have to go into that drawer to retrieve anything.

Email

Email probably causes more angst than any other form of communication apart from other people's mobiles on the train. Although a boon to communication across great distances, it can be a great time waster. I recommend the following strategies.

- Do not check your emails more than twice a day, unless something is a matter of urgency.
- Do not have 'you have mail' alerts – you will be tempted to stop what you are doing and review them.

- Approach email communication like a traditional letter. Write fully, with proper greetings, constructed sentences, punctuation and courtesy. Nothing is more irritating that curt communication. Nothing is more confusing than ambiguous emails, and their clarification makes more work.
- Read and check before sending.
- Ask, 'Would I say this to this person's face?' If you are unsure, keep it as a draft for a day and go back to it.

Organising other people

Delegating appropriately

An important way of managing time and stress is to identify the right people to do a task, brief them and then support them appropriately. A good practical way is to treat them like adults and after the task has been delegated be available to support and answer queries. Do not look over their shoulders and harass them.

Many people hesitate to give up tasks because they are concerned about giving up some of the jobs they like doing or are afraid of losing control and authority. But it is important to delegate so that you can be effective by doing the right things. It is important to remember that, as a leader or manager, you may be able to delegate the task but you cannot delegate authority as, in the end, the leader or the manager will have to take the responsibility.

Identifying the task and the person

When delegating it is important to consider which exact task is being delegated and to whom it is being delegated. Communication has to be brief and to the point (Bird, 1992). Transmission of ideas is critical. It is important that it is clear what the parameters of the delegation are and also that other members of the team are aware of the delegated tasks.

The first step is to ensure that the people who have to perform the task are capable of (have the strength and skills to deliver) the task. If they do not have the skills, it may be possible for them to learn the task but the question is then whether they have the right amount of time available to learn the skills. Is the person capable of handling it?

Make a training plan

Good leaders and managers will be able to pre-empt some of the issues emerging and have people in their teams ready to take on the tasks.

Monitoring progress

Having delegated, as mentioned above, it is important that the managers takes their hands off but be available to advise and keep an eye on progress.

433

Specific issues for psychiatrists

For individuals who are dealing with patients and their crises or dealing with relatives and families of patients (with their queries and requests), it may be difficult to prioritise. One way is to set some time aside or have emergency slots available in clinic times to deal with emergencies. It is important to learn how to differentiate between what is urgent and what is important, as they are two very different things, and both urgency and importance change, depending upon a number of factors.

Another effective aspect of managing time is learning to say 'no'. Doctors in general, by virtue of their training and world view, find it difficult to say 'no' but it is important, otherwise saying 'yes' carries no meaning.

Finally, it is important to have the right team, so that according to their skills tasks can delegated. Delegation means that the person the task is delegated to should be allowed to get on with it, but the delegator must be available to advise if needed.

Conclusion

I hope this chapter has presented you with some practical ways to manage your time more effectively. Remember that you will not get it right all the time! With the time saved, treat yourself by doing something you really enjoy. Good luck.

References

Bird M (1992) *Effective Leadership*. BBC Books.

Covey S (1989) *The 7 Habits of Highly Effective People*. Simon & Schuster.

Hill KSE (2007) Team leadership. In *Leadership: Theory and Practice* (ed. PG Northouse): pp 207–36. Sage.

McGrath JE (1986) Leading groups in organisations. In *Designing Effective Work Groups* (ed. PS Goodman): p 76. Josey–Bass.

Teal T (1998) The human side of management. *Harvard Business Review on Leadership*, 147–70.

CHAPTER 30

Developing effective leaders in the National Health Service

Charles Marshall

The NHS is a huge, complex and heterogeneous organisation with the basic function of taking care of patients in primary, secondary or tertiary care, supported by a series of supportive functions which carry with them a number of managerial and leadership roles. Leadership therefore has different facets and aspects which vary according to the organisation or the team one works in. There remain key differences between managers and leaders (also see Chapter 11). To put it simply, managers manage and leaders lead. There is no doubt that in both roles there needs to be a degree of understanding and synergy so that both functions can be carried out. Sometimes these roles overlap and management skills may be embedded in leadership roles. There is a high level of validity to the view that the demands placed on managers in the NHS – be they clinical or non-clinical – are so great that traditional views of management and leadership need to be drastically overhauled if the service is to survive.

What is traditionally referred to as *transactional* management has been largely consigned to junior managers and administrators. By 'transactional', we mean the process-driven managerial activities, such as monitoring performance on a daily basis and the administration of people and their working lives in order to ensure effective performance. That is not to say that these skills are unimportant: they clearly are, but they are no longer the sole domain of today's leaders. The current agenda forces leaders to think in more *transformational* terms – how the service can be changed to meet the current demands of the population given an ever-decreasing level of resource. This requires individuals to be encouraged to think radically and to have the courage and opportunity to create original solutions, often requiring acknowledgement that they are part of a wider system, beyond the organisation they are working for. Unfortunately, many organisations within the NHS are transactional by nature and as such can be internally focused on short-term measures and fixes which simply delay the inevitable.

Organisational structures and leadership development

The result is 'organisational compression', which creates an environment of command and control, micro-management and the inevitable cultural background of stress, resentment and reluctant compliance (see Fig. 30. 1).

To release the potential needed to drive the kind of change the service is looking for requires organisations to step back from the transactional methodology and create space for a more distributed form of leadership at every level within the organisation. The motor industry has shown that solutions to apparently intractable problems often arise from the shopfloor if people there are given the space and opportunity to step back. Of course there is a need to provide structure and frameworks for individuals to operate within, but there is a growing need to create more freedom within those frameworks to allow individuals to have a greater say in how the organisation is run (see Fig. 30.2).

To create this culture of distributed leadership requires a major re-evaluation of the leadership within NHS organisations, and a move away from simply 'managing people' to enabling and empowering them.

Research surrounding the nature of leadership is exhaustive. Our understanding of the component parts of leadership has increased dramatically over recent years and a far more complex picture has emerged that has moved us away from the 'Great Man' concept of the last century to a much more comprehensive understanding.

Disappointingly, however, even modern theory has remained one-dimensional in its approach, in that it focuses primarily on the role of the

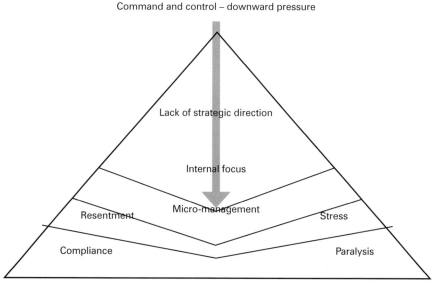

Fig. 30.1 Organisational compression

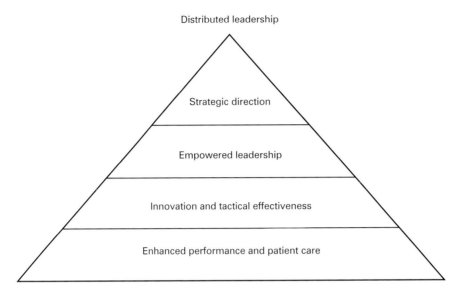

Fig. 30.2 Freedom within a framework

individual and the characteristics an individual needs to display in order to perform as an effective leader. Interestingly, concepts such as situational and transformational leadership carry strong references to a wider set of influences on leadership, yet still focus on individual characteristics, competencies and behaviours.

Providers of leadership development with a wide range of leaders, primarily in healthcare, have for many years focused on individual development, the hope being that these individuals are then able to return to their place of work and instigate, support and encourage positive change within that work environment. There has been a tendency to concentrate on personal attributes, qualities, behaviours, skills and knowledge – in other words, the development of 'human capital' as a means of improving 'social capital', defined as a 'collective capacity or efficacy – the quantity and quality of connections and relationships in a system' (Pedler & Artwood, 2010). Experience would suggest, however, that there is no such relationship and that the considerable investment which has been made in the development of individual human capital has done little to create the 'active connections among people where trust, mutual understanding, shared values and behaviours act as links making cooperative action possible' (Prusak & Cohen, 2001).

While partially successful, the 'human capital' approach has never really achieved the kind of significant and transformational organisational change that was initially envisaged. In-house programmes incorporating work-based projects have gone a long way towards this but very few have led to significant, lasting change in the way in which healthcare is provided.

437

Organisational development

As one of those providers of leadership development, our understanding has recently begun to shift from an approach to leadership which focuses on the individual to one which embraces a much wider, multidimensional framework. Central to this lies a model of organisational development rather than one of leadership. Burke and Litwin's approach to organisational development places leadership at the heart of a process which creates linkages between a complex set of external and internal causal factors necessary to create transformational organisational change (Fig. 3.30) (Burke & Litwin, 1992).

Organisational culture and performance in the NHS can no longer be viewed as one-dimensional. Clinical and non-clinical leaders in the NHS have traditionally tied themselves to their own organisation and focused on internal change and improvement. This has been exacerbated by the political emphasis on the 'purchaser–provider' split, in the hope that never the twain shall meet. In recent years, however, that divide has been challenged. The Health and Social Care Act 2012 created a new commissioning model which, in order to work effectively, requires a different approach of 'joined-up thinking' between primary and secondary care, as the emphasis has swung towards better community care, fewer admissions and shorter episodes of acute care. More recent attempts to extend this joined-up approach have seen a need to include social care in the commissioning agenda, reflecting the need to extend our understanding of patient care beyond the traditional medical model.

To assume that any of this can be achieved without leaders who possess a thorough understanding of the 'big picture' and the ability to create cooperative and productive inter-organisational relationships is naive and doomed to failure. The entire leadership map within the health and social

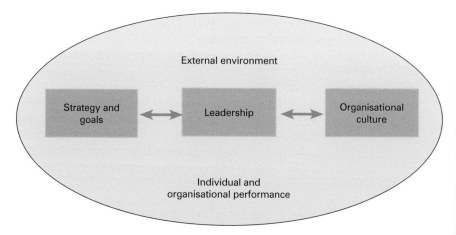

Fig. 30.3 Burke & Litwin's approach to organisational development, with leadership at the heart of a process leading to transformational organisational change

care sector is much more abstract and complex than ever before and, as such, requires an approach to leadership which recognises a diversity of interests as opposed to fixed, vested interests. It requires an approach which recognises a series of loose coalitions as opposed to clear organisational boundaries, a plurality of power holders who draw their power from a variety of sources inside and outside their own organisations.

Integration is therefore the current mantra in the NHS and its related organisations in social care, and while this may seem the obvious way to go, the route is not well defined. If leadership is unable to provide the vision, the understanding and the energy to create significant change, then inertia will be the result and the tendency will be to revert to traditional practices and silo-based thinking.

It is, however, a journey and it is difficult to claim that the service is ever 'fully integrated'. The importance for leaders is the recognition that the journey must be undertaken, and they need to be able to understand and facilitate that process. This requires the development of a new type of leader, who possesses the ability and aspiration to achieve more than just the introduction of a successful CIP within their clinical directorate, or a cost reduction on the commissioning budget. They need to be visionary and transformational in their approach to the service they represent and make connections throughout the system with all partners and stakeholders. This requires them to connect with the system at every level and begin to view the service from the patient's or client's perspective rather than that of the organisation.

Leadership and context

This understanding is taken a stage further by Karan Janman (2009), who suggests that leadership cannot effectively exist without context, as it is the context within which individuals operate that tends to dictate the opportunity for them to lead.

The objective is twofold: to develop a new understanding of leadership development based on a multidimensional approach, and to move away from a theoretical understanding to a practical application. This could then form the basis of a forward-looking leadership development programme.

At the heart of this new approach lies a framework which effectively mixes aspects of the more conventional approach to leadership with less-conventional thinking and the wider components of effective organisational development. The driving force is the critical link between the need for system change and the leadership which is required to make it happen (see Fig. 30.4).

Each part of the framework requires some understanding and, as such, becomes a component part of any leadership development process. People management is integral to this but presents itself in a different guise to the traditional approach.

439

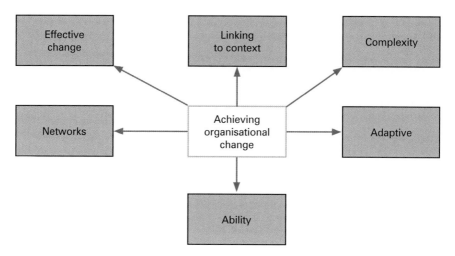

Fig. 30.4 A framework which mixes aspects of the conventional approach with the wider components of organisational development

Effective change

Before we go on to examine the components outlined above, it is important to establish a methodology for developing managers into effective leaders. Any intervention which develops leaders must have a purpose and a clearly described outcome and must be built around a large enough cohort from within the system or organisation to form a guiding coalition which can then go forward to instigate *change within the system*. Taking people out of their work environment and 'teaching' them leadership will not have a significant effect on the organisation. The Warwick model for whole-system leadership supports this (Bennington & Harvey, 2009) (see Table 30.1).

The size and nature of the cohort is also important. To achieve critical mass, the leadership cohort needs to be a significant number, ideally between 50 and 100, and drawn from the entire breadth of the system, as this adds depth to the quality of the group and ensures that a wide range of perspectives are taken into account during group sessions within the programme.

Linking to context

The fact that it is no longer acceptable in today's healthcare system to adopt a myopic view of service or system redesign seems to be widely understood but seldom practised. It is a basic requirement for anyone leading change in this sector to have a full understanding of the context in which they operate and to start with an organisational or inter-organisational network as the unit of analysis rather than the individual.

Table 30.1 Comparison of the traditional approach to leadership development and a whole-system approach

	Traditional approach	Whole-system approach
Unit of analysis	The individual	The workgroup / team
Starting point	Theory	Practice / problem
Location	The retreat	The front line

One of the key elements of this whole approach is to emphasise the importance of context as a focus for leadership. Only by doing this will individuals develop a more strategic outlook, which will be essential to the organisation's success in the future.

Effective leaders must have an understanding of the 'golden thread' which links up-to-date policy and legislation with the practical aspects of the day-to-day operation of the service and what it is trying to achieve. A key difference between managers and leaders is that managers tend to have authority and status.

Leadership differs from management but a good leader needs to know what a manager can and should do so that tasks can be delegated. Managers produce order and consistency by planning and budgeting resources and controlling as well as problem-solving. Leaders, on the other hand, produce change and movement by establishing direction for the organisation or the team and aligning people as well as motivating and inspiring them. Aligning people is best done by clear communication, and seeking commitment and building teams and coalitions. Team members can be motivated and inspired by identifying and meeting their unmet needs, and by providing rewards through recognition and support.

Complexity

The application of ready-made solutions to recurrent problems is primarily the domain of the manager. Facing 'wicked' problems – those that are hugely complex (Grint, 2008) and have no clear solution – is the domain of the leader. Today's leaders in health operate in an environment of high ambiguity.

So-called adaptive leaders need to be encouraged to make connections across systems, where the solutions may lay in the hands of the stakeholders. Leadership may often involve helping stakeholders to realise they are part of the problem and therefore part of the solution rather than providing magical solutions to complex problems.

Key priorities for any leader must be to incorporate a direct approach to these problems within the organisation and not shy away from issues which are either too complex or too large to provide an immediate solution within the bounds of current ideology.

Adaptive

Taking the concept of the adaptive leader a stage further builds on the basic qualities of emotional intelligence and requires individuals to react appropriately within the changing environment. This demands resilience, capability, credibility and a broad knowledge base outside a particular field of specialty. It forms the bridge between the more organisational-based elements of the framework and the personal qualities of the individual leader.

Self-awareness is therefore only part of this; individuals need to understand not only the impact of their behaviour on others but also the role of their organisation and its impact on the rest of the system. Opportunities for a more collaborative approach, as opposed to the more traditional adversarial approach, need to be sought and a recognition is needed that solutions may sit outside the confines of the organisation.

John Edmonstone takes this a stage further in his comparison of two views of professional practice (Table 30.2) (Edmonstone, 2014). This is particularly interesting in the heavily regulated environment of the NHS, where Monitor and the Care Quality Commission undoubtedly place a huge emphasis on the left-hand column of Table 30.2 (technical/rational). The expectation is that leadership is there to monitor, regulate and repair

Table 30.2 Two views of professional leadership practice

Technical/rational view	Professional/artistry view
Follows rules, laws, routines and prescriptions	Starts where rules fade; sees patterns and frameworks
Uses diagnosis and analysis	Uses interpretation and appreciation
Wants efficient systems	Wants creativity and room to be wrong
Sees knowledge as graspable and permanent	Sees knowledge as temporary, dynamic and problematic
Theory is applied to practice	Theory emerges from practice
Visible performance is central	There is more to it than surface features
Setting out and testing competence are vital	There is more to it than the sum of the parts
Technical expertise is all	Professional judgement counts
Emphasises the known	Embraces uncertainty
Measurable standards must be fixed	What is most easily fixed and measurable is controlled and often trivial
Emphasises assessment, appraisal, inspection and accreditation	Emphasises investigation, reflection and deliberation
Professional activities can be mastered	Mystery is at the heart of professional practice

faults in the system rather than to experience, reflect and take a creative approach to solving problems.

Networks

Represented within the previous aspects of the framework is a strong case for the understanding and development of solid professional and social networks. The value of networks is now well established, but is often an area of anxiety for aspirant leaders. Modern leaders need to take a multidisciplinary approach, particularly regarding the involvement of clinicians, and encourage the development of inter-organisational networks via learning scts or task-based work groups. This forms an excellent base from which to develop wider, system-based networks.

Cross-boundary working or collaboration with associated organisations can develop strong links to alternative sectors and provide a good basis for networks as well as insights into best practice. As we move towards a more integrated approach, then new organisational forms start to emerge, built on networks – strategic alliances, clinical networks, joint ventures, partnership arrangements, remote working, teams and projects, all giving rise to the blurring of organisational boundaries and the loss of the more command and controlled self-contained environment (Bolden & Gosling, 2006).

Ability – developing leaders

It is only now, having addressed the previous five elements of this framework, that we finally arrive at the point of focus, which has been the traditional approach to leadership development, the individual and the ability to lead.

Underpinning the need to accommodate the wide range of change and leadership components is the need to develop a well equipped toolbox of *leadership behaviours*, based on an equally well equipped set of beliefs and values. This development at the individual level is critical in creating effective leadership within organisations and it is important to understand some of the key elements which underpin 'effective leadership'.

Kouzes & Posner (2012) describe five key elements of 'exemplary leadership' and have developed methods to measure, support and develop these behaviours for individuals across a multitude of different organisations.

Model the way

In order to be effective as a leader it is essential to develop mindfulness around our own values and how these connect to our behaviour. Leaders are constantly under scrutiny and are often remembered more for what they do than what they say. Are our beliefs and values reflected in our behaviour? Are we true to ourselves as leaders and authentic in the moment?

Leaders establish principles concerning the way people should be treated and the way goals should be pursued. They create standards of excellence and then set an example for others to follow. Because the prospect of complex change can overwhelm people and stifle action, they set interim goals so that people can achieve small wins as they move towards their larger objective. They unravel bureaucracy when it impedes action; they put up signposts when people are unsure of where to go or how to get there; and they create opportunities for victory.

Inspire a shared vision

Having the ability to develop vision and clarity in leadership is not just the domain of politicians and the heads of organisations. People are affected most significantly by those they work with closely and the impact of the immediate manager on individuals can be profound. This proximity of influence provides great opportunity for positive influence and personal growth. Northouse (2007) provides a very helpful theoretical and practical outline of the leadership skills needed in various settings.

Leaders passionately believe that they can make a difference. They envision the future, and create an ideal and unique image of what the organisation can become. Through their magnetism and quiet persuasion, leaders enlist others in their dreams. They breathe life into their visions and get people to see exciting possibilities for the future.

Challenge the process

An essential characteristic of any leader is a questioning nature. Being critical of existing systems and methodology is essential for change. Strong leaders challenge in every direction and have the assertiveness and confidence to avoid defensiveness and blame when things go wrong.

Leaders search for opportunities to change the status quo. They look for innovative ways to improve the organisation. In doing so, they experiment and take risks, and because leaders know that taking risks involves mistakes, they accept the inevitable disappointments as learning opportunities (Kotter, 1995).

Enable others to act

Building effective teams is perhaps the single most important ability for leaders to possess in healthcare, as teams form the basis of most systems within health and social care. Several studies have established the link between effective patient care and well-run teams, and the process of team development, staff retention and consistent provision of care is an essential component of leadership and managing people.

Leaders foster collaboration and build spirited teams. They actively involve others and understand that mutual respect is what sustains extraordinary effort. They strive to create an atmosphere of trust and human dignity. They strengthen others and make each person feel capable and powerful. Bird (1992) suggests that setting clear aims and recruiting the right people and right skill mix are critical aspects of managing and leading teams.

Encourage the heart

People need to feel valued and the successful management of people should always incorporate meaningful recognition. Leaders need to be constantly on the lookout for opportunities to exploit this and actively seek out good performance.

Accomplishing extraordinary things in organisations is hard work; to keep hope and determination alive, leaders must recognise the contributions that individuals make. The members of every winning team need to share in the rewards of their efforts, so leaders celebrate accomplishments. They make people feel valued. Clinical leadership (Stanton *et al*, 2010) allows clinicians to move out of their clinical comfort zone and help develop services. Bhugra *et al* (2013) provide an overview of what leadership means and how to learn about leadership and provide it.

Conclusion

Traditionally, the skills required to manage people have been documented and structured to form the basis of training programmes and personal competency maps, and these allow people to tick the box when that particular aspect of their development has been satisfied. More recently, we have moved towards a more holistic model which puts the emphasis on leadership and a whole range of capabilities which reach outside the organisation in which the individual operates.

Managing people is a complex process which demands a greater range of skills, personal awareness and system-wide understanding than the traditional model supported. Greater levels of clinical engagement are essential to this and clinicians need to have more influence over how the system runs. To achieve this, however, requires them to be leaders, not managers, and this in turn requires a greater understanding of a broader set of issues than before.

References

Bennington J, Harvey J (2009) *Whole Systems Go*. National School of Government.

Bhugra D, Gupta S, Ruiz P (2013) *Leadership in Psychiatry*. Wiley-Blackwell.

Bird M (1992) *Effective Leadership*. BBC Books.

Bolden R, Gosling J (2006) Leadership competencies – time to change the tune. *Leadership*, 2: 147–63.

Burke W, Litwin G (1992) A causal model of organisational performance and change. *Journal of Management*, **18**: 523–45.

Edmonstone J (2014) What is wrong with NHS leadership development? *British Journal of Healthcare Management*, **19**: 531.

Grint K (2008) Wicked problems and clumsy solutions. *Clinical Leader*, 1: 54–68.

Janman K (2009) *The Leadership Illusion*. Palgrave Macmillan.

Kotter J (1995) Leading change. *Harvard Business Review*, March–April.

Kouzes J, Posner B (2012) *The Leadership Challenge* (5th edn). Wiley.

Northouse PG (2007) *Leadership: Theory and Practice*. Sage.

Pedler M, Artwood M (2010) Does action learning generate social capital. *Action Learning Research and Practice*, **8**: 27–39.

Prusak L, Cohen D (2001) Invest in social capital. *Harvard Business Review*, **79**(6): 86–93.

Stanton E, Lemer C, Mountford J (2010) *Clinical Leadership: Bridging the Divide*. Quay Books.

CHAPTER 31

Mental health informatics

Martin Baggaley

Health informatics can be defined as:

> 'The knowledge, skills and tools which enable information to be collected, managed, used and shared to support the delivery of healthcare and to promote health'. (Department of Health, 2002*a*)

Mental health informatics applies to mental health services. Smartphones, social media, iPads, personal computers and the electronic transfer of information are now part of normal day-to-day life. Psychiatrists need to understand the key principles of mental health informatics, both to be able to work effectively now and also to appreciate the opportunities for more effective ways of working in the future which modern information technology (IT) affords.

To use IT successfully requires a certain level of personal competency, although it is not necessary to understand the technology or how the software or 'app' is written. (A mobile app is a software program designed to run on tablets and mobile phones.) Technology moves on at great pace and it is likely that personal computers themselves will become obsolete before too long. Many people are using tablets and smartphones to browse the internet and access electronic patient records without a personal computer. The majority of trusts in the NHS use a version of Microsoft Office and all psychiatrists need to be able to use a word processor, an internet browser (e.g. Microsoft Internet Explorer) and an email client (e.g. Microsoft Outlook). A basic understanding of a spreadsheet (e.g. Microsoft Excel) is helpful.

Trusts use email as a standard communication tool but increasingly social media and various related apps are becoming important tools too. Trusts have a Twitter and Facebook presence which medical managers may contribute to. Trusts are keen to move to mobile working because it potentially offers savings in expensive buildings and clinics and is more convenient to patients. Videoconferencing will become more widely used in the future, to speak with both colleagues and patients.

Electronic patient records

The majority of mental health trusts are now largely paperless or at least 'paper light' and use an electronic patient record (EPR) system. One of the successes of the now abandoned National Programme for IT has been the widespread provision of EPRs for mental health trusts, with systems such as RiO. There are significant potential safety gains in implementing a full EPR, particularly with electronic prescribing and decision support, although most systems are not as advanced as this yet.

An EPR also should improve the availability of information for both service users and carers, as it is possible to print off or even email copies of care plans, drug information leaflets and so on.

Most trusts, as they move towards a paperless system, will still keep paper records for a transitional period. This requires careful management and may in itself represent a risk, as vital information may remain in the paper records while the clinical teams look only at the up-to-date electronic information, unaware of the existence of relevant past material.

EPRs have inevitably changed the way psychiatrists practise. Unfortunately, in many trusts the EPR is effectively an electronic version of a folder of paper notes and many of the potential benefits offered by an electronic system are not realised. It can be quicker to flick through a paper folder than search through a complex system. In addition, much time and effort is put into entering data in and much less in getting information out. Also, electronic systems allow management to ensure the collection of and completion of information in a far more comprehensive way than with paper. As a result, clinicians can find that they are spending more and more time at their computers and less time with patients. Links to external systems such as general practice records or acute hospital records are rare but as integrated healthcare becomes more important such interfaces will be required.

Email

Email has largely replaced letters and written memos as the standard way of communicating. To get the most out of email, it is important to understand how to use the software effectively and to be aware of the basic rules of etiquette (see below), which unfortunately are rarely taught.

Microsoft Outlook

Most NHS computers have Microsoft Office as a standard suite of programs which includes Outlook as the standard email application. Outlook is like a postbox but it needs a mail system to operate. Many trusts will use an application such as Microsoft Exchange to distribute email around the system.

NHSmail

NHSmail is a fully integrated email, calendar and directory service for use by all NHS employees throughout their careers in the NHS. It allows for transmission of patient-sensitive data to another NHS user on NHSmail using secure encrypted messages. It has a huge flexible database of contact details, which, provided trusts and other NHS organisations keep it up to date, will prove to be a very useful way to contact other people in the NHS. NHSmail can be used from any computer connected to the internet and it is compatible with Microsoft Outlook. Individual NHS clinicians can register to use NHSmail and many NHS organisations have migrated across to use NHSmail instead of their own email server. The advantage of NHSmail is that it offers one address wherever anyone moves in the NHS and allows transmission of patient-sensitive information, both within the system and to other secure domains such as Government Secure Internet (gcsx) and the Police National Network (pnn). One disadvantage is that email addresses cannot be as easily guessed; for example, most trusts use the format firstname.secondname@trustname.nhs.uk, whereas NHSmail uses numbers to distinguish same names, for instance john.smith99.

Email etiquette

Email is a very powerful tool but can easily be misused. It can be all too easy to send angry emails copied to everyone up to chief executive, which are soon regretted. It is sometimes possible to retrieve emails after pressing 'send' but do not rely on this to salvage potential disasters. It is a good rule never to send an email when feeling angry; it is better to calm down and review the matter the next day. It is always a good rule never to send work emails after a glass of wine. It is also easy to appear rude when this was not the intention at all. There are many circumstances when a quick telephone call is better than an email. Typing in capitals to indicate irritation is rude and should not be done. Avoid sending copies to everybody in the trust. Beware of an email trail – there can be information much further down the trail which can be inadvertently sent to people it was not intended for. Finally, never write an email you would be embarrassed by if it had to be disclosed to a tribunal or if it were published in the *Daily Express*.

Email psychotherapy

There are some psychotherapists who provide psychotherapy by email. The regulation and ethical framework of such services are difficult to determine, especially when the therapist lives in a different country to the patient. A number of studies have demonstrated the efficacy of such treatment. Some service users appear to appreciate such contact and the impersonal nature of the interaction. Service providers charge per email or by time taken over a case. Most internet psychotherapists are based in the USA, although it can be difficult to know exactly where some of them are based.

In the UK, there are few services which offer internet therapy. However, there are therapists and psychiatrists who use emails as a follow-up and as a way of monitoring the progress of patients they also see face to face.

Email is much less intrusive than telephone calls, and therapists and patients can read the message at their convenience. There are some web-based cognitive–behavioural psychotherapy treatment programmes which have been shown to be effective in the treatment of depression and anxiety disorders.

SMS messaging

Short Message Service (SMS) or Multimedia Messaging Service (MMS) are more commonly known as texting. This well-established technology has been used to remind patients of appointments. It is a very convenient means of two-way communication with patients. If a patient did not attend an appointment texts can be automatically sent to both the patient and clinicians involved in the case.

Psychotherapy via videoconferencing

Some trusts and individual clinicians offer clinical sessions for both assessment and treatment via videoconferencing or Skype. This has been demonstrated as convenient and as effective as face-to-face sessions. Patients do not have to travel. Now that it is possible to videoconference easily via tablets and smartphones, it is likely to be become more frequently used.

Trust intranets

An intranet is effectively an internal internet; thus, people use a browser, such as Internet Explorer, to look at web pages, but these are not accessible to those outside the firewall (a firewall is software which prevents unauthorised access to computers connected via a network). A trust can use an intranet to share information which might otherwise clog up the email system. For example, instead of sending an email to everyone, notices of interest can be posted on the intranet.

Patient portals and personalised health records

A central component of the Department of Health's Information Strategy published in May 2012 (see below) was for patients to be given access to their own records. South London and Maudsley NHS Foundation Trust has developed a patient portal accessed securely via the internet to a personalised web page where the patient's mental health electronic records and, in due course, primary care records can be viewed. There is the facility to complete patient-reported outcome measures and to engage in co-production of care plans.

'Cloud'-based computing

This is internet-based computing in which large groups of remote servers are networked to allow sharing of data-processing tasks, centralised data storage, and online access to computer services or resources. It can be cost-effective, although there are restrictions on NHS data being hosted on servers outside the UK.

'Big data'

In 2012, Gartner updated its definition as follows:

> '*Big data* is high volume, high velocity, and/or high variety information assets that require new forms of processing to enable enhanced decision making, insight discovery and process optimisation.' (See Wikipedia at https://en.wikipedia.org/wiki/Big_data)

'Big data' refers to very large, complex data-sets that require great power to analyse (usually using cloud computing) but can reveal new and helpful insights. NHS genomics is involved in projects harnessing the power of big data. There is also the example of the collaboration of five academic health science centres linking five EPRs and using a tool (the Clinical Records Information System) to interrogate an anonymised version of their records.

Knowledge management

Clinicians are faced with an exponential growth of new knowledge, including new research and new guidelines and policy directives. This knowledge is available electronically, which allows clinicians to access it at their desktop, as required, even when seeing service users. Many services can be configured to send alerts when relevant research is published. Online searches can be performed and the relevant abstracts retrieved and saved or printed out. Librarians are changing function from managing books to becoming experts on electronic information management. It is possible simply to use an intranet search engine to try to look up suitable material. However, it is usually more effective to access a site which can act as a gateway to relevant resources via hyperlinks.

National Library for Health

The National Library for Health is a digital library for NHS staff, patients and the public. This includes access to journals and other sources of evidence such as Evidence Search. Access to much of the material requires an Athens account. All NHS employees can apply for an Athens password, which allows access via the internet to a large range of electronic resources, including Medline, the Cochrane database and a specialist library for mental health. This includes many full-text articles of original papers.

Confidentiality and security

All medical data are potentially sensitive and information regarding mental health especially so. The principles of confidentiality and security with regard to medical records are not fundamentally different for electronic notes and paper systems. The former cause greater concern because of the potential ease of browsing vast numbers of records, but in fact most electronic systems can be more secure than the paper equivalent, for example by having an audit trail of who has accessed what page. One principle is that of role-based access (i.e. the access to data is dependent on nationally determined roles, such as doctor or administrator) and having a legitimate relationship to the patient. In some systems, access is controlled by a smart card and password, and is checked once the individual logs on to the system. Other systems typically use password and username access only.

Data protection

The current UK legislation is the Data Protection Act 1998 (a complex piece of legislation). It contains eight principles regarding the handling of personal data. These state that all data must be:

- processed fairly and lawfully
- obtained and used only for specified and lawful purposes
- adequate, relevant and not excessive
- accurate and, where necessary, kept up to date
- kept for no longer than necessary
- processed in accordance with the individual's rights (as defined)
- kept secure
- transferred only to countries that offer adequate data protection.

Freedom of Information Act 2000

The Freedom of Information Act 2000 gives a general right of access to all types of recorded information held by public authorities; full access was granted in January 2005. The Act sets out exemptions to that right and places certain obligations on public authorities. It requires all organisations in the NHS to set up and maintain publication schemes that tell the public what information is held.

Caldicott guardians

'The Caldicott principles and processes provide a framework of quality standards for the management of confidentiality and access to personal information under the Leadership of a Caldicott Guardian.' (Department of Health, 2002*b*)

The name arises from the work of Dr Fiona Caldicott, a past President of the Royal College of Psychiatrists. Chief executives were required to appoint a Caldicott guardian by 31 March 1999 and in 2002 this responsibility was extended to councils with social service responsibility (CSSRs). There are approximately 1000 Caldicott guardians throughout the NHS and in CSSRs. The Caldicott report (Caldicott, 1997) established a clear set of principles, reflecting best practice in the handling of confidential information:

- *Justify the purpose*. Every proposed use or transfer of information within or from an organisation should be clearly defined and scrutinised, with continuing uses regularly reviewed by an appropriate guardian.
- *Do not use patient-identifiable information unless it is absolutely necessary*. Patient-identifiable information should not be used unless there is no alternative.
- *Use the minimum necessary patient-identifiable information*. Where the use of patient-identifiable information is considered to be essential, the use of each individual item of information should be justifiable, and its identifiability reduced as far as possible.
- *Access to patient-identifiable information should be on a strictly need-to-know basis*. Only those individuals who need access to patient-identifiable information should have access to it.
- *Everyone should be aware of their responsibilities*. Action should be taken to ensure that those handling patient-identifiable information, both clinical and non-clinical staff, are aware of their responsibilities and obligations to respect patient confidentiality.
- *Understand and comply with the law*. Every use of patient-identifiable information must be lawful. Someone in each organisation (the Caldicott guardian) should be responsible for ensuring that the organisation complies with the legal requirement.

Royal College of Psychiatrists' Mental Health Informatics Committee

The Royal College of Psychiatrists for many years had a special interest group in informatics which became known as MHISIG (Mental Health Informatics Special Interest Group). In 2014, MHISIG became a Committee of Council. Details of the work of the Committee can be found on the members area of the College website. The latter is a useful source of information for psychiatrists (http://www.rcpsych.ac.uk).

UK government policy

Department of Health Information Strategy

The Department of Health Information Strategy was published in May 2012, under the title *Power of Information: Putting Us All in Control of the Health and Social Care Information We Need*. There was a strong drive to place personal health records in the hands of patients.

Mental Health Minimum Data Set

The Mental Health Minimum Data Set (MHMDS) is an aggregated data-set with the potential to provide useful comparative information for service managers to assess how one service performs compared with another. To date it has been under-used for this purpose.

The MHMDS was developed to improve information on usage and need. It describes the care received by service users during a 'spell of care'. It covers clinical problems, treatments, aspects of social care and outcomes, and records geographical markers. Its prime purpose is to provide information for clinical audit, and for service planning and management. The MHMDS became mandatory for service providers in 2003.

The future

Mental health informatics is a rapidly developing topic, driven by continuing technological advance. There will always be differing levels of enthusiasm for such systems and progress will always seem slower than it might be. However, if psychiatrists can understand the basic principles, they will be in a better position to obtain real benefit from developments in informatics, rather than feeling that the technology is being imposed on them. There is a great challenge to all from constrained resources and increasing demand. Mental health informatics is not a panacea. Nevertheless, the use of IT can make services more effective and less expensive. One way of thinking about this is to use the analogy of retail banks, which, with internet banking, arguably provide a better service without customers ever, or only very rarely, needing to visit a branch.

References

Caldicott F (1997) *Report on the Review of Patient-Identifiable Information.* Department of Health.

Department of Health (2002a) *Making Information Count: A Human Resources Strategy for Health Informatics Professionals.* Department of Health.

Department of Health (2002b) *Implementing the Caldicott Standard into Social Care. Appointment of Caldicott Guardians* (HSC 2002/003-.LAC (2002)2). Department of Health.

Department of Health (2012) *Power of Information: Putting Us All in Control of the Health and Social Care Information We Need.* Department of Health. Available at https://www.gov.uk/government/uploads/system/uploads/attachment_data/file/213689/dh_134205.pdf (accessed April 2016).

CHAPTER 32

Stress, burnout and engagement in mental health services

Jerome Carson and Frank Holloway

This chapter looks at the stresses that mental health workers, particularly psychiatrists, experience and the potential adverse consequences of these stresses. In tune with contemporary psychological thinking, we also look at the positive aspects of working within mental healthcare, sources of resilience and how organisations can better look after their employees. The authors have worked in mental health services in the UK, but the problems and solutions presented have wide relevance across all advanced healthcare systems (Lasalvia & Tansella, 2011). We draw on the empirical evidence and our own experiences as a clinical psychologist with a particular interest in staff stress (J.C.) and a psychiatrist and former medical manager (F.H.). We aim to offer practical suggestions as to how psychiatrists can manage the stresses they inevitably experience. We also highlight the legitimate expectations staff should have of their managers and employers.

There have been recurrent crises surrounding morale, recruitment and retention in psychiatry (Mukherjee *et al*, 2013). Kendell & Pearce (1997) noted that large numbers of experienced psychiatrists were opting for early retirement and explored the reasons for this. The reasons people gave for leaving the profession early were poignant and provide insights into potentially remediable sources of distress (see Box 32.1). They include: the impact of serious adverse events, such as patient suicide, serious violence or homicide; a pervasive feeling of accountability without power to influence the actions of others; and alienation from the edicts of a 'management' that is perceived as remote, critical and unaware of day-to-day clinical reality.

These findings remain relevant (Kumar, 2011). The 1990s were a time of upheaval and radical change for mental health services, marked by severe shortages of acute in-patient beds in the context of rapid, and ultimately successful, deinstitutionalisation. After a decade of rapid growth in mental health services, the 2010s have seen significant disinvestment and increasing stresses on the care system.

In the past, doctors could expect, after considerable early sacrifices in their working lives, to have a high degree of autonomy in their work and to be treated with deference and respect in return for good-quality clinical

---

Box 32.1 Selected reasons for early retirement given by consultant psychiatrists who retired prematurely in 1995 and 1996

- A consultant colleague committed suicide in 1994. I did not want to be next.
- A recurring feeling that I was failing despite working long hours.
- I had no wish to be 'crucified' in a future hospital inquiry into a suicide/homicide.
- Persistent awareness of a disaster about to happen at any time ... I realised it was only a matter of time before I was in the dock (i.e. a homicide inquiry) despite all my best efforts.
- Stress, stress, stress.
- I feel I let a patient down ... with serious consequences.
- I was tired. I had nothing left to give.
- I was unable to give enough time to many needy people because of imposed changes in practice.
- Increasing fears for personal safety.
- The level of violence against staff ... and the level of violence committed by my patients.
- The night work got too demanding.
- A total disregard for the views of the clinical team in planning services.
- An impossible medical director.
- Unable to meet the conflicting demands of NHS work and university work.
- Appointment of a colleague as clinical director for whom I had no respect.
- I was always in cross-fire between medical colleagues and non-medical managers.
- I was deeply disenchanted by the fact that I didn't have any influence over long-term or day-to-day plans, though ultimately I carried the can.
- Only negative feedback from managers.
- The main reason was a feeling of being unappreciated/unsupported by management – an atmosphere of alienation – 'us and them'.
- Appalling attitude (hostility and grossly inadequate funding) to psychiatry of the purchasers.

Adapted from Kendell & Pearce (1997)

---

care. Contemporary medical practice is understandably characterised by an ever-increasing level of accountability, team-working, a 'patient-centred' approach, openness to evaluation by non-professionals and exposure to an increasingly litigious, risk-averse culture. (Concern over the threat of litigation is an even greater worry for American psychiatrists – DeMello & Deshpande, 2011.)

This shift in expectations on doctors may be particularly difficult because of the personality traits that traditionally characterise the medical profession. Consultants characteristically enjoy autonomy and innovation, want their decision-making to be based on logical analysis and need to be able to control their working life (Houghton, 2005). These traits are at apparent odds with the demands of the consumer-oriented, protocol-driven, team-based and undoubtedly chaotic contemporary health service.

Mental health workers face increasing demands to provide treatment for people who experience workplace stress. It is therefore more than a little ironic for psychiatrists as a professional group to be described as being particularly prone to stress, burnout and suicide (Fothergill *et al*, 2004; Kumar, 2011; Heponiemi *et al*, 2014), as are nurses (Mark & Smith, 2012) and mental health social workers (Johnson *et al*, 2012).

Concepts: stress, burnout, engagement and well-being

Stress in the workplace

'Occupational stress' is a fashionable term, defined by the Health and Safety Executive (2009) as 'the adverse reaction people have to excessive pressures or other types of demands they face at work'. It is estimated that 40% of all work-related illness is due to stress. Consequences of stress include high staff turnover, absenteeism, symptoms of depression and anxiety and, ultimately, 'burnout'.

One way of understanding workplace stress is the *job demands–control–support model* (Karasek *et al*, 1998). This identifies three dimensions of any occupation:

- the demands the job makes, for example pressure of work and the emotional demands
- the level of control a person has over work
- the supports available in the workplace from co-workers and managers.

This model has been used to investigate the quality of consultant psychiatrist posts (Mears *et al*, 2007) and in a recent large-scale study of morale within mental health services in England (Johnson *et al*, 2012).

An alternative conceptual approach is the *stress process model* (Carson & Kuipers, 1998). This has three levels: external stressors, moderating factors and stress outcomes (see Fig. 32.1).

External stressors comprise specific occupational stressors, hassles and uplifts and major life events. Psychiatrists face a number of job-specific work stressors. These include responsibilities under the Mental Health Act, the prescribing of psychotropic medications, responsibility for decisions surrounding hospital admission and discharge, and the ever-present fear of criticism following a serious adverse incident. 'Hassles' are the sort of minor irritations that can have a cumulative effect on our sense of feeling stressed. They can range from the problems of commuting and difficulties with secretarial support to arguments with others. 'Uplifts' reflect the positive aspects of personal and professional life. None of us is immune from the effects of major life events such as serious illness, bereavement,

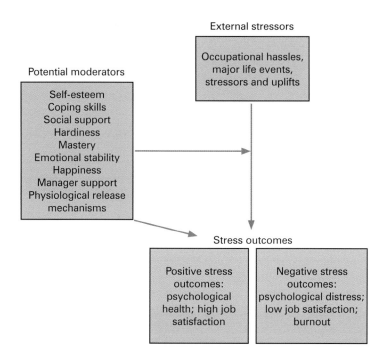

External stressors

Occupational hassles, major life events, stressors and uplifts

Potential moderators

Self-esteem
Coping skills
Social support
Hardiness
Mastery
Emotional stability
Happiness
Manager support
Physiological release mechanisms

Stress outcomes

Positive stress outcomes: psychological health; high job satisfaction

Negative stress outcomes: psychological distress; low job satisfaction; burnout

Fig. 32.1   The revised stress process model

marital breakdown, financial pressures and family problems: cumulatively they take their toll.

Within the stress process model, whether stressors cause positive or negative *stress outcomes* depends on the range of *potential moderating factors* available to us as individuals. These can be *internal factors* such as self-esteem, coping skills and hardiness or *external factors* such as having the support of your line manager and your work colleagues. Hence a member of staff with a robust sense of self-esteem may be better able to deal with external stressors than a more fragile colleague. Someone working in an effective team may be less affected by a stressor than someone who experiences the team as dysfunctional and unsupportive.

Stress outcomes can be positive or negative. The former include psychological health and high job satisfaction, which are characteristics of engagement. The latter can include psychological distress, low job satisfaction and the occupational burnout syndrome.

The *job demands–control–support model* and the *stress process model* provide ways of conceptualising the complex issue of staff stress but are not comprehensive. For instance, while the issue of life events is highlighted in the stress process model, significant stress can also be generated by 'non-events', for example failure to get a job or win a promotion. There are also significant difficulties with the stress literature, which remains largely reliant on cross-sectional rather than prospective studies.

Burnout

The concept of burnout originated in the USA. Schaufeli & Enzmann (1998: p. 36) provide a useful definition:

> 'Burnout is a persistent, negative, work-related state of mind in normal individuals that is primarily characterised by exhaustion, which is accompanied by distress, a sense of reduced effectiveness, decreased motivation and the development of dysfunctional attitudes and behaviours at work. This psychological condition develops gradually but may remain unnoticed by the individual involved. It results from a misfit between intentions and reality in the job. Often burnout is self-perpetuating because of inadequate coping strategies that are associated with the syndrome.'

The main psychometric measure used to assess burnout is the Maslach Burnout Inventory (MBI; Maslach & Jackson, 1986). This has 22 items which assess the degree to which individuals are *emotionally exhausted* by their jobs; their level of *depersonalisation* (their ability to feel for their patients); and their level of *personal accomplishment* (the degree to which they feel they are effective or are rewarded by their jobs).

Engagement

Engagement is the positive opposite of burnout (Maslach, 2011). It has been succinctly defined as 'a positive, fulfilling, work-related state of mind characterised by vigour, dedication and absorption' (Schaufeli *et al*, 2002: p. 74). Engagement is a good predictor of employee performance. It relates to:

> 'a range of constructs that are already known about within organisational psychology, including proactive behaviour, personal initiative and organisational citizenship behaviour, prosocial behaviour and contextual performance.' (West & Dawson, 2012: p. 6)

Fostering engagement rather than avoiding stress and burnout is an example of positive psychology in action (Priebe & Reininghaus, 2011).

Mental well-being

If engagement is the positive opposite of burnout then mental well-being is the positive opposite of stress. Accordingly there is a Public Health Guideline from the National Institute for Health and Care Excellence (NICE) entitled *Promoting Mental Well-Being at Work* (NICE, 2009), which is actually about decreasing workplace stress. It adopts the following definition of mental well-being:

> 'a dynamic state in which the individual is able to develop their potential, work productively and creatively, build strong and positive relationships with others and contribute to their community.'

Implications

Medical and service managers must take the issue of staff morale and stress seriously, since a distressed workforce will be an ineffective workforce (Firth-Cozens, 2003). On the positive side, an engaged workforce is an effective workforce: within healthcare, levels of engagement predict patient satisfaction, patient mortality and hospital infection rates (West & Dawson, 2012).

It is sobering to note that how we experience our job in terms of its demands and the latitude we have over decisions has a very significant effect, independent of other risk factors, on the occurrence of fatal coronary heart disease (Kuper & Marmot, 2003). High demand and low decision latitude are potentially dangerous – and increasingly characterise the lot of the mental health professional. If taken seriously, this finding and the clear benefits of engagement have profound implications for the responsibilities of the employer and specifically for job design.

Psychiatrists and the stress process

There is a diverse body of literature investigating aspects of the stress process as experienced by psychiatrists. The international evidence is that psychiatric specialists experience higher levels of stress than those working in other specialties, despite their lower objective workloads (Deary et al, 1996a; Heponiemi et al, 2014). Psychiatric trainees in the UK have reported higher levels of stress than consultants (Guthrie et al, 1999); subsequent uncertainties surrounding medical career pathways have added to this stress (Rathod et al, 2011). It is also now recognised that the transition from trainee to consultant is commonly experienced as particularly difficult. This has led to the development of mentoring programmes for newly appointed consultants (Royal College of Psychiatrists, 2008). There is some evidence that psychiatric trainees experience less burnout than general medical trainees (Sochos & Bowers, 2012). Psychiatric trainees also found their trainers to be more supportive.

A wide range of stressors have been identified. These include recurrent changes within health services, changes in community care, personal stresses, management and resource issues, and lack of time. Working across complex service interfaces has recently emerged as an issue for consultant psychiatrists in England (Rathod et al, 2011). Some studies have identified patient characteristics, particularly the management of a violent or potentially violent patient, as a major stressor (Guthrie et al, 1999). Indeed, one London study found that 12.4% of psychiatrists had been assaulted by a patient in the previous 12 months (Dhumad et al, 2007). In practice, looking after risky individuals with severe personality disorder is very demanding. Psychiatrists are, understandably, distressed by patient suicide. The process of investigation of serious untoward incidents, which is required as part of governance structures, can be both very prolonged and deeply distressing. Relationships with work colleagues, both psychiatrists and those from other disciplines, can be another source of distress. Staff may feel bullied by their seniors and their managers.

Moderating factors

The moderating factors most explored in the stress outcome literature for psychiatrists relate to what might loosely be termed personality factors. Low self-esteem and neuroticism have been, rather predictably, associated with poor stress outcomes (Deary *et al*, 1996*b*). Work climate and workload have a profound impact on stress outcomes. Perceived support, being able to participate in the organisation and good leadership have a positive effect (Thomsen *et al*, 1998). There is some evidence that different styles of working are associated with different stress outcomes (Mears *et al*, 2004).

An important moderating factor is the coping strategies that a person uses. A recent study identified both 'positive' and 'negative' coping strategies (Rathod *et al*, 2011). Among the positive were seeking support, engaging in leisure activities, exercising, socialising and managing one's time more effectively. Reported negative strategies included worrying, ignoring the problem, losing sleep, being anxious and working ever harder. (This study did not mention use of alcohol or non-prescribed drugs – there is abundant evidence that harmful alcohol use is a problem among mental health professionals.)

Stress outcomes

Despite the comparatively high levels of stress that psychiatrists report, there are some positive indicators. Compared with other mental health disciplines, job satisfaction among German and British psychiatrists was found to be higher, as was the 'personal accomplishment' domain of the MBI, while emotional exhaustion and depersonalisation were lower (Priebe *et al*, 2005). An Israeli study found that while psychiatrists were not as 'happy' as some of their multidisciplinary colleagues, they had higher scores on seeing work as a 'calling' and as contributing to the greater good (Baruch *et al*, 2013). Less positively, a study of over 700 psychiatrists working in academic departments in Japan found that 70% experienced a low level of personal accomplishment on the MBI (not feeling themselves to be personally effective in their work roles or deriving much satisfaction from them) (Umene-Nakano *et al*, 2013); protective factors were status and perceived social support.

Managing stress and burnout

Cooper (1996) identified workplace stress interventions as fitting into a model of primary, secondary or tertiary prevention. In the primary prevention of workplace stress, the aim is to reduce or eliminate stressors and positively promote a supportive and healthy work environment. Secondary prevention is concerned with the prompt detection and management of depression and anxiety by increasing self-awareness and improving stress management skills. The aim here is to help workers evaluate the psychological effects of stress and to develop their own personal stress control plans. Tertiary prevention is concerned with the rehabilitation and recovery process of those individuals who have suffered or are suffering from stress-related disorders. The main forms of help at the tertiary level are workplace counselling and employee assistance programmes.

The majority of reported workplace stress management interventions are at the secondary level (Richardson & Rothstein, 2008). Stress management interventions commonly include the following elements: (1) changing, increasing or enhancing coping responses and resources; (2) teaching arousal-reduction techniques, such as relaxation or meditation; (3) changing perceptions or appraisals of work stress via cognitive restructuring (Dollard & Winefield, 1996). A meta-analytic review suggested that stress management interventions based on cognitive–behavioural therapy were the most effective (Richardson & Rothstein, 2008).

While there are many empirical studies of the stress process in mental health professionals, few intervention studies have been reported, and those that have tend to be of low methodological rigour or have a negative outcome. Nurses form the focus of most studies and there are no published studies of stress management interventions solely for psychiatrists. A conventional stress management programme proved difficult to recruit to (Kunkler & Whittick, 1991) and 'stress-busting' groups for psychiatrists proved hard to maintain (Murdoch & Eagles, 2007). The published literature on stress in psychiatrists focuses on assessment of stress, coping and burnout, and not on interventions. Papers dealing with stress reduction tend to be advisory (Firth-Cozens, 2007) or commentaries on the stressful nature of the work (Lachter, 2013). In an unconventional case study, consultant psychiatrist Dr Tom Harrison wrote a personal account of his own occupational health problems, with commentaries from both his secretary and his wife (Harrison *et al*, 2006).

In a review of the stress management literature, Reynolds & Briner (1994: p. 75) stated that:

> 'Occupational stress reduction is … one of the many fads initiated by academics, commercialised by consultants and embraced by managers but that ultimately fail to deliver the panacea-like solutions which they promise.'

Two decades later the disappointing results to date from stress management interventions underline the need for further research in the area and the likely value of primary prevention as opposed to therapeutic strategies. In the words of Christine Maslach (2011), 'preventing burnout is a better strategy than waiting to treat it'.

Reducing stress and enhancing engagement: what can be done?

Primary prevention

Maslach (2011) noted that 'building engagement is the best approach to preventing burnout'. Quite simple managerial actions can serve to buffer the effects of objective job demands on resulting employee stress and potential burnout (Buttigieg *et al*, 2011). Within the NHS, those working within well-structured teams (characterised by an effective system of appraisal, clear team objectives that team members worked closely together to achieve and regular team meetings) were significantly more likely to show engagement than those who worked in 'pseudo-teams' or were not working in a team (West & Dawson, 2012). An effective mental health team has clear goals, is well led, is adequately resourced and is characterised by mutual respect between professional colleagues (West *et al*, 2012).

The generic occupational literature identifies a wide range of interventions that might decrease stress in the workplace (see Box 32.2). Five issues are discussed in some detail: working styles; effective working within teams; achieving a work–life balance; relationships with medical colleagues; and training.

Working styles

The practice of psychiatrists, like that of all doctors, is changing rapidly. Traditional models of working within adult psychiatry, which involved both high individual case-loads within out-patient settings and responsibility for all patients on the case-load of the team, are associated with higher levels of stress than those adopting a more 'progressive' role (Mears *et al*, 2004). This

---

Box 32.2 Potential areas for intervention in the workplace to decrease stress

- *Role characteristics:* issues of clarity of role and workload
- *Job characteristics:* attending to the design of the job
- *Interpersonal relationships:* improving communication in the workplace
- *Organisational climate and structure:* encouraging decentralisation and participation by the workforce in decision-making
- *Human resource management:* recruitment and selection policies that select staff for the task in hand; effective mechanisms for supervision, appraisal and performance management
- *Physical aspects of the work environment:* quality of the physical environment, safety issues, adequate personal space

'progressive' working style is characterised by limited personal case-loads, protected time for professional development, ability to react to unforeseen situations and much scope for delegation within the team. Clarity over the consultant role and perceived levels of support from the multidisciplinary team and service managers are also associated with lower levels of stress and burnout.

The potential roles and responsibilities of the consultant psychiatrist are discussed in detail elsewhere in this book. Having some form of boundary around one's workload is important. This has obvious implications for the design of consultant jobs. However, a job that was so well designed that it offers little or no direct patient and carer contact, makes no intellectual demands or does not require post-holders to feel responsible for the service within which they work is unlikely to attract high-quality applicants (or much in the way of remuneration).

Working within teams

For mental health staff in general, their colleagues within the multi-disciplinary team are the major perceived source of support (Reid *et al*, 1999). Mutual support and respect from colleagues can buffer the adversities that inevitably occur within the life of a mental health professional. Effective teams can offer a valuable sounding board for discussing problematic cases and have subtle ways of supporting a colleague who is temporarily finding things difficult. Good teams do not, however, tolerate or condone established poor performance. This partly reflects team culture, but also follows from the fact that good teams tend to have good managers.

A core skill of the contemporary consultant is the ability to work effectively within the multidisciplinary team. Some consultant behaviours will encourage good team-working, while others will consistently erode the support potentially available from the team (see Chapter 13 of this book, on team-working). Although an adequate degree of technical competence, effective decision-making and specialist expertise are important to mental health teams, it is the 'softer', interpersonal competencies that dominate the relationship between psychiatrists and their teams. Putting the issue another way, it is the experience of most medical managers that their consultant colleagues rarely cause problems because of lack of technical competence. Issues much more commonly arise because of personality difficulties or personal style and subsequent emerging conflicts with their teams or consultant colleagues. Supporting and managing the 'problem psychiatrist' of whatever grade requires rather specific skills that in part relate to the local regulatory regime (Margerison, 2008).

Much more difficult than working well within an effective team is to support the transformation of a failing team. The failing team will increase the burden on the consultant in a number of ways, for example by colleagues refusing to share responsibility for the case-load, engaging in poor decision-making and not carrying out agreed tasks. Management must support the consultant where teams are failing, although the remedies will largely lie with the team leader and service manager. One particularly important but much neglected aspect of team functioning is the administrative support to the team.

Work–life balance

In the past, a male-dominated consultant workforce generally relied on a support system comprising a wife and family. Women entering higher levels of the profession were required to make choices between their role as a parent and their role as a professional, either by forgoing parenthood altogether or by depending on domestic support. One core demand of doctors is to achieve an appropriate balance between work and other aspects of life (Dumelow *et al*, 2000) and there is some evidence that women physicians who work their preferred hours have the best family and work outcomes (Carr *et al*, 2003). Doctors are seeking jobs that can offer a reasonable work–life balance, and part-time posts are becoming increasingly popular for both women and men. Unless premature retirement is to become the norm, career pathways should allow for less physically demanding jobs to be available towards the end of one's working life (which is set to become significantly longer than in the past).

Job planning offers an opportunity to introduce flexibility into the consultant job description. Medical managers also need to consider developing more part-time posts that will be attractive to those seeking to improve their work–life balance. Part-time posts do, of course, have implications for the organisation of the service, raise the issue of providing continuity of care and are, because of the negotiated structure of the job plan, more expensive than full-time posts.

Relationships with medical colleagues

In contemporary community-based practice, consultant psychiatrists tend to have much more regular and frequent contact with their multidisciplinary teams than their consultant colleagues. This may be the explanation for the surprising finding that consultants frequently reported their contacts with their colleagues as being a source of stress (Guthrie *et al*, 1999). There are a number of drivers to improving the links between consultant colleagues working within a service.

Appraisal and revalidation are based on a model of the 'good doctor', who will be in regular communication with peers to discuss and review standards of practice and clinical outcomes. Accreditation for continuing professional development (CPD) and revalidation require the doctor to participate in a peer group, which should be both supportive of and challenging to its members. Simple measures, such as grouping consultant offices together and meeting colleagues regularly, in both a work and a social context, can improve working relationships. Traditionally, case conferences and academic meetings have offered opportunities for consultant medical staff to meet. Regular informal meetings at which clinical issues are discussed (cases that consultants are finding problematical – a 'risk forum') can be helpful and also contribute to CPD.

Medical managers need to be aware of interpersonal difficulties occurring within a consultant group, although effective interventions are extremely difficult. There are particular sensitivities where consultants share medical responsibility for a team or service, which is likely to become increasingly common as part-time working increases. Working within a job-share or with a co-consultant can be experienced as enjoyable and supportive or on a spectrum towards the deeply dysphoric. The Psychiatrists' Support Service offers specific advice about dealing with difficult colleagues (Royal College of Psychiatrists, 2010).

Training issues

The literature on stress provides no clear guidance on how training for the consultant role and CPD could help improve stress outcomes. The stresses that trainees experience are subtly different from those that consultants identify (Guthrie *et al*, 1999; Rathod *et al*, 2011), although patient suicide, hostility from patients and carers, complaints and serious untoward incidents are significant stressors for all psychiatrists. Training should provide all staff with the technical competence for the roles they undertake, and the ability to identify when they must seek additional expertise. All staff should have a thorough grounding in the ethical aspects of clinical practice. Many of the most stressful situations psychiatrists experience are products of the ethical dilemmas that are an inevitable part of working within mental health services.

Our experience suggests that a thorough grounding in the theory and practice of the assessment and management of risk is helpful, but in a much more thoughtful way than mere familiarity with the local risk assessment documentation (Holloway, 2004). Discussion during training about how to deal with a patient suicide, both practically and emotionally, might help staff manage a situation that is almost inevitable, even during the most exemplary professional lifetime (Foley & Kelly, 2007). Specific training for appearing in a coroner's court, often a peculiarly distressing experience, may also be useful (St John-Smith *et al*, 2009).

All psychiatrists must develop an understanding of how teams work and how they can work effectively within a team (see Chapter 13). These 'soft' competencies are not commonly formally taught, but deficiencies are often picked up on by trainers.

Conclusion

Difficulties with management are frequently identified as sources of stress for psychiatrists. This book, which seeks to provide an insight into the management process, should help psychiatrists learn to use their managerial colleagues more effectively. Health services are undergoing continual change: specific training in leading processes of service redesign and change management can allow psychiatrists to feel empowered rather than disoriented and distressed.

The Health and Safety Executive (2009) has developed management standards for work-related stress which set out what is expected of employers. The standards cover sources of stress at work: *demands* (workload, work environment); *control* (how much say people have in their work); *support* (from managers and colleagues); *relationships* (including how to manage unacceptable behaviour); *role* (clarity regarding expectations); and *change* (communication and management of organisational change). Implicit is the development of an organisational climate that is seeking to both get the best out of its workforce and do the best for them.

The stressors that psychiatrists experience are largely external to any particular mental health service and the propensity to experience stress (and to attract stressful experiences) seems to relate significantly to personality factors. However, there are many ways in which psychiatrists can ensure their long-term professional survival. Individual clinicians need to identify whether they prefer the stimulation of the varied professional life of the generalist to the usually more boundaried role of the specialist, and recognise when they need to change from one to the other. In psychiatry the pace of service change is such that one can expect to undertake a number of roles within a professional lifetime, adapting generic skills to each new role and learning additional skills as necessary.

In an era obsessed with risk assessment and risk management, consultants need to adopt effective strategies that do not leave them paralysed by fear or vulnerable to criticism should disaster strike: the simplest strategy is, if in doubt, 'phone a friend'. Discussion with colleagues is an under-used resource, although some psychiatrists have found it helpful as a peer supervision tool (Mason & Hayes, 2007). New technology, such as Skype and FaceTime, offer additional ways of communicating with colleagues.

A degree of humility in the face of complex situations is a valuable trait. Humility also helps one embrace the processes now in place to review serious untoward incidents and complaints by looking honestly for lessons that can be learned. It is also valuable for the consultant to have particular areas of interest for which there is protected time and which boost the individual's self esteem and sense of autonomy. These may, for example, be clinics that require specific expertise, medical management roles, teaching, research or even private practice. In choosing jobs, consultants need to think carefully about their working environment, and to pay at least as much attention to the quality of medical and multidisciplinary colleagues and service management as to simple workload parameters.

The literature clearly shows that medical managers can contribute to psychiatrists' stress (Kendell & Pearce, 1997). Service modernisation, which implies job redesign, offers the opportunity for reducing work pressures. Setting up mentorship schemes can be helpful for the younger consultant, who will benefit from the opportunity to discuss frustrations and difficulties with a more experienced colleague (Roberts *et al*, 2002). Above all, medical managers need to promote an open, respectful and positive organisational culture that offers all staff the opportunities to experience a sense of autonomy in their working lives and that ensures that staff have the skills to undertake their tasks and roles.

References

Baruch Y, Swartz M, Sirkis S, *et al* (2013) Staff happiness and work satisfaction in a tertiary psychiatric centre. *Occupational Medicine*, **63**: 442–4.

Buttigieg SG, West MA, Dawson JF (2011) Well-structured teams and the buffering of employees from stress. *Health Services Management Research*, **24**: 203–12.

Carr PL, Gareis KC, Barnett RC (2003) Characteristics and outcomes for women physicians who work reduced hours. *Journal of Women's Mental Health*, **12**: 399–405.

Carson J, Kuipers E (1998) Stress management interventions. In *Occupational Stress: Personal and Professional Approaches* (eds S Hardy, J Carson, B Thomas). Stanley Thornes.

Cooper C (1996) Stress in the workplace. *British Journal of Hospital Medicine*, **55**: 569–73.

Deary I, Blenkin H, Agius R, *et al* (1996*a*) Models of job related stress and personal achievement among consultant doctors. *British Journal of Psychology*, **87**: 3–29.

Deary I, Agius R, Sadler A (1996*b*) Personality and stress in consultant psychiatrists. *International Journal of Social Psychiatry*, **42**: 112–23.

DeMello T, Deshpande S (2011) Career satisfaction of psychiatrists. *Psychiatric Services*, **62**: 1013–8.

Dhumad S, Wijeratne A, Treasaden I (2007) Violence against psychiatrists by patients: survey in a London mental health trust. *Psychiatric Bulletin*, **31**: 371–4.

Dollard M, Winefield A (1996) Managing occupational stress: a national and international perspective. *International Journal of Stress Management*, **3**: 69–83.

Dumelow C, Littlejohns P, Griffiths S (2000) Relation between a career and family life for English hospital consultants: qualitative, semistructured interview study. *BMJ*, **320**: 1437–40.

Firth-Cozens J (2003) Doctors, their well-being, and their stress. *BMJ*, **326**: 670–1.

Firth-Cozens J (2007) Improving the health of psychiatrists. *Advances in Psychiatric Treatment*, **13**: 161–8.

Foley SR, Kelly BD (2007) When a patient dies by suicide: incidence, implications and coping strategies. *Advances in Psychiatric Treatment*, **13**: 134–8.

Fothergill A, Edwards D, Burnard P (2004) Stress, burnout, coping and stress management in psychiatrists: findings from a systematic review. *International Journal of Social Psychiatry*, **50**: 54–65.

Guthrie E, Tattan T, Wiliams E, *et al* (1999) Sources of stress, psychological distress and burnout in psychiatrists. *Psychiatric Bulletin*, **23**: 207–12.

Harrison T, Cook C, Robertson M, *et al* (2006) Work-related stress and the psychiatrist: a case study. *Psychiatric Bulletin*, **30**: 385–7.

Health and Safety Executive (2009) *How to Tackle Work-Related Stress* (leaflet INDG430). HSE.

Heponiemi T, Aalto A-M, Puttonen S, *et al* (2014) Work-related stress, job resources, and well-being amongst psychiatrists and other medical specialists in Finland. *Psychiatric Services*, **65**: 796–801.

Holloway F (2004) Risk: more questions than answers. *Advances in Psychiatric Treatment*, **10**: 273–4.

Houghton A (2005) The importance of having all types in a workforce. *BMJ Careers*, **5** February: 56–7.

Johnson S, Osborn DP, Araya R, *et al* (2012) Morale in the English mental health workforce: questionnaire survey. *British Journal of Psychiatry*, **201**: 239–46.

Karasek R, Brisson C, Kawakami N, *et al* (1998) The Job Content Questionnaire (JCQ): an instrument for internationally comparative assessments of psychological job characteristics. *Journal of Occupational Health Psychology*, **3**: 322–55.

Kendell RE, Pearce A (1997) Consultant psychiatrists who retired prematurely in 1995 and 1996. *Psychiatric Bulletin*, **21**: 741–5.

Kumar S (2011) Burnout and psychiatrists: what do we know and where to from here? *Epidemiology and Psychiatric Sciences*, **20**: 295–301.

Kunkler J, Whittick J (1991) Stress management groups for nurses: practical problems and possible solutions. *Journal of Advanced Nursing*, **16**: 172–6.

Kuper H, Marmot M (2003) Job strain, job demands, decision latitude and risk of coronary heart disease within the Whitehall II study. *Journal of Epidemiology and Community Health*, **57**: 147–53.

Lachter B (2013) The stress of work with bonus vaudeville section. *Australasian Psychiatry*, **21**: 486–9.

Lasalvia A, Tansella M (2011) Occupational stress and job burnout in mental health. *Epidemiology and Psychiatric Science*, **20**: 279–85.

Margerison N (2008) Problem psychiatrists? *Advances in Psychiatric Treatment*, **14**: 187–97.

Mark G, Smith AP (2012) Occupational stress, job characteristics, coping, and the mental health of nurses. *British Journal of Health Psychology*, **17**: 505–21.

Maslach C (2011) Burnout and engagement in the workplace. *European Health Psychologist*, **13**: 44–7.

Maslach C, Jackson S (1986) *Maslach Burnout Inventory*. Consulting Psychologists Press.

Mason R, Hayes H (2007) Telephone peer supervision and surviving as an isolated consultant. *Psychiatric Bulletin*, **31**: 215–7.

Mears A, Pajak S, Kendall T, *et al* (2004) Consultant psychiatrists' working patterns: is a progressive approach the key to staff retention? *Psychiatric Bulletin*, **28**: 251–3.

Mears A, Pajak S, Kendall T, *et al* (2007) Consultant psychiatrists' working patterns. *Psychiatric Bulletin*, **31**: 252–5.

Mukherjee K, Maier M, Wessely S (2013) UK crisis in recruitment into psychiatric training. *The Psychiatrist*, **37**: 210–4.

Murdoch J, Eagles J (2007) 'Stress-busting' groups for consultant psychiatrists. *Psychiatric Bulletin*, **31**: 128–31.

NICE (2009) *Promoting Mental Well-Being at Work*. NICE.

Priebe S, Reininghaus U (2011) Fired up, not burnt out – focusing on the rewards of working in psychiatry. *Epidemiology and Psychiatric Sciences*, **20**: 303–5.

Priebe S, Fakhoury W, Hoffmann K, *et al* (2005) Morale and job perception of community mental health professionals in Berlin and London. *Social Psychiatry and Psychiatric Epidemiology*, **40**: 223–32.

Rathod S, Mistry M, Ibbotson B (2011) Stress in psychiatrists: coping with a decade of rapid change. *The Psychiatrist*, **35**: 130–4.

Reid Y, Johnson S, Morant N, *et al* (1999) Improving support for mental health staff: a qualitative study. *Social Psychiatry and Psychiatric Epidemiology*, **34**: 309–15.

Reynolds S, Briner R (1994) Stress management at work: with whom, for whom and to what ends? *British Journal of Guidance and Counselling*, **22**: 31–43.

Richardson KM, Rothstein HR (2008) Effects of occupational stress management intervention programs: a meta-analysis. *Journal of Occupational Health Psychology*, **13**: 69–93.

Roberts G, Moore B, Coles C (2002) Mentoring for newly appointed consultant psychiatrists. *Psychiatric Bulletin*, **26**: 106–9.

Royal College of Psychiatrists (2008) *Mentoring and Coaching* (OP66). Royal College of Psychiatrists.

Royal College of Psychiatrists (2010) *Information Guide: On Dealing with Difficult Colleagues.* Web page at http://www.rcpsych.ac.uk/workinpsychiatry/psychiatristssupportservice/informationguides/difficultcolleagues.aspx (accessed April 2016) .

Schaufeli W, Enzmann D (1998) *The Burnout Companion to Study and Practice: A Critical Analysis.* Taylor and Francis.

Schaufeli WB, Salanova M, Gonzalez-Roma V, *et al* (2002) The measurement of engagement and burnout: a two sample confirmatory factor analytic approach. *Journal of Happiness Studies,* **3**: 71–92.

Sochos A, Bowers A (2012) Burnout, occupational stressors and social support in psychiatric and general medical trainees. *European Journal of Psychiatry,* **26**: 196–206.

St John-Smith P, Michael A, Davies T (2009) Coping with a coroner's inquest: a psychiatrist's guide. *Advances in Psychiatric Treatment,* **15**: 7–16.

Thomsen S, Dallender J, Soares J, *et al* (1998) Predictors of a healthy workforce for Swedish and English psychiatrists. *British Journal of Psychiatry,* **173**: 80–4.

Umene-Nakano W, Kato T, Kikuchi S, *et al* (2013) Nationwide survey of work environment, work–life balance and burnout among psychiatrists in Japan. *PLoS ONE,* **8**: e55189.

West M, Dawson JF (2012) *Employee Engagement and NHS Performance.* King's Fund.

West M, Alimo-Metcalf B, Dawson J, *et al* (2012) *Effectiveness of Multiprofessional Team Working (MPTW) in Mental Health Care. Final Report.* NIHR Service Delivery and Organization Programme.

CHAPTER 33

How to get the job you *really* want

Dinesh Bhugra and Sabyasachi Bhaumik

In order to get any job that you really want, a number of factors have to be considered. Becoming a consultant is a culmination of training in the right specialty and the right type of experience in training, teaching and research. Getting a consultant job is not impossible provided you have the right aptitude, knowledge and skills. The number of vacancies at the consultant level in the NHS is limited, and hence job interviews are becoming highly competitive. For this reason, you have to prepare yourself at a very high level to get the right job. Geting the job you *really* want requires technique and background work. This chapter aims to help the trainee look at a job and apply the right skills to obtain it.

It will be helpful to consider the kind of job as well as the environment you would like to pursue your career in. Within the NHS, there are teaching and non-teaching trusts as well those that have already achieved a foundation status or are aspiring to do so. The NHS posts are primarily based in either the community or in-patient settings but they can also have combined responsibilities. The growth of the independent sector has led to the offer of a considerable number of jobs within it. Increasingly, it is being seen that trainees are taking up these jobs quite early in their careers. However, jobs in the independent sector can be in highly specialised areas, mostly in in-patient services. Academic jobs with university tie-ups have dwindled in number in recent years.

There is little doubt that for those in psychiatric practice, becoming a consultant is important: if not a pinnacle of achievement, it is at least a stopover to bigger achievements. Assessing a job and going after the one you really want must be approached as a professional task. The art of getting such a job is not a battle that has to be won but courtship, in which potential employers and colleagues have to be wooed. When planning to go out on a date, you decide whether there is any long-term potential in the relationship and prepare accordingly (where to go to, what to wear, what food to order, what wine to drink). Similarly, applying for a consultant job requires careful thought, preparatory work and rehearsal, all of which should make the actual performance of the task easier. This should enable you to show yourself in a strong light in the pre-interview visits and reflect your glory in the actual interview.

Failure to secure a job is often due to inadequate preparation, not being clear about why you would like that particular job and about your own career plans, and poor performance at the interview. Appearing for an interview and becoming a consultant require long-term and short-term planning.

In relation to long-term planning, most candidates for consultant jobs in the UK will have done exactly the same period of training in similar rotations, although their management, teaching and research experiences will be more varied. For this reason, in addition to having the MRCPsych examination or equivalent and the CCT (Certificate of Completion of Training)/CESR (Certificate of Eligibility for Specialist Registration), having other research diplomas or degrees, such as an MD or PhD, will make you a more attractive candidate. (You have to make sure that you have a CCT or are eligible for it within the relevant period – for the latest guidelines consult the Royal College of Psychiatrists.)

The focus of this chapter is on short-term planning. Once you know your date of completion of training and the date on which you will obtain the CCT, you should start to look around for jobs. You may find it helpful to break down the process of gaining a consultant job into the following steps:

- starting a job folder
- applications and preparing an up-to-date curriculum vitae (CV)
- preparatory visits and homework
- preparing for the interview.

In addition, if you are offered the job, there will be negotiations over the contract, but these are beyond the remit of the present chapter.

Starting a job folder

The job folder should become the repository for every bit of information that you need to prepare for a particular job and will likely be a combination of information stored on your computer as well as hard copies and clippings of materials. You should bear in mind that the application process adopted by most NHS trusts these days is online and through the NHS Jobs website. It is important to familiarise yourself with what the website offers: from searching for jobs and setting email reminders, to filling in applications and saving draft versions before final submission. Having identified an advertisement that interests you, it may be helpful to make a note of the application deadline and plan your application process accordingly. You can then decide on what other specific information may be helpful. Within such a folder or ring binder you could include specific questions and proposed answers, and relevant documents and papers.

The job file should also be the place where you list reasons why you want the job, what problems you envisage in the job, what the responses of various people (whom you have been to see) are, what your plans will be and what your CV's strengths and weaknesses are. You may wish to include recent medico-political documents as well as the responses to those from the Royal College of Psychiatrists and the British Medical Association (BMA), for example.

Other material that you may find useful to gather would include:

- general information about the trust
- its business development plan
- its quality strategy/quality accounts
- an organisational flowchart (the who's who of the trust)
- the vision and mission statements, and
- (last but not least) information available on other websites such as those of the Quality Observatory, the Care Quality Commission (CQC) and Monitor.

Thus, the file will give you comprehensive information even when you need it in a hurry. During this phase, talk to others who may have participated in recent interviews either as an interviewer or a candidate. This will give you an idea of the questions likely to be asked and also of how to deal with pressures and different styles of interviewing. It is not likely that you will be asked the same questions but at least this may give you some hints.

Applications and preparing a curriculum vitae

You cannot be interviewed unless you are shortlisted, and your shortlisting depends on the quality of your application, the attached CV and how you have managed to sell yourself. The shortlisting is on the basis of all of these factors and helps employers to distinguish between definite candidates and probable candidates.

The role of the CV has become secondary to the online application, where information traditionally included in a CV has already been asked for. While completing an online application, make sure that every section is completed in a lucid style. The answers should be personalised to a degree, and where possible replete with clear illustrative examples from your actual clinical work as well as other areas of interest, to influence the shortlisting panel to lean in your favour. It cannot be overemphasised that this is a task that takes time, effort and creativity and may require several draft versions, at least for your first application.

The emphasis is on keeping the CV concise, and definitely not exceeding 8–10 pages. Different people have different ideas about the layout and the contents of the CV. Most word processing software offers ready-made CV and résumé templates and these can add to the visual aesthetics of the document. Make an effort to tailor the CV for the job in question and use it as a platform to highlight your strengths and achievements that may not

---

Box 33.1 Suggested contents and ordering of a curriculum vitae

- Name
- Address
- Other contact details (including mobile phone number and email address)
- Gender
- Qualifications (year/school/degree)
- Distinctions
- General education
- Current post (also note experience – clinical, administrative, research and teaching)
- Previous posts
- Management experience
- Teaching experience (medical – undergraduate and postgraduate – and also non-medical)
- Research (current experience)
- Publications (peer reviewed, invited, commentaries, editorials, chapters, abstracts)
- Membership of learned societies
- Career plans
- Other interests
- Referees

---

have been asked for in the main application. The aim is to impress your potential colleagues sufficiently to make it on to the shortlist. A suggestion for the ordering and content of the CV is presented in Box 33.1.

All institutions have equal-opportunity policies and no discrimination on the basis of ethnicity, age, gender, marital status or sexual orientation is allowed. Thus you do not need to give these details unless specifically asked.

Training and education

Undergraduate training and education should be mentioned briefly, as should basic schooling. Dates of entry, graduation and any awards, distinctions and prizes should be mentioned. A complete list of qualifications with the years in which they were obtained should be given, followed by details of posts. Giving a list of all the posts in a tabular form with details of overall experience gained in the text below the table is often helpful.

Work experience

Previous posts should be in chronological order. The most common format is to give the most recent job first and then to work backwards to foundation-year jobs. Try to highlight your relevant experience in each job, as this allows you to draw the reader's attention to your suitability for the job on offer.

Management, teaching and research

The sections on management, teaching and research should give a succinct summary of your relevant experience. Depending on the type of job applied for, you may need to detail the relevant experience accordingly. For example, if applying for an academic job, academic components (i.e. research and teaching) will take precedence over clinical experience. Management experience may well be more useful for jobs that contain clinical lead roles.

The list of publications should be up to date and accurate. Either the Vancouver or the Harvard style may be used, but consistency of style is important. For multi-authorship papers your name should be underlined or in bold letters. A long list of publications can be divided into those in peer-reviewed journals, reviews, editorials and book chapters; or it could be divided according to subject. Details of membership of learned societies may be given if these reflect appropriate experience. Scientific communications or presentations may be added if required. For management experience, it is not sufficient simply to state that you were a member of however many committees: your roles and responsibilities must be stated. Similarly, teaching and supervision experience can be divided into undergraduate, postgraduate, non-medical and so on, rather than simply listing lectures.

References

You will be required to provide names and contact details of two or more referees. It is important to have the right referees for each application. If you are applying for an academic job or a job in a teaching hospital, you should give the professor's or academic head's name if you have worked with him or her directly; otherwise, you may need to give the names of other academics in the department with whom you have worked. All jobs will require a referee from your current placement and unless there are exceptional circumstances you should provide those details. A third referee could be another person you have worked for. Thus, one clinical and one academic referee are helpful and if the job is clinical the third referee could be a clinician, or an academic if the job is academic. It is advisable to name referees you have worked with in the past 5 years. You must obtain your referees' permission before giving their names and keep them informed by sending them an up-to-date copy of your CV and the job description of the post you have applied for, so that they can tailor the reference accordingly.

Within the CV you should have no more than a paragraph stating what your career plans are and how this particular job fits in with those.

Before submitting your application and CV, show them to the scheme organisers, to your clinical/educational supervisors, training programme

475

director and other senior consultants and colleagues who have had experience of shortlisting. Get their advice and do not leave any editing or updating to the last minute. A slovenly written, misspelt, shoddy application and CV will certainly lose you the shortlisting, no matter how brilliant you are.

Covering letter

A covering letter should accompany your application. Some trusts use standard application forms which will be used for recruiting other members of staff as well, and therefore will not be adequate for your purpose. Under these circumstances, fill in all the sections as appropriate and if there are gaps that cannot be filled you can draw the employer's attention to the relevant sections in your CV. Some employers may ask that the accompanying letter be handwritten, in which case do so on plain paper and not on hospital headed notepaper.

Preparatory visits and homework

After you have read the job description, get others – colleagues, consultant or scheme organiser – to cast an eye over it to identify areas of potential problems, such as office space, secretarial support and potential changes in service development.

You need to be clear as to why you want this particular job in this particular area and why the appointments committee should take you seriously. You have to be certain that you meet all the essential and most of the desirable criteria and person specifications.

You should try to get hold of trust annual reports. You should explore your fixed session commitments and resources. The actual contract will be issued only after you have been offered the job, which you should discuss with representatives of the BMA.

Use both formal and informal channels to gather information about the job. Informal visits before the interview are encouraged, although some hospitals prefer that this occurs only after shortlisting. You may, of course, need to make more than one or two visits. Have a list of questions with you, some of which will be suitable only for medical colleagues, others for managers and some for both. When you arrange a visit by contacting the relevant clinical director or human resources people, you should arrange to see as many people as possible or, if it is impossible to do so, at least talk to them by telephone or correspond via email. If you are visiting, it is essential that you meet the clinical team members besides the medical director, clinical director and consultant colleagues.

You need to find out if it is a new job or a replacement. If the latter, find out how long the post has been vacant and whether there have been problems in recruitment and, if so, what the reasons are. You may get some of the information from the regional advisor of the Royal College of Psychiatrists, who can also tell you whether the post is approved for placement of trainees. You must explore the number of sites that you will be expected to work at and the distances involved. You need to know about staffing levels and whether there are trainees in post and any impending changes. You may wish to find out about further education, study leave, details of relocation and travelling expenses, research facilities and support. You should have your own list of priorities and arrange to see all those who may give you an overview. You should attempt to visit the site and talk to members of the multidisciplinary team. You may find it helpful to talk with some trainees, who may be able to tell you things which are pertinent to your application. You must arrange to see the chair of the trust, the chief executive and managers who are responsible for the specialty or sector. These managers will be able to give you details of potential changes which may affect the job in the long run. You should review the retention/attrition rate in the trust, which will give you a clear idea of what the trust's priorities and attitudes are.

The visit is for mutual appraisal, in that you need to find out about the job and the people, and the employers need to ascertain your strengths and weaknesses. The visits also serve another purpose, in that you may feel less anxious during the interview as you have already met your potential interviewers and eventually this may benefit you in the interview, especially if your performance is below par. Take extra copies of your CV and the job description with you and arrive in plenty of time for your appointment.

Also make sure that the secretary and the individuals concerned are aware of your arrival. It is acceptable to take notes but this may be distracting. If you do not, try to do so as soon as possible after the visit, as you are likely to forget vital information. After finishing your visit, you may wish to drive around to get a feel for the area if you are not familiar with it. You may also wish to take your family around and may choose to discuss the visit with your referees. Always ask the people you are seeing whether there is anyone else they think you should be seeing.

The interview

The interview is a vital process, which, although meant to select the best candidates, does not always do so: it selects those candidates who are good at being interviewed.

View the interview as another stage in the courtship ritual: you have to show yourself to be confident, enthusiastic, honest and charming.

The consultant appointment procedures are enshrined in law (with the exception of foundation trusts) and you can find the most up-to-date information on the structure of the panel by checking relevant websites. For consultant appointments, committees usually include a lay member (often the chair of the trust or another non-executive director), a College representative, the chief executive (or a board-level executive or associate director), the medical director, clinical director, a consultant from the trust and a university representative (especially if teaching and/or research commitments are part of the job description). These are core members and the committee may not proceed if any core member (or an appointed deputy) is not present. Trusts are free to add additional members but the balance of the committee is usually tilted towards a medical majority. Further details of the actual procedure can be obtained from the Department of Health (2005) document *The NHS (Appointment of Consultants) Regulations*. For academic appointments, the head of the department, one or two external assessors and at least one other member of the department should be on the committee. A representative of the human resources department is also in attendance.

The committee is looking for a competent, dedicated and sensible individual and it has been known for committees to appoint a more suitable candidate over a 'preferred' or favoured candidate.

You should appear neat and well dressed, relaxed and assertive. Even if you feel anxious (which you should be and are entitled to be), try to hide it. As a consultant, you will be expected to contain other people's anxieties and to try to deal with them in a non-pharmacological way. Ensure that you are properly dressed – old school ties may prove disadvantageous. For women, jewellery should be unobtrusive and make-up minimal. Before you are called in, ensure that your mobile phone is switched off and set your watch so that it does not beep.

When you are called in, greet the chair politely; the chair will then introduce the panel and set the rules for the interview. Try to relax and control your nervousness. Do not flop in the chair; sit erect and maintain eye contact with members of the panel.

Mock interviews and use of video may make you aware of your good and bad points. A good interview combines preparedness with spontaneity and naturalness. Most trusts ask you to do a 10-minute presentation before the interview or at a separate time. The topic for your 10-minute presentation may vary from trust of trust; however, it is likely to focus on improving quality of care and medical leadership. Prepare your subject carefully. Avoid jargon. Do mock presentations. Avoid having too many slides. Leave time for questions. Some trusts may ask you to appear before a user or carer panel, where you may be asked questions about your attitudes to different types of treatment and your empathic approach to personalised care.

In the interview, the questions will be quite sophisticated and divided broadly into general, training/research/teaching, management and clinical categories (Boxes 33.2–33.5). Different panel members tend to ask questions from different areas; for example, the Royal College representative is likely to ask you questions about your training and competencies. The university representative usually asks questions on research, audit and teaching. The management representatives are likely to focus on leadership, team working and clinical governance; in addition, they may ask you questions related to

---

Box 33.2   Examples of general interview questions

- Why do you want this job and what will you bring to it?
- Tell us about your strengths and weaknesses. How are you going to address any weaknesses that you have?
- What will be your key targets to achieve in your first year as a consultant?
- What are your plans over the next 5-10 years? (Talk about both professional and personal aims).

Box 33.3   Examples of interview questions on your research and training

- Please go through the competencies you have acquired at different stages of your training.
- Do you think you have any gaps in your training and if so how are you going to address these?
- Tell me about key lessons learnt during your training period.
- Can you tell me the difference in skills and competencies between a higher psychiatric trainee and a consultant?
- Please describe an audit or a research project that you have completed and please tell us what impact it has made in terms of clinical care.
- Why do you think trainees' research tends not to get published? What would you do about these barriers?
- Please describe the teaching methods you are going to use for the medical students and the reasons why.
- What in your opinion is the best method of learning?
- How do you contribute to the improvement of recruitment to psychiatry?

---

recent national policies and the benefits of becoming a foundation trust. The consultant colleague is more likely to ask you questions focused on clinical areas. If there is more than one candidate, each panel member is expected to ask the same questions. The first few questions are designed to set you at ease. A list of questions you may be asked is given in Boxes 33.2–33.5. There is no fixed length of the interview, but it is rare for it to exceed 1 hour.

The chances are that your output related to audit and research will be assessed formally in the interview. The output must include peer-reviewed publications, either in press or published. The role and utilisation of special-interest sessions may also be explored, especially in the context of the job for which you have applied.

Box 33.4 Examples of interview questions on management issues

- Please tell us about the clinical governance process and its current pitfalls. How are you going to address the existing problems?
- What are the key problems in learning from a serious untoward incident investigation? How are you going to resolve these?
- Care Quality Commission visits carry a high degree of significance for the trust. What is your view about improving our performance in relation to Care Quality Commission performance indicators?
- Real-time data is an important area for growth and development in the NHS. Why do you think that is the case?
- Payment by results in mental health comes with its own problems. Describe your concerns and give us some idea about the way forward.
- Have you heard of the term 'ward to board'? Why is it important?
- How will you address the issue of a poorly performing colleague?
- How are you going to improve staff engagement?
- Team working in mental health service is the norm. What will be your contributions to team-building and development?
- Tell us about your plans for improving the quality of service and creating efficiency at the same time.
- How do you balance finance and quality at your workplace?
- Do you think doctors should be involved in management and if yes please tell us the reasons why.
- What leadership style will you bring to this organisation and why?
- A consultant is not considered anymore to be a leader automatically. Why do you think that view prevails? What will be your view in relation to this vexed topic?
- What in your opinion are the pitfalls of the Health and Social Care Act? What will be your contributions to improving the commissioning process?
- The commissioners are keen to take 10% away from the budget for the next year as efficiency savings. How will you tackle this situation?
- What will be your strategy for engaging commissioners?
- Why do you think it is important for our trust to become a foundation trust? What will be your contribution towards this?

When the panel has finished asking questions, the chair will ask you if you have anything to add or have any questions for a member of the panel. This is your opportunity to clarify major points, but ask no more than one or two. This is not the time to ask questions that can be answered by human resources personnel separately (e.g. pay protection or relocation expenses). It may be worth stating that you have already been to the place and seen relevant people, who have been very helpful in answering all the questions you had. Indeed, if you have done your homework, you should have had all your questions answered by the time of the interview.

Box 33.5 Examples of clinical interview questions

- What will be your contribution as a consultant in response to Sir Francis' Report?
- What is your view about improving user/carer engagement for the trust?
- Give us an example of innovation in psychiatric practice. How are you going to promote innovation in your work environment?
- What will be your contribution in improving the quality of care that you provide to our patients?
- Tell us about cases where you felt you have not done well and where you felt your input has brought on positive change.
- New Ways of Working has caused controversy. What are the concerns and how would you address these concerns?
- What will be your strategy to improve interface working? Why is it important?
- Patient experience and outcomes are considered to be important parameters in measuring quality. How would you ensure that these get routinely captured in your day-to-day clinical practice?
- Revalidation is being rolled out to all medical practitioners. How prepared are you for it and why is it important?
- Do you have any particular area where you want to develop your subspecialty skills?

At the end of the interview, thank the chair and the panel before leaving. You may be asked to wait for the decision or the chair may ask you to provide contact details so that the committee can let you know their decision. The committee is advisory and they will make a recommendation to the trust board.

The procedure of interviewing has problems of its own. The important factor to bear in mind is selling your uniqueness. For women and doctors trained overseas, there may be additional factors that come into play. Questions about personal circumstances and private lives have to follow guidelines for equal-opportunity legislation and conform with the code of good practice. It is unacceptable to ask a woman any questions which are not asked of men. In the event of a complaint regarding ethnic or gender discrimination, members of the panel may be required to give evidence.

It is important to be clear about the job you are applying for, the reasons for your choice and the commitment required.

Be yourself and you cannot go far wrong. Good luck!

References and further reading

Asbury A (1985) Assess a job. In *How To Do It* (Vol. I) (2nd edition) (ed S Lock): pp 81–5. BMA Publications.

Department of Health (2005) *The NHS (Appointment of Consultants) Regulations.* Department of Health.

Drife J (1985) Be interviewed. In *How To Do It* (Vol. I) (2nd edition) (ed S Lock): pp. 92–5. BMA Publications.

Gray C (2005) Fair interviewing is harder than it looks. *BMJ Careers,* **331**: 68–9.

Hobbs R (1985) The interview. *British Journal of Hospital Medicine,* **33**: 220–2.

Naeem A, Rutherford J, Kenn C (2005) From specialist registrar to consultant. Permission to land. *Psychiatric Bulletin,* **29**: 348–51.

Poole A (2005) What not to do at an interview. *BMJ Careers,* **331**: 65–6.

Rhodes P (1983) Applying for jobs. *BMJ,* **286**: 618–20.

Rhodes P (1983) Interviews: sell yourself. *BMJ,* **286**: 706–7.

Rhodes P (1983) Interviews: what happens. *BMJ,* **286**: 784–5.

Rhodes P (1983) Women doctors. *BMJ,* **286**: 863–4.

Rhodes P (1983) Overseas doctors. *BMJ,* **286**: 1047–9.

CHAPTER 34

Surviving as a junior consultant: hit the ground walking

Mark Salter

Whatever the quality of your higher specialist training, or the resourcefulness and resilience of your personality, the early years of your first substantive post as consultant psychiatrist will be a time of challenge and more than a little stress. Nothing can fully prepare you for this. Upon starting work, you will encounter a sudden hike in the range and complexity of your responsibilities, and the demands made of you by others, senior and junior, in terms of decisions, actions and calls for leadership and support. You will need to balance your responses to these demands against the seemingly ever-changing motives and agendas of countless other individuals from many backgrounds, clinical and managerial. Many of these people will be total strangers, and will bring with them all the unpredictable quirks and foibles that human nature is heir to. In the early months, you will also need to assimilate a large amount of critical, need-to-know information – names, places, forms, faces, phone numbers and so on – while at the same time handling a vast increase in seemingly less crucial information that reaches you, via meetings, phones, pigeonholes, text messages and emails. Much of this will prove useless; some of it will be invaluable. Few people will tell you which is which. Against this blooming, buzzing backdrop, you will also need to continue to practise the clinical psychiatry for which you have trained, and grapple with the ever-present problems of work in an under-resourced and stigmatised service. Occasionally, you will need to make quick decisions about high-risk situations, possibly involving suicide or even homicide, with incomplete information. If you have any energy left, you might even try to maintain a life outside work.

None of this need be half as forbidding as it sounds, provided that you think about these matters before and during the first months of the job. All of the key issues have been well described elsewhere in this book. It is useful to reiterate them here in a simple maxim: surviving as a junior consultant can be made easier – fun even – by looking after six things: objects, time, systems, information, people and yourself. Return to the opening of this chapter and see how these themes define that entire paragraph.

Get the hardware to work the way that you want

Never start work without at least the bare essential tools of the job. Think about this well before the start date. Research into the availability of a personal office, dedicated administrative support and access to the rest of the world, by phone, post and email, should form an essential part of your pre-interview reconnaissance. It is also handy filler for that 'Is there anything that you want to ask?' part of the job interview. The reply will say much about the department. Mental health services are usually cash-strapped and many consultant posts, especially new ones, are created with scant thought for administrative support, in spite of the massive expansion in paperwork and electronic communications in recent decades. Your own private space is an absolute must. Never agree to share, let alone 'hot-desk', with a colleague: if they really want you, they can hire a Portakabin. See Box 34.1 for a full list of the essential items that you should demand on, or before, the first day of the job.

Having secured these tools, learn to use them properly. Of all the skills that can transform your consultant life, confident use of a keyboard, dictation software and ten-finger typing are by far the most valuable. If you aren't already literate in Word, Outlook, PowerPoint and Dragon, arrange for your trust to send you on a course. The computer and the mobile phone are essential tools for controlling the flow of information through to you, but make sure you control these devices and not vice versa. Technology allows you to manage a crucial aspect of consultant life: availability. Be available, but not too available.

The only piece of kit more essential than the computer is the humble diary. Never keep more than one and make sure your secretary keeps a regular backup. It is debatable whether this should be of the paper or electronic variety, but only one will survive a drop down a flight of stairs

---

Box 34.1   Essential items from the start of the job

- Dedicated office
- Dedicated secretary
- Telephone
- Fax
- Computer, with full internet and intranet access
- Dictating machine
- Mobile phone
- Signed contract
- Pension agreement
- Clear understanding of annual leave, study leave, sabbatical allowance

on a council estate. Cultivate the art of diary husbandry from day one: a well-kept diary is the secret to mastery over time and systems.

Know your network: the teams they are a-changin'

A disconcerting aspect of life as a new consultant is the impression that everyone else seems to have a much better idea of how things work. This is largely an illusion. Instead, they are just a little more familiar with the chaos and unpredictability inherent in any large system. The NHS, with its burgeoning management and ever-shifting arrangement of teams, is no exception. The truth is that no one, anywhere, really knows how best to make it work. A useful lesson that derives from this inherent chaos is to ask not *how* various teams, clinics, managers and meetings function, but *why*. Although people tend to do things better with familiarity, it also blinds them to alternatives. It may seem hard to believe on day one, but your lack of familiarity with the way things work is an asset. Try to keep the 'why' question alive in your head throughout the early months of the job, and never accept 'That's just the way it is' as a reasonable answer.

Your timetable is a case in point. If everything can change, then so can your timetable. Never commit yourself to a fixed timetable in the early months, whatever it said in the job description. No matter what you are told about the immovable nature of this clinic or that ward round, ignore it. Devising your own timetable – which usually means changing someone else's – is essential for your survival. It is hard to overstate the importance of customising your timetable early in the job. Every clinical session generates about two-thirds as much work again in phone calls, dictation, proofing and countless other tasks. Build these into your timetable from week one and make sure that you allow at least two weekly sessions for personal time. This means time dedicated to whatever activity you wish: study, read, talk, lecture, visit, anything. If you find yourself doing routine work in this time, stop and ask yourself how you intend to move it to a more appropriate place in your working month. A useful rule of thumb is the ratio of 3:3:2 for clinical, administration and personal sessions. Defend those last two sessions as though your life depended upon them. In a year or two, it possibly will.

At the outset, your clinical work will not be at full pressure, and so these carefully carved spaces may have an uncomfortably cavernous feel to them. Do not fall into the trap of filling them with other people's problems. All of us, in our first consultant job, arrive with a blend of energy, insecurity and ingenuousness that is both the pity and the envy of more experienced colleagues. This makes it easy to rush in and offer too much in attempt to make a favourable impression. Resist this urge at all costs – do as little fixed work as possible in the first month of the job.

Instead, spend this precious time and clarity of vision learning about the local terrain. No clinical service functions in isolation. Rather, we all work in a rich lattice of teams, roles and organisations. The ubiquity of mental

---

Box 34.2 Sensible things to do – and not to do – early on in the job

- Check your contract is signed and agreed
- Check that you exist in the eyes of payroll, pension and human resources
- Go on an induction course
- Get yourself a mentor, enrol with a peer group and attend case-based discussions
- Pay a visit to the chief executive of your trust
- Check out the local non-statutory services
- Do not commit yourself to a fixed timetable in the first 2 months
- Watch more experienced colleagues in action
- Do as little clinical work as possible

---

illness means that there is much overlap between the work of many services both inside and outside the trust. These overlaps are important: they are a common source of border conflict, as well as an opportunity to pass work on to others. Pay special attention to the work done by local non-statutory organisations in your area. A sensible investment of early energy is to pay a visit to your local day centres, hostels, homeless units, Samaritans, MIND, counselling services, or anyone else you think may be useful to meet. If there are leaders of important minority groups living on your patch, go say hello. A list of sensible things to do in the early weeks is given in Box 34.2.

Within your trust, you can afford to familiarise yourself with systems and faces a little more slowly. You should have visited the human resources offices within days of starting, but also attend early on to those facets of the department that are usually invisible: the security office, the front desk, the switchboard, the cleaners and every other organ of that vast creature that is a mental health trust. It always repays itself in time.

Information overload: hello real world, goodbye perfection

We are drawn to psychiatry because it reflects the richness of human nature; psychiatry is the one branch of medicine that touches upon politics, biography and philosophy as much as biology. Non-psychiatric colleagues tease us for the detail of our letters and summaries; what they are really doing is acknowledging the bewildering complexity of mental illness. Psychiatry is a data-rich specialty. Above, we observed how we all work within a lattice of teams and organisations. It is also useful to view our work in terms of information flowing between points in a complex, abstract system. Learning how to control this vast flow is a major challenge to the new consultant. There are two key aspects to all of this information: its quantity and its objective quality.

The way we gather, consider and act upon clinical information varies greatly with experience. Medical training teaches us to abandon data quantity in favour of quality. Medical courses start 'bottom up', encouraging students to accumulate large amounts of information – most of it redundant – through which we then sift for significance. By the time we reach the level of specialist registrar, most of us have this sifting down to a fine art, but the habit of wanting to know everything dies hard. The catch comes with the move to consultant level, because a massive hike in the things that we think we need to know inevitably accompanies this move. Much of this is non-clinical. It is difficult at first apply our well-honed sifting skills to such strange new material, and so we fall back on the habits of our training. Probably the greatest challenge in surviving as a junior consultant lies in learning how to stop thinking and acting like a specialist registrar. Or, put another way, the secret of survival as a junior consultant lies in learning that you do not need to know everything. There are many ways to do this, some more drastic than others.

First, get technologies working for you. Set your computer to filter incoming data, for example. Emails addressed to you alone and copied to no one are often the most important. The rules wizard in Outlook allows you to create an 'inner inbox' that receives only such emails. Some incoming calls require a more swift and tactful reply than others. Keep your secretary up to date with this important who's who and why. It will not only improve your service but it can also work wonders for your secretary's job satisfaction. Second, surround yourself with reliable people and make sure that you share a clear understanding of exactly what you want and expect from each other. Third, ration your availability to less experienced staff. You have been appointed as a consultant because you can do the job better than most of the people around you, but this does not mean you should do it. Instead, start delegating from day one, and make a habit of it. This skill is not easy to acquire, for good reason: one of the hardest things in the world is to give an important job to someone else knowing that they will screw it up.

Having learnt to handle the torrent of information that reaches you, next turn your attention to the issue of quality. What do you really need to know? In clinical terms, this usually relates to matters of risk, capacity and responsibility. Despite 5000 years of human civilisation, mental illness has remained perplexing; if there were simple answers to the questions posed by madness, sadness and consciousness, we would have found them by now. Part of the job of a consultant lies in helping people feel less uncomfortable with the truth that there are no easy answers to the big questions that psychiatry considers as stock in trade. Get used to answering the unanswerable.

Fortunately, deciding what non-clinical information is worth knowing is usually easier, and derives from a combination of common sense and spotting the key players in your network, great and small. Meetings are a good place to gather large amounts of this information in one swoop, but *caveat salutor*, seven out of every ten meetings are a waste of time, and you cannot tell which is which until you have been. In the early months, it is sensible to attend as many meetings as possible – this is also a useful way to start practising non-availability – but attend, listen carefully and no more. Try to say as little as possible, and never, ever volunteer to do anything. Afterwards, ask yourself whether the meeting really changed anything. If it did, return, but never attend a meeting whose sole purpose is to decide whether or not to have a meeting.

Hell is not necessarily other people

Whoever said 'liking your colleagues is a bonus' was a curmudgeon, but probably right. We choose psychiatry for many reasons, but a decent social life should not be top of our list. Mental health attracts an extremely wide range of professions and personalities, and it is unrealistic to expect to get on with all of them all of the time, but attention to the way we relate to all of our colleagues is always rewarded. Of course, much of the way we act towards others relates immutably to our own personality, but much besides remains under our control.

Pay careful attention early on to the standards that you demand from junior medical staff. Decades of under-resourcing have overstretched the workload of many senior house officer posts, especially on in-patient units and in teams battered by the latest round of clinically irrelevant reorganisation. As a junior consultant, it is tempting to allow for this by lowering your expectations. Instead, work to raise resources, rather than lower standards. Supervision of juniors is another source of discomfort for some. Lack of familiarity with your post can create the illusion that you really know little more than an experienced senior house officer, and that your senior status is somehow as yet unjustified. The wisdom gap with specialist registrars is, of course, even narrower. Fortunately, the rules do not allow you to train such colleagues until you have worked for a year or two.

Aside from the fact that your own secretary is a form of minor deity, treat all admin staff like royalty. Although much of what they do may seem so uneventful as to be taken for granted by many, their memories are a precious repository of data that can transform your working life. Identify and pay special respect to those who have been around for much longer than you. Take time to identify their likes and dislikes. Machiavellian perhaps, but if you want a permit for that new parking zone outside your office, it helps to be on good terms with the person who fills out the application forms. Similarly, cultivate relations with your local managers. Try to think of the key issues in your service from their point of view and work out what lines of compromise might be reasonable in the event of conflict. Most importantly, in these litigious, risk-averse times, read and reread your local protocols on untoward incidents and discuss them with your managers before, rather than after, your first near miss. Try to build storm-proof bridges with management before it starts to rain. Most management work is effectively invisible when it is done well. If you think a piece of admin work has been well done, or made a particular difference, say so. Wherever you see excellence, it is your responsibility as a consultant to nourish it.

Of all the managerial staff worth getting to know, none is as important as the chief executive of your trust. It is a good idea to pay him or her a visit a month or two after you have settled into the job. When you go, do not take along a particular agenda. Have a few points to talk about, certainly, but try to make 'getting to know each other' the primary purpose of the meeting. Surprisingly few consultants actually do this. Your chief executive will certainly remember you, and will usually welcome the meeting as a chance to pick up news from the front line. When the brown stuff hits the fan during a tricky case in the years to come, that visit can prove very useful indeed.

As a junior consultant, you should also consider the way that you relate to your colleagues for reasons beyond duty, common sense and human civility. Your transition from specialist registrar to consultant brings with it an ineluctable progression to a leadership role, for which no amount of training can truly prepare you. People will look to you for certainty and clarity in the face of the inexplicable and will make demands – some of them unreasonable – unaware that you are simultaneously dealing with many similar requests from other quarters. Few jugglers begin their practice with five balls, standing on a log, but this is roughly what it feels like in the early years of your consultancy. Of course, each of us deals with these first anxious moments differently, but by far the commonest way is to look to others around us for reassurance.

Be very careful whom you turn to in these moments. Be no less careful about the way you reveal your discomfort. Some, in a rush to obtain positive affirmation, go to lengths to prove that they are still 'just one of the lads'. Others may inadvertently offer to take on work of others. More cynical colleagues – often those closer to burnout – may exploit this. Take on extra work if you must but only ever do so if there is more in it for you than a shoulder to lean on. Another urge to resist when things get tough is pouring your heart out to junior staff, especially if this involves criticism of others. The urge to let off steam can sometimes be very strong, particularly when your listener seems sympathetic but, ultimately, such reassurance-seeking behaviour will inhibit your growth as a leader. Leaders must display a greater degree of strength, confidence or skill (or a combination of all three) than those whom they choose to lead.

The stark truth is that you are no longer one of the lads. The sooner you incorporate this into your working style, the easier it is to survive as a consultant. A valuable way to spend time in the early weeks of the job is to sit in on the clinics or rounds of several more experienced colleagues, who are doing broadly similar work to your own. Watch someone you respect, as well as someone you don't, and think about what it is that makes them different.

Take me to your leader – the rise of mindless managerialism

There has been an interesting shift in the way our culture views authority. Not long ago, leadership brought with it automatic respect. This respect is nowadays qualified, and rightly so. The emphasis on equality in multidisciplinary teams and 'flat management structures' is a laudable response to the arrogant paternalism of the past, but these shifts have raised new problems, which are acutely felt by junior consultants.

One problem is that management has become *the* dominant profession in the NHS over the past 20 years. When the NHS was created, its core values of public service and trust were taken for granted. Back then, 'cuts' were made only by surgeons on living flesh. Nowadays, clinicians of almost every kind must face a crueller kind of cut, better known in managerialese (they too have their jargon) as CRES, or 'cash release efficiency savings'.

At some point you will face the fact that in a world of increasing demand and shrinking resources, clinicians and managers often face irreconcilable priorities. Increasingly, budgets, productivity evaluations and reorganisations will take priority over patient care, whatever the local 'trust policy' declares. This in part reflects the shift away from blind faith in these mistrustful times, but it also reflects the way people respond to uncertainty in interesting times (and mental illness is about as uncertain and interesting as it gets), namely to retreat from values to the false comfort of measurement. This explains not only the move towards so-called 'evidence-based' treatments, in other words drugs and short-term relationships offered by 'functional teams', but also the use of diagnostic 'clusters', which have everything to do with money and little to do with the kindness and care we hold central to our work. It takes effort to identify this often subtle shift from valuing to costing. It takes courage to say it clearly in meetings. But, like it or not, the consultant psychiatrist is one of the few people in the service with the wit, power and influence to point this out. It is a responsibility that we shirk at our peril.

Another problem is that the *Zeitgeist* of egalitarianism obscures the undying truth that humans will always need leaders in any tough job; working with mental illness in our culture is about as tough as it gets. Another problem is the modern tendency to view a leader as a victim of the situation. This is reflected in current talk about burnout, early retirement and other gloomy themes. The job *should* be tough and sometimes thankless. But it should also be enjoyable, and it should never be lonely. The shift of consultant work away from the time-honoured familiarity of the hospital base to community teamwork can lead to isolation. An important goal in the early months of the job is to establish a vestigial network to counter this. There are many ways to build such a support system: regular academic, clinical or management meetings, mentoring, peer groups, sharing the occasional breakfast or drink after work, or whatever. Clearly, some are more formal than others, but whatever method, choose it and use it.

Conflict

Another interpersonal challenge concerns conflict. Most of us dislike and avoid confrontation, but the status that comes with consultancy usually obliges us, sooner or later, to impose our will on something that needs to stop, start or change. Asserting oneself in the early years of the post, especially with senior colleagues, can be uncomfortable and is easily mishandled. Successful assertion requires confidence and experience, commodities that are often in short supply early on. In this state, it is easy to make two errors. The first is to confuse the personal with the professional. The second is to act prematurely. The first is an error of emotion; the second is an error of rationality. To put it another way: keep your powder dry and don't shoot till you can see the whites of their eyes.

Many of us mistakenly assume that conflict is an emotional process. It isn't. Try to confine the basis of your challenge to purely factual matters, and make sure well in advance that your information is high in quality and quantity. It is pointless confronting someone simply because you do not like what they are doing, or when you are basing your argument on only a few instances. If you manage to score against someone who annoys you, then fine, but that must never be your primary objective. Try to amass adequate grounds before making a move. Pay careful attention to your language, too. Successful negotiation is always phrased in verbs and nouns rather than adjectives; be especially careful when putting your assertiveness into writing. Pages of passionate complaint may or may not achieve their aim, but they can be stored easily and used to weaken the objectivity of your argument at a later stage. Angry letters can become hostages to fortune so do not write them. Instead, cultivate a cool, calm and succinct style, especially for the things you feel strongly about. This is how experienced negotiators get results.

Look after yourself: charity begins at home

Of all the things that require your care and attention from day one, none is as important as your own head. Doctors make lousy patients, and it is a curious irony that we spend much of our working day asking about the very things that we ignore in ourselves. The medical profession is renowned for its dark humour, its myths of indefatigability and excessive partying. Pay close attention to the predominant emotional themes of your workaday thinking, and keep a low threshold for the auto-diagnosis of tetchiness and gloom. Irritability in the workplace is almost always abnormal, and best defined as disagreeing with more than one colleague in any one 24-hour period. Watch your sense of humour – assuming you have one, that is – for signs of drift towards the gallows. Don't only watch what comes out of your mouth; watch also what goes into it. The early years of consultancy can be a taxing time for the hardiest of souls, and more than a few of us bump up our intake of booze and other substances in the early years. Disconsolation born of fatigue or frustration is an insidious thing, like gas in a coal mine. It can creep up on you subtly, in a way that is often hard to notice. Try to be as honest as you can with yourself regarding your thoughts and feelings about your work and make sure that you share these thoughts, light or dark, with someone. Your peer group, or mentor, or whatever should provide a helpful – and private – yardstick for deciding when enough is enough in these matters.

Don't just listen to your peers: listen also to what your body tells you. Be honest with yourself about your pattern of sleeping and eating, and if it is even a little out of kilter, ask yourself what you would say to a patient in that situation. Most of us have a musculoskeletal weak point in our bodies that twinges whenever we are overdoing it. If that left eyelid doesn't stop twitching after a weekend off, then it is time for a holiday.

Holidays, from the occasional well-crafted bunk to the fully declared three weeks of annual leave, are an essential part of the job. You will have familiarised yourself with your annual and study leave entitlement in the first days of the job. Make sure you use it; only fools fail to take their full quota. Be careful, too, about what you get up to on holiday. Taking work on holiday is absolutely contraindicated. A good holiday should pass Taub's test: it should require an effort to recall the code for the office door on return to work.

Holidays, however, should not become the only way to recover from the accumulated angst of months on the clinical front line. Pay scrupulous attention to your work–life balance. Think very carefully before taking work home. Of course, psychiatry would not be the fascinating job that it is if we didn't carry some aspects of it over into the rest of our life, but just make sure that there is a rest of your life to bring it home to. Work taken home is less mentally toxic if it differs in some way from day-to-day clinical tasks. Some take the view that coming home with work of any kind is a first step on the road to burnout, and many, looking back over their working lives, often date the start of their consultant life as the point at which they gave up those Serbo-Croat evening classes. Whatever you do, make sure work comes through your front door only when you want it to. Make sure you are ex-directory and, having made sure that the hospital switchboard can always contact you in an emergency, switch off your work phone if you aren't on call.

Having learnt to monitor yourself and your life for the signs of work-related distress, keep an eye out for the same in your colleagues, senior and junior, especially after near misses and serious incidents. Occasionally, you will spot someone who displays some quiet, early sign of buckling under the weight of it all. A hint of excess irritation, bags under the eyes, a sustained loss of sparkle or the faint whiff of booze on a Monday morning. No matter how tired you are, be good to them. Listen to them. Young consultant or old, it is your job to help them if you can.

Conclusion

The entirety of this chapter has tried to emphasise how successful adjustment to a consultant lifestyle lies in setting out the skeleton of a balanced working life early on. Strive to keep this skeleton bare at first. You will definitely put on the flesh as the years go by. A well-kept diary, well-honed connections with the key players around you and a firm grip on the flow of data in and out of your head should allow you to read the road ahead, long term and short. But above all, don't go in search of work. Let it find you, as it surely will. What truly separates the tyro from the veteran is the knowledge that time and nature are the greatest allies a doctor will ever have. Until you learn this for yourself, make sure you hit the ground walking.

CHAPTER 35

Working with the media – many benefits but some risks

David S. Baldwin and Peter G. Conradi

The importance of public education about psychiatric illness

Misunderstandings about the nature of mental disorder, its origins and consequences, and its prevention and treatment are widespread among our patients, their carers, our colleagues and the general public. Reducing ignorance and misgivings about psychiatric illness, and tackling unhelpful and discriminatory attitudes towards people with mental health problems, are important parts of the workload of all psychiatrists.

The Royal College of Psychiatrists actively engages with all forms of national and local media, using the expertise and goodwill of health professionals and patient organisations in liaising with journalists and broadcasters in efforts to improve the situation of people with mental health problems, and to reduce the stigma that is still so damagingly associated with mental disorder. This is achieved through:

- the College Media Centre, which supports the College's divisional public education officers and media spokespersons by providing them with detailed information about particular mental health problems
- the activities of the Public Education Committee, including the development and publication of books, factsheets and web-based resources
- a series of public education campaigns, such as 'Defeat Depression', 'Changing Minds', 'Partners in Care' and 'Fair Deal'.

The College's *Public Education Handbook (2013): Practical Advice on Working with the Media* includes much helpful advice on the benefits and risks of media engagement (available on the College website).

For psychiatrists interested in improving public understanding of mental illness, the College has the experience and resources needed to optimise the impact of educational activity, although many psychiatrists might wish to undertake this role locally, working in collaboration with university or NHS trust press offices and local patient support groups. Many other organisations also work to confront stigma and to provide accurate information to the media about the nature of mental health problems and their treatment.

Are you the right person for the job?

This is a simple question. We all want to do our bit to increase public understanding and reduce stigma, but there is a world of difference between undertaking these roles within the setting of clinical practice and attempting to address these matters through liaison with local, regional and national media. Reflect on whether you have the necessary communication skills, time and personal resources to undertake an additional role in public education. Consider how your overall workload may be affected, and imagine the sentiments that could be aroused through being misquoted or ridiculed, with little opportunity for redress.

The problem is that if you are a talented communicator your name will become known, with progressively more calls for your opinion. Speaking with journalists is at first rather exciting, compared with the often dull nature of some aspects of your work, and quite reinforcing. It may become easier for a journalist to contact you than to seek out the opinion of others with potentially greater knowledge, but this is to the detriment of all concerned: you can acquire the reputation of being a 'rent-a-quote' doctor, the scientific accuracy of the story may be compromised, and the target audience could be misinformed. This damages the reputation of you and the journalist, and our discipline, and may have untoward consequences for patients.

What is your area of expertise?

Define and limit your area of expertise. Journalists may sometimes cast around for anyone available to comment on a current news story, but most want the opinion of someone familiar with the subject and able to place study findings, policy initiatives or emerging controversies within a wider context. It is clearly foolish to comment on a story relating to Alzheimer's disease when you work as a child psychiatrist and have not seen a patient with a dementing illness for over 20 years, but defining the boundaries of your expertise can be difficult. For example, you might feel tempted to answer a query relating to a particular new pharmacological treatment, but if your clinical practice is predominantly psychotherapeutic it would be hard to place the relative benefits and drawbacks of this drug in the correct context. Think about the clinical situations in which your colleagues come to you for advice, as it is in these areas that you are considered expert. Avoid taking on activities outside your area of expertise, and feel confident in stating that probing questions should be addressed elsewhere if you begin to feel you are straying into unfamiliar territory.

Do I need to undergo media training?

With a reasonable degree of self-awareness, you should know whether you can communicate clearly and effectively, as any problems should have been addressed at medical school and during your training as a psychiatrist. Reflect on whether you can make simple, accurate and interesting statements, delivered in a way likely to engage an audience. If you have no problems in this area, there is no need for media training. But attending a brief course can be instructive in revealing any behavioural peculiarities or verbal idiosyncrasies that might interfere with effective communication. Are you so perfect that media training is unnecessary? Most people enjoy the experience and find it surprisingly helpful.

How can I prepare for a media interview?

If you are speaking on behalf of an organisation, you will probably have been told who made the initial contact, the nature of their enquiry, the format for the interview and whether others are also involved. You may have already been provided with a prepared press briefing and a summary of relevant facts and figures. Most journalists work to tight deadlines and often hold unrealistic expectations of having almost immediate access to a nominated spokesperson, but it is essential to have at least some time to prepare for an interview.

Think about what you want to say, how you intend to say it and what might follow. Identify the overall message – it is best to have just one – and the two or three specific points to be conveyed, and think about their relevance to the target audience. Anticipate potential questions and prepare your answers. Journalists differ in the way they work, but it could be useful to provide some written material they can read prior to the interview and to which they can refer back afterwards. This could be the abstract of the scientific paper when describing research findings, or a public education leaflet when discussing a particular medical condition. If you have time, you might even want to draft some basic points and quotes from yourself setting out the essence of the 'line' you want to get across – similar to an informal press release. If the subject matter is complex and likely to be unfamiliar to the journalist, this will help make your point and reduce the scope for misunderstanding. You may be able to express yourself more succinctly in writing than you can verbally. If the journalist has little time, is unsure of his or her ground – or is just plain lazy – you may find the resulting story can bear a very strong resemblance to what you have written.

Do you have a conflict of interest?

It is common to preface presentations in scientific meetings with a disclosure regarding sources of funding, and press releases relating to research findings typically acknowledge sources of financial support. These explicit statements acknowledge the often considerable investment from the funding agency, and so can enhance the appraisal of the scientific information. Such declarations usually relate to research support from the pharmaceutical industry, although most who work in leadership roles in professional bodies will have many potential conflicts of interest, through allegiances or hostilities to particular groups or organisations that might influence judgements or actions. It is wise to be guided by the Nolan principles of public life when offering your personal views and professional opinions to others (see Table 35.1).

Table 35.1 Application of the Nolan principles of public life to engagement with the media

Principle	Application to working with the media
1. *Selflessness*. Holders of public office should act solely in terms of the public interest. They should not do so in order to gain financial or other benefits for themselves, their family or their friends	Ensure your activity aims to improve general public understanding of mental disorder, rather than to push your individual interests
2. *Integrity*. Holders of public office should not place themselves under any financial or other obligation to outside individuals or organisations that might seek to influence them in the performance of their individual duties	Avoid payments or other inducements. If a fee is payable for your work, direct it towards a related medical charity
3. *Objectivity*. In carrying out public business, including making public appointments, awarding contracts, or recommending individuals for rewards and benefits, holders of public office should make choices on merit	Evaluate the quality of the supporting scientific evidence, including its strengths and limitations
4. *Accountability*. Holders of public office are accountable for their decisions and actions to the public and must submit themselves to whatever scrutiny is appropriate to their office	Consider any potential wider unintended consequences of expressing specific personal views
5. *Openness*. Holders of public office should be as open as possible about all the decisions and actions that they take. They should give reasons for their decisions and restrict information only when the public interest clearly demands it	Be prepared to justify your statements and acknowledge areas of uncertainty or disagreement
6. *Honesty*. Holders of public office have a duty to declare any private interests relating to their public duties and to take steps to resolve any conflicts in a way that protects the public interest	Consider all potential conflicts of interest and preface your opinions with a clear declaration
7. *Leadership*. Holders of public office should promote and support these principles by leadership and example	Strive for excellence and inspire your colleagues through these activities, as in all areas of your professional work

Think about your position, its roles and responsibilities, and how these could affect any comments you make on emerging stories. Potential conflicts may not be immediately obvious. For example, it might be tempting to comment adversely on the impact of certain mental health services on clinical outcomes when you have been arguing forcefully for a different pattern of resource distribution. Remember that you are a clinician, whose first concern should be to improve health, and that unacknowledged conflicts might mislead colleagues or prejudice patient welfare. Consider carefully whether you should preface your comments with a statement of interests: it is sensible to declare anything that might cause embarrassment if currently undeclared but revealed in the future. Write down what you declared, for your records.

How is a press briefing organised?

Busy clinicians do not have the time or expertise to organise what is typically a complex operation: this task is normally undertaken by the parent institution (for example, the Royal College, a university press office, or an interposed public relations or communications company). Typically, the date of a briefing will be chosen to avoid similar news events and the timing selected to ensure the maximum press coverage. Journalists will have been lured to the meeting by the promise of individual discussions with 'key opinion leaders', so it is important to ensure you can remain at the venue for a while after the initial presentations have been done, to avoid disappointing them.

It is often helpful to rehearse the presentations before the meeting, but the final presentations should be delivered in a fairly spontaneous and flexible way. The chair will identify each speaker in turn, refer the attending journalists to the written material (the press release) and will encourage each speaker to talk for only a few minutes, to allow plenty of time for questions. The chair should ensure that any patient representative is treated courteously and sympathetically, and that questions are not monopolised by a specific journalist. It is sensible to record the proceedings, partly to verify what was said should there be inaccurate or misleading coverage after the meeting.

How should I conduct myself during the interview?

Be certain the journalists know your name and affiliation, and whether you are speaking on behalf of an organisation such as the Royal College of Psychiatrists, or whether you are giving only your personal view. Ensure that you will not be interrupted and do not be tempted to undertake another activity (such as reading your emails) during the course of a telephone interview. When speaking, remember that you are the expert, not the journalist. Do not let yourself be interrupted or intimidated: but keep the message simple and verifiable, and wherever possible ensure it is relevant to clinical practice. Do not be tempted to digress into areas that were not specified in advance of the interview and be sure to avoid rampant speculation.

Be careful when asked to comment on the views of others. Journalists, whatever their discipline, are always on the lookout for a row – or something that can be portrayed as such to the reader – even if to those involved it can often seem little more than a normal difference of opinion between professionals. This can be the case as much in covering medical matters as in politics. By going along with this, you may help to give the story more prominence, but at the cost of losing control of it and potentially alienating those on the other side of the argument by seeming to question their judgement in public.

Bear in mind that the journalist is coming to the interview with a different agenda from yours. The journalist's role is not simply to convey your professional opinion in a balanced manner to a waiting world, but to come up with a story. The 'stronger' the story the better, since this will determine how prominently it is carried in the newspaper, on the television or radio bulletin, or on the website. A journalist may also have a clear idea in advance of what he or she would like that story to be.

The definition of what constitutes a good story depends on the subject area and on the publication. For non-specialist media, a good medical story will typically be something that challenges the status quo (or at least what appears to lay readers to be the status quo), or has a strong 'human interest' component. In the case of a scientific study, this may lead to the tendency to exaggerate the significance of findings, to downplay the various caveats that you are careful to highlight, to push them to the end of the story (where they may be further cut during the editing process) or to leave them out completely. If the story centres on a perceived failure by health professionals, the journalist will be keen to 'name and shame' the guilty and perhaps to give the story a wider political resonance by identifying failures in the system that could be blamed.

This is all par for the course. If, however, you get the impression from the journalist's question that he or she is trying to take the story too far in a questionable direction then put extra emphasis on the various caveats. Also correct any inaccuracies – it is perfectly acceptable to use phrases such as, 'I'm afraid that is quite wrong. The real situation is ...'). Otherwise restrict the discussion to what you had intended to say. Even if you are strapped for time, try not to cut off the interview if you feel the journalist still has not grasped the point.

Should I comment on individual case stories?

No. The Royal College of Psychiatrists believes it is unethical for a psychiatrist to offer a professional opinion on someone unless he or she has conducted an examination and has been granted proper authorisation for such a statement, and organisations such as the American Psychiatric Association have given similar advice. It might be tempting to speculate on the psychological motivations of celebrities caught in the glare of publicity, but without personal knowledge of the person and her or his permission this is highly inadvisable, and could prove damaging to you and to the profession. The most you can do is to make a general statement about the problem being discussed, while stressing that it would be unprofessional to comment on specific aspects of the case.

Most dealings with the press relate to less sensational matters. Professional bodies usually maintain a list of former or current patients who are willing to speak about their experience of illness, and journalists will often accompany an otherwise rather dry account of research findings or health service changes with an illustrative personal-interest story. If you feel the impact of a news item might be increased through illustration with a relevant clinical case, keep the account simple and make sure the patient cannot be identified.

What happens if I am misquoted?

You should expect to be misquoted occasionally. Good preparation prior to an interview and clarifying any uncertainty during the discussions reduces the chance of this happening, but oversimplifications and factual errors can creep into articles, given the need to keep them brief and punchy. You may be tempted to ask the journalist to send for your approval a draft version of any material intended for print, especially if you feel during the course of your interaction that he or she has not understood the points you are trying to make or is trying to put a particular 'spin' on the story. Your concern may be well founded, but beware: you are straying into potentially dangerous territory. Most journalists will be reluctant to do so, and asking them risks antagonising them. They could be affronted at what seems like an attempt to control what they are planning to write and will be reluctant to launch into what could be a protracted process of negotiation with you over the content of the article that could mean they miss a deadline. It may also get them into trouble with their boss: many national newspapers refuse as a matter of principle to grant 'copy approval' to interviewees and discipline employees who allow themselves to be browbeaten into providing it.

If you are really concerned, however, you could ask the journalist to grant you 'quote approval', that is, to email back to you any direct quotes that are attributed to you. If that is agreed, then make sure to respond quickly and try to confine any suggested changes to matters of substance rather than minor quibbles. Do not be taken aback if a long conversation has been reduced to a few sentences. If you have done your job well, you will have helped shape the angle of the story. There will never be as much space devoted to the article as you – or the journalist – might like. However important the subject is to you, there are many other things competing for limited space.

If you discover that some aspects of a report are incorrect, pause to reflect on whether this inaccuracy is inadvertent, and if so whether it adversely affects an otherwise helpful article. Keep a record of what you said, and what appeared, and note the differences. If you feel that you have been deliberately misrepresented, it may be worth contacting the editor of the newspaper (not the journalist who wrote the article) to arrange a prompt 'correction'. Make your complaint as succinct as possible, concentrating on the main problem. No newspaper likes to print corrections but will do so if you demonstrate that a factual error has been made. Send in your complaint as soon as possible as any delay substantially reduces the chance of your correction being printed.

Try also to draw lessons for future interviews. Were you not as clear as you should have been? Thinking back, was there a moment when you could see things were heading in the wrong direction but did not do enough to put the interview back on course? If you think the journalist deliberately misrepresented your views, then think carefully before talking to him or her again. If that journalist does approach you about another story, then first make clear your concerns about the last one – but do not be surprised if she or he blames sub-editors. This may actually be true, especially in the case of tabloid newspapers, where stories will be rewritten and 'hardened up' by sub-editors in search of a good headline far more than is the case with broadsheets or specialist publications. Console yourself with the memory of all the other times when liaison with the media went well, and rest assured that the opinions of your valued colleagues will not be swayed by partisan and antagonistic news reports.

Should I do live interviews?

The audiences for many radio and television programmes far outstrip the circulation of even national newspapers and if the message is really important it should be addressed to as many people as possible. But particular care is needed when preparing for live interviews. Establish who will be interviewing you, the questions likely to be raised, the duration of the transmission, and who else is being asked to comment on the story. It is rare to be given the chance to speak to the interviewer before 'going live' but editorial staff should provide this information, and will often let you know the likely gist of the first question. Whenever possible, make yourself familiar with the news events of the day, as an interviewer may well seek to put a topical spin on an otherwise worthy but dull press release.

During the interview, do not be disappointed if the questions seem rather elementary. Take the opportunity to make simple statements of broad relevance to the audience. When asked detailed questions on specific problems, reply in kind but try to place your comments in a broader context, as the audience will not be interested in endless discussion of minor points. Be certain when the interview has ended: do not make statements 'off the record', as programmers may find it hard to resist the temptation to broadcast any contentious comments.

How should I appear on television?

Before a television appearance, most people experience some anxiety about what to wear. Communication companies offer much advice about how to dress for television interviews. 'Dressing down' is risky, particularly if you are discussing serious matters such as suicide or homicide. The most important considerations are to dress smartly but not too flashily. Avoid checks and stripes as these 'fuzz' distractingly on the screen. Remember that you may perspire a lot in the studio environment. Men should shave to avoid the impression famously conveyed by Richard Nixon during his doomed 1960 television debate with John F. Kennedy that helped lose him the presidential election. Expect a shiny forehead to be powdered. Women will be made-up in a fashion that would be considered rather scary in other environments.

Do not have a drink before the interview 'to steady the nerves': an inebriated psychiatrist is not a good advertisement for the profession. During the interview, look at the presenter and not the camera; sit back in your chair; smile when appropriate; and remain engaged and polite, despite hostile questioning.

This all seems quite daunting – is it worth it?

Working with the media has its occasional irritations and carries some potential hazards. Most of these will be avoided by remembering that you are a clinician, not a celebrity. The most tiresome aspect of media liaison is being asked the same recurring questions, by journalists who have clearly not bothered to read a press briefing, only to find your efforts sidelined in an article which appears driven by another agenda. Excessive cynicism about the media is not conducive to the effective delivery of the message, so if ennui starts to characterise your dealings with journalists, it is time to stop.

Do not undertake public education activity about mental disorder in the hope of raising your personal profile, for that is a waste of opportunity, a squandering of limited resources, and a perversion of its aims. Remind yourself of the overall aim. The greatest reward for your efforts should be to read a sympathetic account of the experience of those with mental disorder, in which the good efforts of mental health professionals have resulted in substantial and sustained improvements for their patients: and to learn some time later that it was articles such as that which encouraged others with the same condition to seek psychiatric help, after avoiding doing so for many years.

CHAPTER 36

Consultant mentoring and mentoring consultants

Bryan Stoten

What is mentoring?

Surprisingly, at a time when the evidence base for clinical practice has never been so eagerly sought after within the NHS, an approach to continuing professional development has emerged which seems to be not susceptible to measurement and to be subject to a wide variety of definitions.

The concept of 'mentoring' has been interpreted across a continuum from a remedial or therapeutic intervention to 'buddying' and the entirely informal. Specific benefits are hard to identify within the available literature. However, Rodenhauser *et al* (2000) do refer to the kind of outcomes that can be obtained from the process:

> 'guidance with socialisation into the profession, assistance with stresses along the way, help with the choice and fulfilment of a career path and inspiration for meaningful involvement in activities such as research and administration.'

However difficult it is to measure the benefits of mentoring in a quantifiable way, there has nonetheless emerged, over the last decade, a consensus among the healthcare community that the encouragement of mentoring schemes is good practice and adds value.

The trend in recent years to hold professionals to account for their practice has seen the adoption of a number of management innovations. In the NHS, the development of appraisal schemes, often associated with discretionary awards, has become universal. Similarly, together with appraisal, coaching schemes, mentoring programmes and similar interpersonal development initiatives for hospital doctors have become increasingly common. Statutory revalidation, while independent of such developmental initiatives, has nonetheless added to the idea that clinical practice requires ongoing reflection and assessment.

A consensus has emerged around the definition of mentoring produced by the Standing Committee on Postgraduate Medical Education of the British Medical Association (BMA):

'[mentoring is] the process whereby an experienced, highly regarded empathic person [the mentor], guides another individual [the mentee] in the development and re-examination of their own ideas, learning and personal and professional development. The mentor, who often, but not necessarily, works in the same organisation or field as the mentee, achieves this by listening and talking in confidence to the mentee.' (Oxley, 1998: p. 1)

Not surprisingly, there are a variety of other definitions which have more or less congruence with this approach. For example Roberts *et al* (2002) describe mentoring as 'the offer of a confidential, professional supportive relationship, by an experienced colleague, able and willing to share his or her knowledge and experience to a protégé or mentee'. It is interesting that Roberts *et al* use the term protégé as equivalent to mentee, having as it does a sense of 'sponsorship' and even 'preferment'. Although such covert patronage has always played a part in the career development of some successful – and indeed unsuccessful – managers it may be seen to challenge a fair-employment policy and the whole nature of an equal-opportunities culture. That tension, present also in the concept of succession planning, requires management attention. In handling such tension the benefits to the organisation and the benefits to an individual demand maximum transparency in the distribution of career development opportunities and preferment decisions. We should be only too aware that mentorship takes a variety of forms and that such forms can range from the specifically remedial through to a privileging of one colleague over another as a result of that person acquiring a mentor possessing particular authority, status and power.

Mentoring, then, is clearly susceptible to a number of interpretations. In consequence, a variety of attitudes have emerged regarding the appropriateness of mentoring in organisations and the kinds of relationships it is appropriate to support through a mentoring scheme. The Royal College of Obstetricians and Gynaecologists (2005) answers the question 'who needs a mentor?' with the response 'every obstetrician and gynaecologist throughout training and career'. The variety of situations in which mentoring is seen to be valuable by the College includes: career change; appointment to a consultant post; returning to practice after absence; returning following sickness or maternity leave; during or after suspension or exclusion; and generally at times of personal development and stress. Clearly, each of those situations requires a rather different mentoring relationship and presents the mentor with very different challenges and expectations. Nonetheless, it accords with the BMA's general advice that 'mentoring should be encouraged at all levels throughout one's medical career' (BMA, 2004).

Not all professional bodies endorse formal mentoring at different career points, however. Some are especially relaxed about the mentoring role. The Faculty of Public Health (FPH), for instance, favours a far less rigorous style:

'FPH is launching a buddy scheme for new consultants ... a friendly ear.... It's informal: no training, no legal liability, no travel expenses. Just the voice of experience to help you along.' (Faculty of Public Health, 2014)

Who should do it?

There is perhaps unsurprisingly, given such attitudes, little discussion in the literature about the characteristics of mentors and, consequently, little consideration given to their training needs. Perhaps the most common approach, several notches away from the 'friendly ear' however, is that of the Royal College of Obstetricians and Gynaecologists (2005), which specifies:

- a good listener
- respected as a professional
- approachable and accessible
- non-judgemental
- enthusiastic, encouraging
- wise, experienced
- challenges but not destructively
- ethical, honest and trustworthy
- good interpersonal and communication skills.

Rather more definitively, Gupta & Lingam (2000) state:

'[mentors] need formal training in communication skills, the laws related to education and training [particularly involving the specialty in which the mentor is working], current immigration rules, GMC [General Medical Council] rules in relation to registration, performance procedures, self regulation etc.'

They conclude that there are indications that the training of mentors significantly improves the satisfaction which both mentors and mentees have from the mentoring encounter, and, indeed, some evidence that the training of mentees before they enter the mentoring relationship adds even more satisfaction.

An approach based upon personality type theory

The Health Partnerships organisation, with the guidance of experienced health service managers, clinical leaders and senior business leaders, has offered a training programme specifically for experienced hospital consultants preparing themselves to offer mentoring to newly appointed consultants within their own hospital organisation, although not necessarily within their own discipline. This approach was informed by Sir Ian Kennedy's Bristol Royal Infirmary Inquiry (2001).

The approach developed was responsive to the demands of both the Royal Colleges and the BMA, for, as they rightly point out, the evidence suggests that more informal mentoring arrangements tend to be more successful. However, if such success is to be generalised there need to be some formal structures in place to increase the likelihood that those wishing to have access to a mentor will be successful in finding one, while the approach adopted by the mentors needs to be recognisably similar and use materials that have both face validity and a common theoretical underpinning.

A framework for consultant mentoring

Not all mentoring schemes assume benefit derives from 'the wisdom of experience' counselling the enthusiasm of the neophyte. The literature contains many references to the idea that 'co-mentoring' and 'non-hierarchical mentoring' offer a useful variant on the common types of mentoring, the definition of which this chapter started with. At the heart of a consultant's practice lies the principle of collegiality and peer relationships. Notwithstanding the reality that some consultants will have more experience than others, and hold positions of greater responsibility than others, such hierarchical factors may often be balanced by the up-to-date sapiential authority of more recently qualified younger colleagues.

Mentoring between fellow consultants, then, must start with an implicit understanding that the mentor–mentee relationship is based on a voluntary desire, on both sides, to improve practice by sharing the experience and insight the mentor has and, often, the familiarity with research and current practice in the given discipline possessed by the newly qualified consultant.

Health Partnerships was anxious in its approach to avoid any suggestion that the mentoring relationship involves teaching, counselling, remedial development or therapy. Rather, the purpose was to accelerate the personal and professional development of newly appointed consultants by allowing them to 'embed' into the organisation, providing support in relation to sources of stress not encountered in a training grade, and offering a 'sounding board' able to protect new entrants to an organisation from organisational pressures, while bringing to their notice opportunities and developments of which they might otherwise be unaware.

In developing this approach Health Partnerships was aware of the general exhortations made in the literature that the role of mentors should not be simply to give instructions on performance. Rather, both the mentor and mentee will do better in a relationship based on personality type preferences (Myers, 1995) . For example, Freeman (1997) calls for:

> '[a] mentor ... deep enough and brave enough to support both the professional and the personal self of their mentee, not to make false divisions between the two dimensions in order to keep the mentoring relationship comfortable – making the task easier for the mentor but short changing the mentee.'

While we can observe that for some mentors such behaviours will be both natural and easily accomplished, for others this may go against their own personality type. Furthermore, it will certainly be the case that such an ability to move easily between the personal and the professional, while positively sought after by some mentees, may appear alarmingly intrusive to others.

The mentoring training developed in this programme of mentor development has had a central place in it for the notion of personality type preference and the likely behaviours which an understanding of personality type theory will encourage the mentor to accommodate. The model adopted, the Jungian-based Myers–Briggs Type Indicator (MBTI), was used by the Health Partnerships team in a variety of coaching and mentoring settings over a 15-year period of professional practice.

Establishing the ground rules of a mentoring relationship is fundamental to ensuring that the relationship starts off with a reasonable chance of longer-term success. Any successful mentoring relationship must be voluntary (on both sides) and all our experience of such schemes in NHS trusts has adhered to that principle. Furthermore, within the requirement to make patient safety paramount, the confidentiality of the exchanges between mentor and mentee has always been treated as sacrosanct.

Other issues, however, are likely to be determined by the personalities of the mentor and the mentee. These issues might include:

- the extent to which the mentor feels able to engage with the personal as opposed to the professional aspects of the mentee's concerns
- the availability of the mentor to the mentee
- the context within which the mentoring relationship is conducted
- discussion of the mentor's wider social ambit within the mentoring relationship.

The Myers–Briggs Type Indicator

The success of mentoring relationships which involve extensive extramural socialisation, engagement with the participant's family and the choosing of informal settings within which the mentoring relationship takes place appears self-evident to some commentators, and yet it is clearly dependent on the personality type preferences of the individuals involved. The MBTI was chosen as a means of legitimising differences in mentoring styles and relationships and as a tool for exploring the different demands that mentors and mentees can place upon the relationship as it develops.

The MBTI is widely used throughout the NHS; a number of large acute providers routinely offer it to their clinical staff as part of a wider organisational development programme. The MBTI offers four dimensions, as set out under the subheadings below.

Introversion/extraversion preference

This is the extent to which an individual engages with the world 'out there' or the world in one's head. Extraverts may accord with the popular use of the term and introverts appear aloof, but this dimension enables access to more subtle aspects of this dichotomy. An extravert mentor may feel an introvert mentee is unenthusiastic, reluctant to engage with or even approach the mentor except when scheduled. On the other hand, an introvert mentor may find an extravert mentee demanding and intrusive.

Sensing/intuiting preference

This dichotomy identifies the way in which information is obtained about the world through our five senses or through an additional or intuitive 'sixth sense'. Mentees with a sensing preference will seek factual information and precision, and live in the 'here and now'. Those with an intuitive preference will be much more interested in exploring the possibilities of the situation rather than the actuality. Matching mentor and mentee may lead to either too much 'blue sky thinking' or too much unchallenged acceptance of the world as it is rather than an exploration of the developmental possibilities. However, mentors with a sensing preference may have difficulty in relating to the intuitive mentee who is focused on the possibilities in the future rather than the practicalities of the present. On the other hand, a mentee with a sensing preference may find an intuitive mentor too non-specific about actual dilemmas and practical information to be worth taking seriously. At least an understanding of such differences may make it easier, perhaps within a framework of humour, to gain benefit from complementary or differing preferences between mentor and mentee.

Thinking/feeling preference

Making decisions about the world using a thinking or feeling preference does require considerable self-awareness and the ability to reflect on how people with a different preference will make crucial decisions about their work and professional development. The thinking/feeling dichotomy may be of particular importance in determining whether or not a mentor and mentee can form a productive relationship. The critical, analytical mode of thinking exhibited by those with a thinking preference can seem harsh and unappreciative to mentors with a feeling preference, while mentors with a thinking preference may be uncomfortable with the amount of personal exposure which a mentee with a feeling preference may wish to offer in the mentoring relationship. Particularly where discussion of the relationships developed by the mentee may form a crucial part of a mentee's early induction into a professional role and practice, a mentor with a thinking preference may be unhelpful and may lack the kind of insights necessary. Conversely, a mentor with a feeling preference may, if able to establish a good rapport with a mentee with a thinking preference, help that mentee to develop the interpersonal skills to which the thinking preference will initially give little priority.

Judging/perceiving preference

Finally, the extent to which one wishes to feel in control of one's world is a function of the judging/perceiving preference. Those with a judging preference will seek an ordered, predictable process lacking in ambiguities and uncertainty. Perceiving types are much more prepared to 'go with the flow', seeming to their mentor possibly more lackadaisical and uninvolved in the relationship, failing to observe a clearly scheduled process of meetings and failing to provide any ordered agenda or specific purpose. For mentors with a judging preference this may be particularly frustrating. Indeed, Grainger (2002) argues that 'the key to choosing a mentor is first deciding what you want to achieve and whether mentoring is the most appropriate way to achieve it'. In reality, for perceiving types, no such clarity is likely when they embark on the mentoring relationship. For those with a perceiving preference, the goals and purpose are likely to emerge over time and be 'retrofitted' to their circumstances rather than providing the framework for their future professional development. Nonetheless, a mentoring relationship between two consultants with a perceiving preference may well flounder, with no particular direction. It is circumstances like these which encourage us to recommend the use of the GROW framework (see below), which, while being of less immediate attraction to 'perceiving types', does at least enforce a framework which is purposeful and future directed.

Using the MBTI

The MBTI is capable of affording complex and subtle appreciation of individual and group interactions. Mentor training for hospital consultants, however, is unlikely to allow highly sophisticated development of these insights. Nonetheless, by making consultants aware of the broad parameters of the taxonomy and the four key dimensions it becomes possible to offer two key insights:

- A failure to establish an appropriate 'chemistry' between mentor and mentee becomes easier to handle and removes 'blame' from the decision to withdraw from such a relationship.
- Knowing something of the characteristics of the eight preferences gives the more experienced mentor a better understanding of both how their own preferences can be used positively and how the mentee's preferences may need to be accommodated in order to obtain the best from the relationship. We are struck again and again by the enthusiasm with which hospital consultants fall upon the MBTI taxonomy to inform not merely their approach to mentoring but their interpersonal behaviours more generally.

Active listening

The well-worn aphorism that 'God gave us two ears and one mouth, but they are rarely used in those proportions' is especially relevant when observing the training of mentors. For many potential mentors, active listening is the most difficult skill to acquire. For mentors who are themselves introverts and preoccupied with their own thoughts and priorities, those who are intuitives living in the 'there and then' rather than the 'here and now', and those who have a thinking preference, which is constantly analytical and critical, the suspending of their own thought processes until sufficient information has been derived from the mentee is especially difficult.

Despite setting off with the best of intentions, active listeners may be sidetracked by:

- looking for congruence between what they hear and their own values
- testing the content of what they hear against their own empirical observations
- constructing their response and advice
- completing the mentee's thought processes by anticipating what will be said next
- developing an awareness of stimuli outside of the setting
- succumbing to the distraction of a busy agenda and diary.

However, having the undivided attention of another is startlingly motivational and enhances self-esteem. Successful politicians understand this and frequently elicit the response 'He seemed completely focused on what I was saying'.

Whether a technique or genuine, such active listening is enormously empowering for the mentee. Nonetheless, in practical sessions in which such active listening is modelled we find that the greatest difficulty expressed by most participants lies in not succumbing to the interruptions, distractions and interjections mentors employ to break up their periods of listening. Perhaps for clinicians it is especially difficult to be non-directive, withholding guidance and advice and rather encouraging self-expression and exploration. Clinicians are trained to take a medical history in as time-efficient and ordered a way as possible, and it may be that such socialisation hampers a listening mode which is less controlling and directional.

Practical exercises in which meaning is sought not merely in the content of the words but also in expression and body language do appear to increase the ability of mentors in training to encourage mentees to say what they want to say, not what the mentor appears to want to know.

The GROW model

The combination of clinical experience, organisational maturity, some insight into the typical behaviours of different personality types and a restraint on the natural clinical urge to advise and prescribe may all contribute to establishing some rapport and mutual confidence in the coming together of mentor and mentee. However, if mentoring is to be purposeful, a basic framework for development seems to be helpful. Milestones in the mentoring process usually help, and the GROW model – goal, reality, options and wrap up – creates a shared process which enables both mentor and mentee to 'keep on track'.

Goal

Establishing what the mentoring session is to focus on – however broadly – gives purpose and direction. Answering the question 'What would you like to get from this session?', particularly if asked a day or two in advance, places the responsibility for the direction which the mentoring relationship takes firmly in the hands of the mentee – where it should be!

Reality

Establishing the 'facts', such as they are, allows for some ground-clearing in the earlier period of the mentoring relationship and establishes the differences between the perceptions and feelings of a mentee and the mentee's goals and aspirations as against the perceived constraints, problems, and opportunities which can be empirically tested by the mentor.

Options

The best courses of action are the product of the mentee's intelligence rather than the mentor's experience. The mentor's job is to facilitate the sifting of wheat from chaff and the quantification of subjective judgements ('Would that be twice as difficult, three times as difficult, or no more difficult?'). The mentor has licence to go on asking the crucial question, 'And what else could you do?', beyond the point when the mentee might reasonably cease enquiry.

Wrap up

Finally, no mentoring session should end without testing what it is that the mentee intends to do following the session. If the mentoring process is to be purposeful and the mentoring relationship to flourish, then a key part of the process must be testing the preparedness of the mentee to take something of the mentoring encounter into professional life. In general, we discourage note-taking during mentoring – at least by the mentor – but when testing the preparedness to act positively following the mentoring session, a single line which records 'the next step' reinforces the importance of the session and provides a starting point for the next one.

Conclusion

Mentoring opportunities now abound within the NHS. The accelerated rate at which junior hospital doctors can now expect to pass through their training grades into a consultancy post, together with the increasing managerial complexity which intrudes on clinical practice, means mentoring by the experienced 'grey heads' in the profession is endorsed by all the professional bodies.

It is appropriate to issue some warnings. Mentoring as a rehabilitative or remedial activity will bring the process into disrepute. Mandatory mentoring schemes do not merely fall foul of BMA guidelines but will simply reduce some schemes to a tick-box routine. Schemes which offer maximum choice to mentees and encourage the emergence of informal mentoring arrangements will be more successful than those which simply allocate mentor to mentee. Schemes in which mentors are first trained and schemes where both mentors and mentees are trained prior to entering the mentoring relationship will have more success. Peer mentoring and non-hierarchical mentoring – as we have found with our consultant mentoring schemes – will have higher satisfaction levels than schemes which encourage the mentoring of trainees by faculty members and senior staff.

Roberts *et al* (2002) made the following observation:

> 'the progressive dispersal of consultant psychiatrists into multi-disciplinary, locality-based teams, has simultaneously been accompanied by relative isolation from their peers.... Nearly 70% of consultants attending our study days on mentorship stated that they no longer have time for coffee or lunch with their colleagues owing to work pressures – times when "continuing professional development" occurred naturally.'

Such is the pressure in the NHS generally now, and the target culture is so all-pervasive, that this description of the situation in psychiatry might be applied across many more disciplines in medicine. Never before has it been so important for newly appointed consultants, entering the consultant grade at unprecedentedly early points in their career, to be offered a supportive framework for their professional development as a matter of course and good management practice throughout the NHS.

Satisfying the oversight of the Care Quality Commission, Monitor or the NHS Trust Development Authority makes the establishment of sound professional development crucially important for any mental health service provider seeking the flexibility and freedom to innovate which clinical professional staff demand. This approach to establishing formal mentoring skills within a planned environment of induction can do just that.

References

BMA (2004). *Exploring Mentoring*. BMA.

Bristol Royal Infirmary Inquiry (2001) *Learning from Bristol: The Report of the Public Inquiry into Children's Heart Surgery at the Bristol Royal Infirmary 1984–1995* (Command Paper CM 5207). TSO.

Faculty of Public Health (2014) *FPH Bulletin*, issue 109, March.

Freeman R (1997) Toward effective mentoring in general practice. *British Journal of General Practice*, **47**: 457–60.

Grainger C (2002) Mentoring – supporting doctors at work and play. *BMJ*, **324**: S203.

Gupta RC, Lingam S (2000) *Mentoring for Doctors and Dentists*. Blackwell Science.

Myers I (1995) *Gifts Differing*. Davies-Black.

Oxley J (ed) (1998) *Supporting Doctors and Dentists at Work: An Enquiry into Mentoring*. BMA.

Roberts G, Moore B, Coles C (2002) Mentoring for newly appointed consultant psychiatrists. *Psychiatric Bulletin*, **26**: 106–9.

Rodenhauser P, Rudishill JR, Devorak R (2000) Skills for mentors. *Academic Psychiatry*, **24**: 14–27.

Royal College of Obstetricians and Gynaecologists (2005) *Mentoring For All*. RCOG.

Index

Compiled by Linda English